EVIDENCE-BASED NURSING

AN INTRODUCTION

Editors

Nicky Cullum PhD, RGN

Professor and Director of the Centre for Evidence-based Nursing,
University of York,
UK

Donna Ciliska PhD, RN

Professor, School of Nursing,
McMaster University,
Canada

R. Brian Haynes MD, MSc, PhD, FRCPC, MACP, FACMI

Michael Gent Professor and Chair,
Department of Clinical Epidemiology and Biostatistics,
McMaster University,
Canada

Susan Marks BEd, BA

Research Associate, Health Information Research Institute,
McMaster University,
Canada

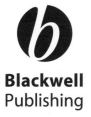

Blackwell
Publishing

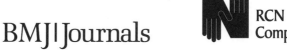
BMJ|Journals

RCN Publishing
Company

© 2008 Blackwell Publishing Ltd, BMJ Publishing Group Limited and RCN Publishing Company Ltd, and American College of Physicians ("ACP") Journal Club

Blackwell Publishing editorial offices:
Blackwell Publishing Ltd, 9600 Garsington Road, Oxford OX4 2DQ, UK
Tel: +44 (0)1865 776868
Blackwell Publishing Inc., 350 Main Street, Malden, MA 02148-5020, USA
Tel: +1 781 388 8250
Blackwell Publishing Asia Pty Ltd, 550 Swanston Street, Carlton, Victoria 3053, Australia
Tel: +61 (0)3 8359 1011

First published 2008 by Blackwell Publishing Ltd

ISBN: 978-1-4051-4597-8

Library of Congress Cataloging-in-Publication Data
Evidence-based nursing : an introduction / editors, Nicky Cullum . . . [et al.].
p. ; cm.
Includes bibliographical references and index.
ISBN: 978-1-4051-4597-8 (pbk. : alk. paper)
ISBN: 978-1-4051-4597-8 (pbk. : alk. paper) 1. Evidence-based nursing. I. Cullum, Nicky.
[DNLM: 1. Nursing Process. 2. Evaluation Studies. 3. Evidence-Based Medicine. WY 100 E93 2007]

RT42.E93 2007
610.73—dc22

A catalogue record for this title is available from the British Library

Set in 10/12pt Sabon by Graphicraft Limited, Hong Kong
Printed and bound in Singapore by Utopia Press Pte Ltd

The publisher's policy is to use permanent paper from mills that operate a sustainable forestry policy, and which has been manufactured from pulp processed using acid-free and elementary chlorine-free practices. Furthermore, the publisher ensures that the text paper and cover board used have met acceptable environmental accreditation standards.

For further information on Blackwell Publishing, visit our website:
www.blackwellnursing.com

CONTENTS

CONTRIBUTOR LIST

Editors

Donna Ciliska PhD, RN
Professor
School of Nursing
McMaster University
Hamilton
ON, Canada
L8N 3Z5

Nicky Cullum PhD, RGN
Professor and Director of the Centre for Evidence Based Nursing
Department of Health Sciences
Area 2, Seebohm Rowntree Building
University of York
York, UK
YO10 5DD

R. Brian Haynes MD (Alberta), MSc (McMaster), PhD (McMaster), FRCPC,
    MACP, FACMI,
Michael Gent Professor and Chair, Department of Clinical Epidemiology and
    Biostatistics,
DeGroote School of Medicine
McMaster University
Hamilton
ON, Canada
L8N 3Z5

Susan Marks BEd, BA
Research Associate
Health Information Research Institute (HIRU)
McMaster University
Hamilton

ON, Canada
L8N 3Z5

Contributors

Joy Adamson PhD
Lecturer
Department of Health Sciences
University of York
Area 2, Seebohm Rowntree Building
York, UK
YO10 5DD

Suzanne Bakken DNSc, FAAN
Alumni Professor
School of Nursing and Professor of Biomedical Informatics
Columbia University School of Nursing
617 West 168th Street
New York
NY 10032
USA

Jennifer Blythe PhD, MLS
Senior Scientist
School of Nursing
McMaster University
Hamilton
ON, Canada
L8N 3Z5

Deborah Braccia RN, MPA
Doctoral Candidate
Columbia University School of Nursing
617 West 168th Street
New York
NY 10032
USA

Esther Coker RN, MScN, MSc
Assistant Clinical Professor
School of Nursing
McMaster University
Clinical Nurse Specialist
St. Peter's Hospital
Hamilton
ON, Canada
L8M 1W9

P.J. Devereaux BSc (Dalhousie), MD (McMaster), PhD (McMaster), FRCPC
Assistant Professor
Department of Clinical Epidemiology and Biostatistics
McMaster University
Hamilton
ON, Canada
L8N 3Z5

Alba DiCenso PhD, RN
Professor, Nursing and Clinical Epidemiology and Biostatistics
CHSRF/CIHR Chair in Advanced Practice Nursing
School of Nursing
McMaster University
Hamilton
ON, Canada
L8N 3Z5

Dawn Dowding PhD, RGN
Senior Lecturer
Hull York Medical School
Department of Health Sciences
University of York
Area 2, Seebohm Rowntree Building
York, UK
YO10 5DD

Ellen Fineout-Overholt RN, PhD, FNAP
Director, Center for the Advancement of Evidence Based Practice
Associate Professor, Clinical Nursing
Arizona State University
College of Nursing
500 N. 3rd Street
Phoenix
AZ 85004
USA

Kate Flemming MSc, RGN
Research Fellow
Department of Health Sciences
Area 2, Seebohm Rowntree Building
University of York
York, UK
YO10 5DD

Ian D. Graham PhD
Associate Professor
School of Nursing
University of Ottawa
51 Gwynne Ave

Ottawa
ON, Canada
K1Y 1X1

David M. Gregory RN, PhD
Professor
School of Health Sciences
University of Lethbridge
AH103 (Anderson Hall)
Lethbridge
AB, Canada
T1K 3M4

Margaret B. Harrison RN, PhD
Professor
School of Nursing
Queen's University
Second Floor
78 Barrie Street
Kingston
ON, Canada
K7L 3N6

Andrew Jull RN, MA
Research Fellow
Clinical Trials Research Unit
University of Auckland
Private Bag 92019
Auckland
New Zealand 1142

Bernice King RN, MHSc
Assistant Clinical Professor (retired)
School of Nursing
McMaster University
Clinical Nurse Specialist
Hamilton Health Sciences
Hamilton
ON, Canada
L8V 5C2

Jo Logan RN, PhD
Adjunct Professor
School of Nursing
University of Ottawa
213 Beech St
Ottawa
ON, Canada
K1Y 3T3

Dorothy McCaughan MSc, RGN
Research Fellow
Department of Health Sciences
University of York
Area 2, Seebohm Rowntree Building
York, UK
YO10 5DD

K. Ann McKibbon MLS, PhD
Associate Professor
Health Information Research Unit
McMaster University
Hamilton
ON, Canada
L8N 3Z5

Bernadette Melnyk RN, PhD, CPNP, FAAN
Dean and Distinguished Foundation Professor in Nursing
Arizona State University
500 North 3rd Street
Phoenix
AZ 85004
USA

E. Ann Mohide RN, MHSc, MSc
Associate Professor
School of Nursing
McMaster University
Hamilton
ON, Canada
L8N 3Z5

Mary Ann O'Brien BHSc (PT), MSc
Research Fellow
Supportive Cancer Care Research Unit
Juravinski Cancer Centre
699 Concession Street, Room 4-204
Hamilton
ON, Canada
L8V 5C2

Emily Petherick MPH
Research Fellow
Department of Health Sciences
University of York
Area 2, Seebohm Rowntree Building
York, UK
YO10 5DD

Jenny Ploeg RN, PhD
Associate Professor
School of Nursing
McMaster University
Hamilton
ON, Canada
L8N 3Z5

Pauline Raynor BA, PGCE, RN, RM
Bradford Health Research Centre
Bradford Royal Infirmary
Duckworth Lane
Bradford
UK
BD9 6RJ

Jackie Roberts RN, MSc
Professor Emeritus, School of Nursing
Systems Linked Research Unit
McMaster University
75 Frid Street
Building T30
Hamilton
ON, Canada
L8P 4M3

Nicole Robinson BA
Research Coordinator
Ottawa Health Research Institute
1053 Carling Avenue
Ottawa
ON, Canada
K1Y 4E9

Joan Royle RN, MScN
Associate Professor (retired)
School of Nursing
McMaster University
Hamilton
ON, Canada
L8N 3Z5

Cynthia Russell PhD, RN
Professor
University of Tennessee
Health Science Center
College of Nursing
877 Madison Avenue
Memphis

TN 38163
USA

Kenneth F. Schulz PhD, MBA
Vice President, Family Health International
PO Box 13950
Research Triangle Park North Carolina
NC 27709
USA

Trevor A. Sheldon DSc
Professor and Deputy Vice Chancellor
University of York
Heslington Hall
York, UK
YO10 5DD

Patricia W. Stone PhD, RN
Assistant Professor of Nursing
Columbia University School of Nursing
617 West 168th Street
New York
NY 10032
USA

Jacqueline Tetroe MA
Senior Policy Analyst
Canadian Institutes of Health Research
160 Elgin St, 9th Floor
Address Locator 4809A
Ottawa
ON, Canada
K1A 0W9

Carl Thompson PhD, RGN
Senior Lecturer
Department of Health Sciences
University of York
Area 2, Seebohm Rowntree Building
York, UK
YO10 5DD

Sally Thorne PhD, RN
Professor
School of Nursing
University of British Columbia
T201–2211, Wesbrook Mall
Vancouver
BC, Canada
V6T 2B5

Jennifer Wiernikowski RN, MN, CON(C)
Chief of Nursing Practice
Juravinski Cancer Program
Hamilton Health Sciences
Hamilton,
ON, Canada
L8V 5C2

ACKNOWLEDGEMENTS

We thank Laurie Gunderman, Sarah Marriott, Sandi Newby and Emily Petherick for their help in preparing material for this book.

DEDICATION

This book is dedicated to those nurses everywhere who are striving to make more informed decisions in order to deliver the best nursing, health care management and policy development that they can.

COPYRIGHT ACKNOWLEDGEMENTS

Chapter 2
© BMJ Publishing Group Limited and RCN Publishing Company Ltd, 2007. All Rights Reserved.

'Implementing evidence-based nursing: some misconceptions' was first published in *Evidence Based Nursing* 1998 **1**: 38–39. See http://ebn.bmj.com/. This reprint (as adapted) is published by arrangement with BMJ Publishing Group Limited and RCN Publishing Company Ltd.

Chapter 3
© BMJ Publishing Group Limited and RCN Publishing Company Ltd, 2007. All Rights Reserved.

'Asking answerable questions' was first published in *Evidence Based Nursing* 1998 **1**: 36–37. See http://ebn.bmj.com/. This reprint (as adapted) is published by arrangement with BMJ Publishing Group Limited and RCN Publishing Company Ltd.

Chapter 4
Haynes RB. 'Of studies, synopses, and systems: the "4S" evolution of the services for finding current best evidence'. Originally published in *American College of Physicians Journal Club* 2001 **134**: A11–A13 and has been adapted and reproduced with permission.

Chapter 5
© BMJ Publishing Group Limited and RCN Publishing Company Ltd, 2007. All Rights Reserved.

'Searching for best evidence. Part 1: Where to look' was first published in *Evidence Based Nursing* 1998 **1**: 68–70. See http://ebn.bmj.com/. This reprint (as adapted) is published by arrangement with BMJ Publishing Group Limited and RCN Publishing Company Ltd.

Chapter 6

'Searching for best evidence. Part 2: Searching CINAHL and MEDLINE' was first published in *Evidence Based Nursing* 1998 **1**: 105–107. See http://ebn.bmj.com/. This reprint (as adapted) is published by arrangement with BMJ Publishing Group Limited and RCN Publishing Company Ltd.

Chapter 7

'Identifying the best research design to fit the question. Part 1: Quantitative research' was first published in *Evidence Based Nursing* 1999 **2**: 4–6 under the title *Identifying the best research design to fit the question. Part 1: quantitative designs*. See http://ebn.bmj.com/. This reprint (as adapted) is published by arrangement with BMJ Publishing Group Limited and RCN Publishing Company Ltd.

Chapter 8

'Identifying the best research design to fit the question. Part 2: Qualitative designs' was first published in *Evidence Based Nursing* 1999 **2**: 36–37 under the original title *Identifying the best research design to fit the question. Part 2: qualitative designs*. See http://ebn.bmj.com/. This reprint (as adapted) is published by arrangement with BMJ Publishing Group Limited and RCN Publishing Company Ltd.

Chapter 9

'If you could just provide me with a sample: examining sampling in qualitative and quantitative research papers' was first published in *Evidence Based Nursing* 1999 **2**: 68–70. See http://ebn.bmj.com/. This reprint (as adapted) is published by arrangement with BMJ Publishing Group Limited and RCN Publishing Company Ltd.

Chapter 10

'The fundamentals of qualitative measurement' was first published in *Evidence Based Nursing* 1999 **2**: 100–101. See http://ebn.bmj.com/. This reprint (as adapted) is published by arrangement with BMJ Publishing Group Limited and RCN Publishing Company Ltd.

Chapter 11

'Statistics for evidence-based nursing' was first published in *Evidence Based Nursing* 2000 **3**: 4–6. See http://ebn.bmj.com/. This reprint (as adapted) is published by arrangement with BMJ Publishing Group Limited and RCN Publishing Company Ltd.

Chapter 12

'Estimating treatment effects: real or the result of chance?' was first published in *Evidence Based Nursing* 2000 **3**: 36–39. See http://ebn.bmj.com/. This reprint (as adapted) is published by arrangement with BMJ Publishing Group Limited and RCN Publishing Company Ltd.

Chapter 13

'Data analysis in qualitative research was first published' in *Evidence Based Nursing* 2000 **3**: 68–70. See http://ebn.bmj.com/. This reprint (as adapted) is published by arrangement with BMJ Publishing Group Limited and RCN Publishing Company Ltd.

Chapter 14

'Users' guides to the nursing literature: an introduction' was first published in *Evidence Based Nursing* 2000 **3**: 71–72. See http://ebn.bmj.com/. This reprint (as adapted) is published by arrangement with BMJ Publishing Group Limited and RCN Publishing Company Ltd.

Chapter 15

'Evaluation of studies of treatment or prevention interventions' was first published in *Evidence Based Nursing* 2000 **3**: 100–102. See http://ebn.bmj.com/. This reprint (as adapted) is published by arrangement with BMJ Publishing Group Limited and RCN Publishing Company Ltd.

Chapter 16
Schultz KF. 'Assessing allocation and blinding in randomized controlled trials: Why bother?' Originally published in *American College of Physicians Journal Club* 2000 **132**: A11–A12 and has been adapted and reproduced with permission.

Chapter 17

'Number needed to treat: a clinically useful measure of the effects of nursing interventions' was first published in *Evidence Based Nursing* 2001 **4**: 36–39 under the title *Clinically useful measures of the effects of treatment*. See http://ebn.bmj.com/. This reprint (as adapted) is published by arrangement with BMJ Publishing Group Limited and RCN Publishing Company Ltd.

Chapter 18

Devereaux PJ, *et al*. 'Double blind, you are the weakest link – good-bye!'. Originally published in *American College of Physicians Journal Club* 2002 **136**: A11–A12, and has been adapted and reproduced with permission.

Chapter 19

'Evaluation of systematic reviews of treatment or prevention interventions' was first published in *Evidence Based Nursing* 2001 **4**: 100–104. See http://ebn.bmj.com/. This reprint (as adapted) is published by arrangement with BMJ Publishing Group Limited and RCN Publishing Company Ltd.

Chapter 20

'Evaluation of studies of screening tools and diagnostic tests' was first published in *Evidence Based Nursing* 2002 **5**: 68–72 under the title *Evaluation of studies of assessment and screening tools, and diagnostic tests*. See http://ebn.bmj.com/. This reprint (as adapted) is published by arrangement with BMJ Publishing Group Limited and RCN Publishing Company Ltd.

Chapter 21

'Evaluation of studies of health economics' was first published in *Evidence Based Nursing* 2002 **5**: 100–104. See http://ebn.bmj.com/. This reprint (as adapted) is published by arrangement with BMJ Publishing Group Limited and RCN Publishing Company Ltd.

Chapter 22

'Evaluation of studies of prognosis' was first published in *Evidence Based Nursing* 2004 **7**: 4–8. See http://ebn.bmj.com/. This reprint (as adapted) is published by arrangement with BMJ Publishing Group Limited and RCN Publishing Company Ltd.

Chapter 1

AN INTRODUCTION TO EVIDENCE-BASED NURSING

Nicky Cullum, Donna Ciliska, Susan Marks
and Brian Haynes

What is evidence-based nursing, and why is it important?

The term 'evidence-based' is really very new. The first documented use of the term is credited to Gordon Guyatt and the Evidence Based Medicine Working Group in 1992.[1] They described *evidence-based medicine* as 'a new paradigm for medical practice', in which evidence from clinical research should be promoted over intuition, unsystematic clinical experience, and pathophysiology.[1] Shortly thereafter, the term was applied to many other aspects of health care practice and further afield. We now have evidence-based nursing, evidence-based physiotherapy,* and even evidence-based policing[2] (see Box 1.1 for more examples)! Definitions vary, and sometimes the central concept becomes diluted, but at its core evidence-based 'anything' is concerned with using valid and relevant information in decision-making. In health care, most people agree that high-quality research is the most important source of valid information, along with information about the specific patient or population under

Box 1.1 Examples of evidence-based everything[2]

Evidence-based medicine
Evidence-based dentistry
Evidence-based physiotherapy
Evidence-based pharmacy
Evidence-based conservation
Evidence-based crime prevention
Evidence-based education
Evidence-based government
Evidence-based librarianship
Evidence-based social work
Evidence-based software engineering
Evidence-based sports

---

* We will use the term 'evidence-based practice' to refer to the application of evidence-based principles in any aspect of health care practice.

consideration. Evidence-based ways of thinking have emerged from the discipline of *clinical epidemiology*, which focuses on the application of epidemiological science to clinical problems and decisions (epidemiological science is the study of health and disease in populations). These roots in epidemiology have enabled the development of a clear-sighted framework for thinking about research and its application to decision-making, and it is these concepts and approaches that we discuss in this book.

Evidence-based nursing can be defined as the application of valid, relevant, research-based information in nurse decision-making. Research-based information is not used in isolation, however, and research findings alone do not *dictate* our clinical behaviour. Rather, research evidence is used alongside our knowledge of our patients (their symptoms, diagnoses, and expressed preferences) and the context in which the decision is taking place (including the care setting and available resources), and in processing this information we use our expertise and judgement. The inputs to evidence-based decision-making are depicted in Figure 1.1. Research has shown, however, that many practitioners simply don't see research evidence as being useful and accessible when making real-life clinical decisions.[3] The grand challenge is therefore showing how this can be achieved, and the quality of care enhanced.

Imagine that, as a community-based nurse, you are responsible for providing care to an otherwise fit 74-year-old man with a chronic venous leg ulcer. Your locally relevant, evidence-based, leg ulcer guideline tells you that high-compression bandaging,

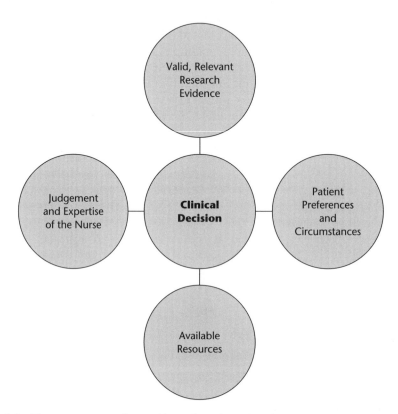

Figure 1.1 The components of an evidence-based nursing decision.

such as the four-layer bandage, should be the first line of treatment, is eminently deliverable in a community setting, and is cost-effective.[4] You have been trained, and are competent, in the application of this bandage and, therefore, proceed to prescribe it for this patient. Contrast this decision with an alternative scenario, one in which all variables are the same, except that you are inexperienced in bandage application. You know that poor bandage application technique can have disastrous consequences for the patient – including amputation. Under these circumstances, you decide to prescribe graduated compression hosiery (stockings) rather than bandages. You know that graduated compression hosiery applies a similar level of compression to the four-layer bandage, and, after determining that the patient is able to apply the stockings himself, you concede that these will also be the safer option given your lack of skill in bandaging. If your patient had arthritic hands and was unable to apply stockings, or did not have the facilities to wash the stockings, your decision would probably have been different (see Figure 1.2). At any given time, the research evidence informing a decision is a constant; however, you must use your professional judgement to determine how you will apply it to the patient in front of you. Obviously, it is also important to remember that, as new research is published, the evidence base will change, and you will need to become aware of important changes in evidence relevant to your practice (see Chapter 5 for information on alerting services).

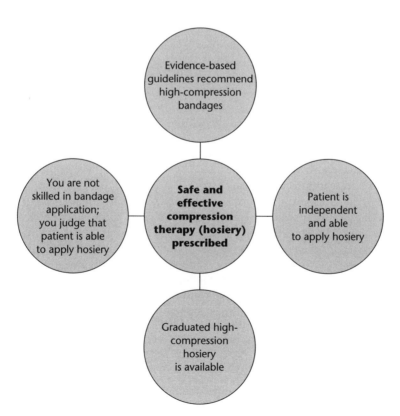

Figure 1.2 Resolution of a decision problem: how research evidence, judgement, patient preferences and circumstances, and knowledge about local resources interplay.

Getting started with evidence-based nursing

There are many ways to begin introducing research evidence into practice. At the simplest level, you might identify an area of practice for which you are responsible, find out if any evidence-based clinical practice guidelines exist, critically appraise them to determine if they are valid, and consider how they might be applied locally. Chapter 26 outlines this very process. In areas where guidelines don't exist, you might, in collaboration with colleagues, identify recurring uncertainties in your clinical area. Next, you would translate your single uncertainty (e.g. *Is it really necessary for people to lie flat for 8 hours after lumbar puncture?*) into a focused, answerable question. Chapter 3 outlines how to develop focused, answerable questions. For the lumbar puncture example, the question might be as follows: *In patients having cervical or lumbar puncture, is longer bed rest more effective than immediate mobilization or short bed rest in preventing headache?* This question is clearly about whether a particular intervention (lying flat for a long time) is better or worse than an alternative (not lying flat or lying flat for a brief time). Chapters 7 and 8 explain how certain types of clinical question demand research evidence from particular research designs because the answers are more likely to be valid, or true. In the above example, where the question concerns an intervention or therapy, the answer is best provided by randomized controlled trials (RCTs) (or, even better, by a systematic review of all relevant RCTs). You would then move into the searching phase to identify relevant RCTs or reviews; Chapters 4, 5 and 6 will guide you through the searching process. The next step is to grapple with assessing the quality of the research you find. We cannot accept the results of research at face value because, irrespective of where research has been published, and by whom, most research is not fit for immediate application. This is best illustrated by the fact that only about 5.4% of the approximately 50 000 articles published in 120 journals, and scrutinized for three evidence-based journals (*Evidence-Based Nursing, Evidence-Based Medicine,* and *ACP Journal Club*), reached the required methodological standard (personal communication, A McKibbon, 20 December 2006).

Fortunately several resources of pre-appraised research now exist, and these are discussed in Chapter 4. If your search does not identify any pre-appraised evidence, you will need to appraise the research you find so that you can judge whether the results are valid and ready for use in practice. Chapters 15–26 lead you through the process of critically appraising reports of study designs you will commonly encounter. Finally, Chapters 27–32 consider different aspects of research utilization: theoretical models (Chapter 27), empirical evidence of interventions aimed at changing professional behaviour (Chapter 28), the influence of the organization on research utilization (Chapter 29), use of research in clinical decision-making (Chapter 30), the emergence of computerized decision support systems in nursing (Chapter 31), and one hospital's experiences of promoting evidence-based nursing (Chapter 32).

Context

The emergence of evidence-based practice could not have happened at a more important time for nursing. The role of the nurse is not a fixed phenomenon; it varies by geography and culture and is heavily influenced by parameters such as the national economy and the supply of doctors. As we write this book at the beginning of the

Box 1.2 The Chief Nursing Officer's 10 new roles for nurses[5]

1. Ordering diagnostic investigations
2. Making referrals
3. Admitting and discharging patients within protocols
4. Managing caseloads of people with chronic conditions such as diabetes or rheumatoid arthritis
5. Running clinics (e.g. dermatology)
6. Prescribing medicines and treatments
7. Carrying out a wide range of resuscitation procedures
8. Minor surgery
9. Triage patients
10. Planning service organization and delivery

21st century, never has the demand for health care been so high, and most countries are struggling to meet this demand. The flexibility inherent in the nursing role is widely used to respond to this demand for health care. For example, in 2000, the United Kingdom (UK) Department of Health's Chief Nursing Officer announced 10 new roles for nurses, and nurses are now adopting these new roles widely (Box 1.2).[5] These new roles were previously held only (formally, at least) by doctors (e.g. prescribing drugs,† ordering diagnostic tests, etc.). It is difficult to imagine how nurses will be able to take on these challenging new roles and responsibilities *without* developing knowledge of clinical epidemiology and adopting an approach to decision-making that is informed by evidence.

At this point, it is probably worth pausing to reflect on how quickly nursing research has developed. The first nursing research journal (*Nursing Research*) was only launched in 1952. Early nursing research mainly used methodologies taken from the social sciences and largely focused on nurse education and nurses themselves. The second issue of *Nursing Research* contained nine research articles, four of which were about nursing students and nurse education. Since these early days, nursing research has developed apace, and there are now more than 1200 journals indexed in CINAHL, with 5400 research articles (identified by the search term 'nurs$') entering the CINAHL index in the year 2005 (searched by N. Cullum, 8 January 2007). In 1998, the *Evidence-Based Nursing* journal was launched, only 3 years after the launch of *Evidence-Based Medicine* (both published by the BMJ Publishing Group).

Early evidence of the impact of evidence-based practice on policy, education and research

Evidence-based practice in general, and evidence-based nursing in particular, can be viewed as complex innovations, and it would be naïve to expect rapid and

---

† Since 1 May 2006, nurses in the UK can prescribe *any* licensed medication for *any* clinical condition in which they have expertise, after a period of 26 days' training plus clinical mentorship.

comprehensive uptake. Nevertheless, there is ample evidence of the impact of 'evidence-based' thinking on policy and education, paralleled by a rapidly growing research evidence base in clinical nursing topics. The Nursing and Midwifery Council, which governs nursing professional practice and nurse education in the UK, outlines in its Code of Conduct an expectation that nurses will 'deliver care based on current evidence, best practice and, where applicable, validated research when it is available'.[6] The Nursing and Midwifery Council standards for nursing curricula demand that 'the curriculum should reflect contemporary knowledge and enable development of evidence-based practice'.[7] Educational establishments all over the world have responded to demands from policy-makers and practitioners and developed educational programmes in evidence-based practice, ranging from half-day courses through to higher degrees. Paralleling these developments, the research evidence base for nursing decisions is also growing and maturing. In 1995, a systematic review of pressure ulcer prevention and treatment by the Centre for Reviews and Dissemination (CRD) at the University of York identified a total of 28 RCTs evaluating different pressure-relieving support surfaces in the entire international literature.[8] The review concluded that '. . . most of the equipment available for the prevention and treatment of pressure sores has not been reliably evaluated, and no "best buy" can be recommended'.[8] More recent reviews completed to underpin UK national clinical practice guidelines show that the number of trials has increased, with 44 RCTs of support surfaces for pressure ulcer prevention and treatment.[9, 10] Importantly, gaps

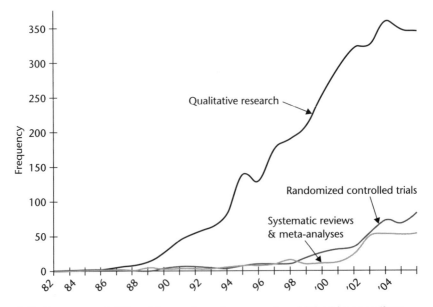

Figure 1.3 Frequency of different types of nursing research published by year (from CINAHL). CINAHL searched using the terms 'phenomenolog$', 'grounded theory', 'ethnograph$', 'randomised controlled trial', 'randomized controlled trial', 'systematic review', 'meta analysis'. Searching was confined to the Nursing Journal subset and research papers (excluding papers *about* research).

Phenomenolog$ + grounded theory + ethnograph$ = qualitative.

in the evidence base have resulted in the UK National Health Service commissioning research on pressure ulcer prevention.[11] Looking at the broader picture, Figure 1.3 shows how the numbers of RCTs and systematic reviews are growing (albeit slowly) as a proportion of the total nursing research indexed in CINAHL. This is important since observational research suggests that decisions about therapies (which, when, and to whom) are the most frequent type of decision made by nurses in acute care and primary care and that these types of decisions are best supported by research from RCTs.[12] We believe that, as evidence-based thinking increases in influence in nursing, the demand for RCTs and systematic reviews will continue to increase, and research funders will respond accordingly.

Why we wrote this book

The idea for this book grew out of our experience of producing the journal *Evidence-Based Nursing* since 1998. In common with other evidence-based journals produced by the Health Information Research Unit at McMaster University, *Evidence-Based Nursing* does not publish new research in full, but rather uses predefined methodological criteria to select, from the published literature, the best original studies and systematic reviews relevant to nurse decision-makers.[13] Full articles are then summarized in new, structured abstracts, which describe the question, methods, results, and evidence-based conclusions in a reproducible and accurate fashion. Each abstract is accompanied by a brief expert commentary written by a nurse, which discusses the context of the article, its methods, and clinical implications. Aside from this important dissemination role, the journal sought to develop evidence-based approaches to nursing through its Notebook and Users' Guides series. We saw these articles as being useful to nurses in clinical practice (who could see real examples of how the evidence-based framework could be applied to nursing decisions), useful to student nurses for the same reasons, and useful to nurse educators who were suddenly expected to teach this stuff with little previous preparation.[7] We regularly receive requests to bring the Notebooks and Users' Guides together as single resource, and so, in producing this book, we have had the same audience in mind: those of you who are somewhat, or completely, new to evidence-based practice, as well as those who are finding it difficult to get to grips with the concept. While the chapters of this book have mainly been developed from editorials already published in *Evidence-Based Nursing*, each has been scrutinized, edited, updated, and in some cases completely re-written. We hope that you will enjoy using the book in a variety of ways. The chapters can stand alone, and therefore you can dip into and out of the book depending on the immediate challenge at hand, or you can work through the book chapter by chapter. We urge you to consider doing this with colleagues so that you can share the learning experience and work through examples that are relevant and meaningful to your practice.

Most chapters include Learning Exercises, which are aimed at reinforcing the chapter material by allowing you to practise the techniques yourself; alternatively, nurse teachers might want to set these as exercises for students. Finally, we have included a comprehensive Glossary of terms that will stand alone as a useful guide to the basic concepts. We are indebted to all of our contributors who have given their time and expertise so freely and helped to bring this material completely up to date. We hope you enjoy reading the book as much as we have enjoyed producing it!

References

1 Evidence-Based Medicine Working Group. Evidence-based medicine. A new approach to teaching the practice of medicine. *JAMA* 1992;**268**:2420–5.

2 Evidence-based management. http://www.evidence-basedmanagement.com/movements/index.html (accessed 12 December 2006).

3 Thompson C, McCaughan D, Cullum N, Sheldon TA, Mulhall A, Thompson DR. Research information in nurses' clinical decision-making: what is useful? *J Adv Nurs* 2001;**36**:376–88.

4 Royal College of Nursing. *Clinical Practice Guidelines. The Nursing Management of Patients with Venous Leg Ulcers.* London: Royal College of Nursing, 2006. http://www.rcn.org.uk/resources/guidelines.php (accessed 12 December 2006).

5 Department of Health. *The NHS Plan.* 2000. http://www.nhsia.nhs.uk/nhsplan/(accessed 12 December 2006).

6 Nursing and Midwifery Council. *The NMC Code of Professional Conduct: Standards for Conduct, Performance and Ethics.* London: Nursing and Midwifery Council, 2004. http://www.nmc-uk.org/ (accessed 12 December 2006).

7 Nursing and Midwifery Council. *Standards of Proficiency for Pre-registration Nursing Education.* London: Nursing and Midwifery Council, 2004. http://www.nmc-uk.org/aSection.aspx?SectionID=32 (accessed 12 December 2006).

8 Effective Health Care. *The Prevention and Treatment of Pressure Sores.* York: Centre for Reviews and Dissemination. 1995. http://www.york.ac.uk/inst/crd/ehc21.pdf (accessed 12 December 2006).

9 Royal College of Nursing. *Clinical Practice Guidelines. Pressure Ulcer Risk Assessment and Prevention.* London: Royal College of Nursing, 2001. http://www.nice.org.uk/guidance/CGB/guidance/pdf/English (accessed 12 December 2006).

10 Royal College of Nursing. *Clinical Practice Guidelines. The Use of Pressure-Relieving Devices (Beds, Mattresses and Overlays) for the Prevention of Pressure Ulcers in Primary and Secondary Care.* London: Royal College of Nursing, 2003. http://www.rcn.org.uk/publications/pdf/guidelines/pressure-relieving-devices.pdf (accessed 12 December 2006).

11 Nixon J, Cranny G, Iglesias C, Nelson EA, Hawkins K, Phillips A, Torgerson D, Mason S, Cullum N. Randomised, controlled trial of alternating pressure mattresses compared with alternating pressure overlays for the prevention of pressure ulcers: PRESSURE (pressure relieving support surfaces) trial. *BMJ* 2006;**332**:1413.

12 McCaughan D. What decisions do nurses make? In: Thompson C, Dowding D, editors. *Clinical Decision Making and Judgement in Nursing.* Edinburgh: Churchill Livingstone, 2002:95–108.

13 Purpose and procedure. *Evid Based Nurs* 2006;**9**:98–9.

Chapter 2

IMPLEMENTING EVIDENCE-BASED NURSING: SOME MISCONCEPTIONS

Alba DiCenso, Nicky Cullum and Donna Ciliska

The past 10 years have seen a strong movement towards evidence-based clinical practice. In 1997, the Canadian National Health Forum, chaired by Prime Minister Jean Chrétien, recommended that 'a key objective of the health sector should be to move rapidly toward the development of an evidence-based health system, in which decisions are made by health care providers, administrators, policy makers, patients and the public on the basis of appropriate, balanced and high quality evidence.'[1] In the United States (US), the Agency for Healthcare Research and Quality (AHRQ) leads national efforts in the use of evidence to guide health care decisions through funding of evidence-based practice centres, systematic reviews, evidence-based practice guidelines, and studies that evaluate strategies to disseminate research findings to practitioners and policy makers.[2] In the United Kingdom (UK), the Department of Health has advocated for evidence-based practice to enhance the quality of patient care, nursing, midwifery, and health visiting.[3]

Specific to nursing, the Sigma Theta Tau International Honor Society of Nursing issued a position statement on evidence-based nursing in 2003 and made a commitment to being a leading source of knowledge and resources that foster evidence-based nursing practice globally.[4] Centres for Evidence-Based Nursing have been established in many countries to provide educational sessions to help nurses learn to use evidence in clinical practice.[5] Journals such as *Evidence-Based Nursing* and *Worldviews on Evidence-Based Nursing* and textbooks such as this one are designed to help nurses to become evidence-based practitioners.

There have, however, been misgivings, sometimes generated by a misunderstanding of evidence-based nursing. Three of these misconceptions will be addressed in this chapter: (1) evidence-based practice isn't new: it's what we have been doing for years; (2) evidence-based nursing leads to 'cookbook' nursing and a disregard for individualized patient care; and (3) there is an over-emphasis on randomized controlled trials (RCTs) and systematic reviews in evidence-based health care, and they are not relevant to nursing.

Evidence-based practice isn't new; it's what we have been doing for years

The plea that 'each nurse must care enough about her own practice to want to make sure it is based on the best possible information' is not new. It was written over 25 years ago. In the same article, Hunt[6] noted that the words 'nursing should become a research-based profession' had already become a cliché. In 1976, Gortner et al.[7] lamented the lack of research evidence in many areas of nursing practice, and one year later Roper[8] spoke of nursing performing 'far too many of its tasks on a traditional base and not within a framework of scientific verifications'.

While recognition of the importance of evidence-based nursing practice is not new, two studies, one conducted in Canada in the mid-1990s and one conducted in the US in 2005, reported worrisome findings about the lack of reliance on research findings in the nursing profession. Estabrooks[9] surveyed 1500 randomly selected staff nurses in Alberta, Canada, to identify the frequency of use of various information sources. The respondents most frequently used experiential information sources (patient data and personal experience), followed by basic nursing education programs, in-service programs and conferences, policy and procedure manuals, physician sources, intuition, and 'what has worked for years'. Articles published in nursing research journals ranked second to last in frequency of usage (15th of 16 ranked sources). Estabrooks[9] identified several troubling issues including the reliance on non-scientific knowledge and on basic nursing education, even though these nurses had graduated from their nursing education programs an average of 18 years earlier.

More recently, Pravikoff et al.[10] surveyed 3000 nurses across the US and found that while nurses reported frequently needing information for practice, they felt more confident asking colleagues or peers and searching the Internet than using bibliographic databases such as PubMed or CINAHL to find information. Fewer than half of respondents (46%) were familiar with the term 'evidence-based practice'. Asked to rank the top three barriers to nurses' use of research in practice from a list of 10 (excluding lack of time, which is a well known barrier), the most highly ranked barriers were lack of value for research in practice, lack of understanding of electronic databases, difficulty accessing research materials, and difficulty understanding research articles. Consistent with the findings of Estabrooks,[9] nurses were relying on what they had learned in nursing school even though they had graduated many years before. Pravikoff et al.[10] concluded that although nurses acknowledged their need for information to guide effective practice, they received little or no education or training in information retrieval, didn't understand or value research, and were generally unprepared for a practice built on evidence.

The reliance on 'human sources' of information found by Pravikoff et al. was also found among nurses in acute care settings,[11–13] nurse practitioners and practice nurses in primary care,[14–16] and physicians.[16–18] These consistent findings suggest that a human dimension to knowledge transfer is important for effective research implementation strategies.[19]

Many researchers have studied the barriers to evidence-based practice and have identified strategies to overcome these barriers. At an individual level, nurses lack skill in accessing research and evaluating its quality,[10, 20] they are isolated from knowledgeable colleagues with whom to discuss research,[21] and they lack confidence to implement change.[20, 22] Organizational characteristics of health care settings are the most significant barriers to research use among nurses.[20–23] Nurses report a lack of time to seek out research information and to implement research findings.[21-25] Mitchell *et al.* found that health care institutions that reported making changes based on the research process were more likely to have at least one nursing research committee and to have access to nurses with expertise in nursing research.[26] Nurses have identified a lack of organizational support for evidence-based nursing and noted a lack of interest, motivation, leadership, and vision among managers.[20]

In a systematic review, Estabrooks *et al.*[27] examined how individual nurse characteristics influenced research utilization and found that, apart from attitude to research, there was little to suggest that any individual determinant influenced research use. The individual nurse cannot be isolated from other bureaucratic, political, organizational and social factors that affect change. The implementation of research-based practice depends on an ability to achieve significant and planned behaviour change involving individuals, teams and organizations.[28]

Ciliska *et al.*[29] suggested strategies to facilitate organizational support for evidence-based nursing practice. These include allowing nurses time for activities that foster evidence-based practice, such as going to the library, learning how to conduct electronic searches, and holding journal club meetings; establishing nurse researcher positions and formalizing nursing research committees; linking staff nurses with advanced practice nurses; linking advanced practice nurses with nurse faculty researchers; ensuring that health care institution libraries have print or online subscriptions to nursing research journals; and making resources such as *Clinical Evidence*, the *Cochrane Library*, and abstraction journals, such as *Evidence-Based Nursing*, available.

Kitson *et al.*[30] proposed that the most successful implementation of evidence into practice occurs when evidence is scientifically robust and matches professional consensus and patient preferences; the environment is receptive to change, with sympathetic cultures; strong leadership and appropriate monitoring and feedback systems exist; and there is appropriate facilitation of change, with input from skilled external and internal facilitators.

Evidence-based nursing leads to 'cookbook' nursing and a disregard for individualized patient care

Those who judge evidence-based nursing as 'cookbook' nursing mistakenly believe that evidence-based practitioners consider only research evidence in the clinical decision-making process. In fact, evidence-based clinical decision-making involves integrating the knowledge arising from one's clinical expertise; patient preferences and actions; patient clinical states, settings, and circumstances; and research evidence within the context of available resources (Figure 2.1).[31] Let's consider an example to illustrate. A nurse practitioner in a cardiology clinic reads a recently published, high quality study that showed that a telephone intervention for people with chronic heart failure reduced admission to hospital for worsening heart failure.[32] Those in the telephone intervention group received an education booklet and frequent, standardized, telephone follow-up by nurses. The purpose of the telephone calls was to educate patients and to monitor their adherence to diet and medication, symptoms, signs of hydrosaline retention, and daily physical activity.

The nurse practitioner shares this *research evidence* with the administrator of her unit, who must decide whether the savings resulting from reduced readmissions are sufficient to cover the costs of the additional nursing time required to make the

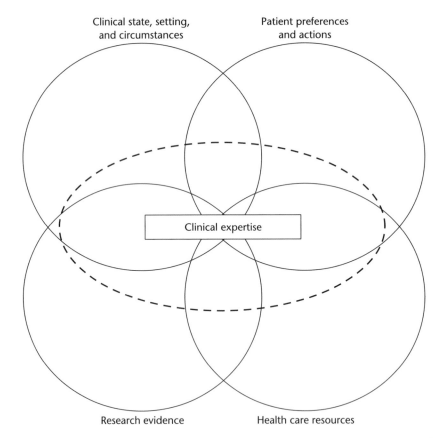

Figure 2.1 A model for evidence-based clinical decisions. Modified and reproduced with permission of the American College of Physicians from Haynes RB, Devereaux PJ, Guyatt GH. Clinical expertise in the era of evidence-based medicine and patient choice. *ACP Journal Club* 2002;**136**:A11–14.

telephone calls (*health care resources*). Assuming that the administrator supports the intervention, the nurse practitioner uses her *clinical expertise* to assess the health state of patients who are potentially eligible for telephone follow-up, their risks, their preferences and actions, and the potential benefits of the intervention; to communicate information about the intervention to patients and their families; and to provide them with an environment they find comforting and supportive. Clinical expertise is the crucial element that separates evidence-based nursing from cookbook nursing and the mindless application of rules and guidelines.

When the nurse practitioner describes the intervention to various patients, those who are feeling very sick or weak, those with hearing problems, or those who do not have a telephone will likely choose not to receive telephone follow-up (*clinical state, setting, and circumstances*), whereas others who do not have these issues may welcome the opportunity for telephone follow-up. Patients who loathe talking on the telephone or who like to sleep during daytime hours because they don't sleep well at night may choose not to receive telephone follow-up even though they have been informed about the benefits of the intervention (*patient preferences and actions*).

Clinical expertise and patient preference may override the other components of the model for a given decision. For example, clinical expertise must prevail if the nurse decides that the patient is too frail for a specific intervention that is otherwise 'best' for his condition, and a patient's preference will dominate when he declines a treatment that clinical circumstances and research evidence indicate is best for his condition. Patients exercise their preferences for care by choosing alternative treatments, refusing treatment, preparing advance directives ('living wills'), and seeking second opinions. Today's patients have greater access to clinical information than ever before, and some, particularly those with chronic conditions, become more knowledgeable about their conditions than their care providers. Although a patient's role in clinical decisions is usually not formalized and is sometimes ignored by care providers, it is an important component of most clinical decisions. Clearly, the best possible scenario is one in which the patient is able to play a full part in making decisions about his or her own health care, having been given an accurate assessment of the current state of knowledge.

When we consider Figure 2.1, the challenge for nursing is to give appropriate weight to research evidence. Nursing training and experience ensure that nurses have clinical expertise. Traditionally, nurses have been respectful and sensitive to patients' clinical circumstances and preferences, and they are frequently reminded about the need to consider limited health care resources. However, based on the research of Estabrooks[9] and Pravikoff et al.,[10] many nurses do not understand or value research and have had little or no training to help them find evidence on which to base their practice. It is the research evidence circle in the figure that requires the most attention from the nursing profession if we are to help patients make evidence-based clinical decisions related to their care.

There is an over-emphasis on randomized controlled trials and systematic reviews in evidence-based health care, and they are not relevant to nursing

Evidence-based health care is about incorporating the best available evidence in clinical decision-making. Nursing practice generates numerous questions related to, for example, the effectiveness of nursing interventions, the accuracy and precision of nursing assessment measures, the power of prognostic markers, the strength of causal relations, the cost-effectiveness of nursing interventions, the meaning of illness, and patient experiences, beliefs, and attitudes. Each of these types of questions can be addressed by different study designs, and an important challenge for evidence-based practitioners is to determine whether the best design has been used to answer the question posed, be it an RCT to evaluate a nursing intervention, a cohort study to examine a question of prognosis, or a qualitative study to learn more about the meaning of illness.

McCaughan et al.[14] found that most decisions made by primary care nurses related to questions about interventions. The rest of this section will focus on the importance of RCTs and systematic reviews in evaluating the effectiveness of nursing interventions. In an RCT, individuals are randomly allocated to receive or not receive an experimental intervention and then followed up over time to determine the effects of the intervention. For example, in an RCT of techniques for intramuscular thigh vaccination, 375 healthy children up to 18 months of age were randomized to the Australian, US or World Health Organization (WHO) technique and followed up for

24 hours to assess local and systemic adverse reactions.[33] The WHO technique resulted in less bruising and infant irritability. The reason that an RCT is the most appropriate design to address this type of question is that through random assignment of study participants to comparison groups, known and unknown determinants of outcome are most likely to be distributed evenly between groups, thus ensuring that any difference in outcome is due to the intervention being evaluated (see Chapters 7 and 15).

There are numerous examples of interventions in both nursing and medicine that initially appeared beneficial but were shown to be of doubtful value or even harmful when they were evaluated using randomized trials. Examples include the use of cover gowns by nurses when caring for healthy newborns in the nursery,[34] and shaving of patients before surgical procedures.[35] Few of us would want to begin a drug regimen that had not been proven safe and effective in an RCT.

Many research questions have been addressed by more than one study. This is a positive development because given the play of chance, any single study, even a methodologically rigorous RCT, may arrive at a false conclusion. However, how does an evidence-based practitioner cope with the myriad of studies addressing the same research question, some with discrepant findings? The first step is to look for a systematic review. A *systematic review* is a process that consolidates the findings of all studies addressing the same research question. In a systematic review, all studies that address a specific research question are identified, relevant studies are evaluated for methodological quality, data are extracted and summarized, and conclusions are drawn. When possible, data from individual studies are statistically combined to, in effect, create one large study. This process, known as *meta-analysis*, results in a more precise estimate of effect than can be obtained from any individual study included in the meta-analysis. Through systematic reviews, nurses are provided with a summary of all methodologically sound studies related to a specific topic. Chapters 5 and 6 describe how to find systematic reviews, and Chapter 19 describes how to critically appraise them.

A rich source of high quality systematic reviews is the *Cochrane Library*, an electronic resource that focuses on systematic reviews of controlled trials of health care interventions. Recent systematic reviews of relevance to nursing have examined whether multidisciplinary interventions reduce hospital admissions and all-cause mortality in patients with heart failure,[36] whether early supported discharge with rehabilitation at home improves outcomes in patients admitted to hospital with stroke,[37] and whether preventive psychosocial and psychological interventions reduce the risk of postpartum depression.[38]

Those who believe that RCTs and systematic reviews are not relevant to nursing need only browse issues of the *Evidence-Based Nursing* journal. Each quarterly issue contains abstracts summarizing 24 studies or systematic reviews, two-thirds of which focus on the effectiveness of nursing interventions. To be eligible for inclusion in the journal, all intervention studies must be RCTs or systematic reviews of RCTs, a strong indication of the number of such studies relevant to nursing that exist.

Summary

While we would like to believe that we have been providing evidence-based nursing practice for years, we are not there yet. What we have been able to do is to conduct research that has identified barriers to evidence-based practice. We must now work to overcome these barriers so that we can create an environment that facilitates evidence-based practice.

Evidence-based nursing does not lead to 'cookbook' nursing and a disregard for individualized patient care. In clinical decision-making, research evidence is integrated with knowledge about a patient's clinical state, setting and circumstances; patient preferences and actions; health care resources; and clinical expertise.

Finally, there are many different study designs, each ideally suited to answering different nursing practice questions. The RCT is the study design of choice when evaluating the effectiveness of a nursing intervention because, through random assignment of study participants to comparison groups, known and unknown determinants of outcome are evenly distributed between groups ensuring that any difference in outcome can be attributed to the intervention. When more than one study has been conducted to address the same research question, one should look for a systematic review. Through consolidation of research findings, a systematic review provides a more definitive answer to a research question.

LEARNING EXERCISES

1. Think about times when you have needed information related to your nursing practice. How did you obtain this information? If you did not seek out electronic databases such as PubMed, the *Cochrane Library*, or *Evidence-Based Nursing* journal, why not? What characteristics of your work setting facilitate the use of evidence in your practice, and what characteristics impede the use of evidence in your practice? What might be changed in your work environment to increase evidence-based nursing practice?
2. Identify some of the clinical decisions you have recently made related to patient care. Refer to Figure 2.1, and consider the role each component in the figure played in your decision-making. Did you consider research evidence, and, if so, how did it influence the decision process? If you did not consider research evidence, why not?
3. Identify three nursing interventions that you carry out in your clinical practice. Conduct a search of *Evidence-Based Nursing* (http://ebn.bmjjournals.com) and the *Cochrane Library Database of Systematic Reviews* (http://www.cochrane.org) to determine if there are any RCTs and systematic reviews evaluating the effectiveness of the three nursing interventions. Are the results of the RCTs or reviews consistent with your current practice? If not, do you plan to change your practice to reflect the study findings, and, if so, what challenges does that present?

References

1 National Forum on Health. *Canada Health Action: Building on the Legacy*. Vol. I. Ottawa: National Forum on Health, 1997:3–43.
2 Titler MG. Use of research in practice. In: LoBiondo-Wood G, Haber J, editors. *Nursing Research: Methods, Critical Appraisal, and Utilization*. 5th edition. St. Louis: Mosby-Year Book, 2002:411–44.
3 UK Department of Health. Making a difference: strengthening the nursing, midwifery and health visiting contribution to health and healthcare. 1999. http://www.dh.gov.uk/assetRoot/04/07/47/04/04074704.pdf (accessed 15 May 2006).
4 Dickenson-Hazard N. Foreword. In DiCenso A, Guyatt G, Ciliska D, editors. *Evidence-Based Nursing: A Guide to Clinical Practice*. St. Louis: Elsevier Mosby, 2005: xxiii–xxiv.
5 Ciliska D, DiCenso A, Cullum N. Centres of evidence-based nursing: directions and challenges. *Evid Based Nurs* 1999;2:102–4.
6 Hunt J. Indicators for nursing practice: the use of research findings. *J Adv Nurs* 1981;6:189–94.

7 Gortner SR, Bloch D, Phillips TP. Contributions of nursing research to patient care. *J Adv Nurs* 1976;**1**:507–18.

8 Roper N. Justification and use of research in nursing. *J Adv Nurs* 1977;**2**:365–71.

9 Estabrooks CA. Will evidence-based nursing practice make practice perfect? *Can J Nurs Res* 1998;**30**:15–36.

10 Pravikoff DS, Tanner AB, Pierce ST. Readiness of U.S. nurses for evidence-based practice. *Am J Nursing* 2005;**105**:40–51.

11 Thompson C, McCaughan D, Cullum N, Sheldon TA, Mulhall A, Thompson DR. The accessibility of research-based knowledge for nurses in United Kingdom acute care settings. *J Adv Nurs* 2001;**36**:11–22.

12 Thompson C, McCaughan D, Cullum N, Sheldon TA, Mulhall A, Thompson DR. Research information in nurses' clinical decision making: what is useful? *J Adv Nurs* 2001;**36**:376–88.

13 Thompson C, Cullum N, McCaughan D, Sheldon T, Raynor P. Nurses, information use, and clinical decision making—the real world potential for evidence-based decisions in nursing. *Evid Based Nurs* 2004;**7**:68–72.

14 McCaughan D, Thompson C, Cullum N, Sheldon T, Raynor P. Nurse practitioner and practice nurses' use of research information in clinical decision making: findings from an exploratory study. *Fam Pract* 2005;**22**:490–7.

15 Cogdill KW. Information needs and information seeking in primary care: a study of nurse practitioners. *J Med Libr Assoc* 2003;**91**:203–15.

16 Gabbay J, le May A. Evidence based guidelines or collectively constructed "mindlines?" Ethnographic study of knowledge management in primary care. *BMJ* 2004;**329**:1013.

17 Covell DG, Uman GC, Manning PR. Information needs in office practice: are they being met? *Ann Intern Med* 1985;**103**:596–9.

18 Tomlin Z, Humphrey C, Rogers S. General practitioners' perceptions of effective health care. *BMJ* 1999;**318**:1532–5.

19 McCaughan D. Commentary on 'Primary care practitioners based everyday practice on internalised tacit guidelines derived through social interactions with trusted colleagues.' *Evid-Based Nurs* 2005;**8**:94. Comment on: Gabbay J, le May A. Evidence based guidelines or collectively constructed 'mindlines?' Ethnographic study of knowledge management in primary care. *BMJ* 2004;**329**:1013.

20 Parahoo K. Barriers to, and facilitators of, research utilization among nurses in Northern Ireland. *J Adv Nurs* 2000;**31**:89–98.

21 Nilsson Kajermo K, Nordstrom G, Krusebrant A, Bjorvell H. Barriers to and facilitators of research utilization, as perceived by a group of registered nurses in Sweden. *J Adv Nurs* 1998;**27**:798–807.

22 Rodgers S. An exploratory study of research utilization by nurses in general medical and surgical wards. *J Adv Nurs* 1994;**20**:904–11.

23 Retsas A. Barriers to using research evidence in nursing practice. *J Adv Nurs* 2000;**31**:599–606.

24 Retsas A, Nolan M. Barriers to nurses' use of research: an Australian hospital study. *Int J Nurs Stud* 1999;**36**:335–43.

25 Thompson C, McCaughan D, Cullum N, Sheldon T, Raynor P. Barriers to evidence-based practice in primary care nursing—why viewing decision-making as context is helpful. *J Adv Nurs* 2005;**52**:432–44.

26 Mitchell A, Janzen K, Pask E, Southwell D. Assessment of nursing research utilization needs in Ontario health agencies. *Can J Nurs Adm* 1995;**8**:77–91.

27 Estabrooks CA, Floyd JA, Scott-Findlay S, O'Leary KA, Gushta M. Individual determinants of research utilization: a systematic review. *J Adv Nurs* 2003;**43**:506–20.

28 Rycroft-Malone J. The politics of the evidence-based practice movements: legacies and current challenges. *Journal of Research in Nursing* 2006;**11**:95–108.

29 Ciliska DK, Pinelli J, DiCenso A, Cullum N. Resources to enhance evidence-based nursing practice. *AACN Clin Issues* 2001;**12**:520–8.

30 Kitson A, Harvey G, McCormack B. Enabling the implementation of evidence-based practice: a conceptual framework. *Qual Health Care* 1998;7:149–58.

31 Haynes RB, Devereaux PJ, Guyatt GH. Clinical expertise in the era of evidence-based medicine and patient choice. *ACP J Club* 2002;**136**:A11–14.

32 GESICA Investigators. Randomised trial of telephone intervention in chronic heart failure: DIAL trial. *BMJ* 2005;**331**:425.

33 Cook IF, Murtagh J. Optimal technique for intramuscular injection of infants and toddlers: a randomised trial. *Med J Aust* 2005;**183**:60–3.

34 Rush J, Fiorino-Chiovitti R, Kaufman K, Mitchell A. A randomised controlled trial of a nursery ritual: wearing cover gowns to care for healthy newborns. *Birth* 1990;**17**:25–30.

35 Hoe NY, Nambiar R. Is preoperative shaving really necessary? *Ann Acad Med Singapore* 1985;**14**:700–4.

36 Holland R, Battersby J, Harvey I, Lenaghan E, Smith J, Hay L. Systematic review of multidisciplinary interventions in heart failure. *Heart* 2005;**91**:899–906.

37 Langhorne P, Taylor G, Murray G, Dennis M, Anderson C, Bautz-Holter E, Dey P, Indredavik B, Mayo N, Power M, Rodgers H, Ronning OM, Rudd A, Suwanwela N, Widen-Holmqvist L, Wolfe C. Early supported discharge services for stroke patients: a meta-analysis of individual patients' data. *Lancet* 2005;**365**:501–6.

38 Dennis CL, Creedy D. Psychosocial and psychological interventions for preventing postpartum depression. *Cochrane Database Syst Rev* 2004;(4):CD001134.

Chapter 3

ASKING ANSWERABLE QUESTIONS

Kate Flemming

Nurses have had to deal with many changes in recent years, one of which is the increased expectation that they will keep their practice up to date by reading and acting upon research reports. This expectation and the pressures of maintaining continuing education requirements come alongside ever increasing workloads and diminishing study time.

So what can be done to ease some of the pressure? Evidence-based nursing (EBN) offers at least some of the answers. In a nutshell, the aim of EBN is to make it easier to move from clinical uncertainty to clinical decisions by incorporating current research evidence into decision-making processes.

What is EBN?

EBN is a five-stage process:

1. Clinical uncertainty from practice is converted into focused, structured questions.
2. The focused questions are used as a basis for literature searching in order to identify relevant external evidence from research.
3. The research evidence is critically appraised for validity and applicability.
4. The best available evidence is used alongside clinical expertise, the patient's perspective, and available resources to plan care.
5. Outcomes are evaluated through a process of self-reflection, audit, or peer assessment.

The purpose of this chapter is to work through stage 1: the formulation of structured, focused questions arising from clinical uncertainty.

Why focus questions?

The types of information needs commonly found in clinical practice arise from questions such as *Why do we do it this way?* or *What is the best way of ... ?* – questions for which neither you nor your colleagues have a ready answer. If you have access to computer databases, the Internet or a library, what efficient strategies exist for finding answers to clinical questions? How do you find high quality, relevant research without wading through hundreds of papers? This chapter and those that follow will provide answers to these questions!

Framing the question in a way that lends itself to searching, while still reflecting a specific patient or service focus, is an important stage to get right. Question framing is a fundamental skill for evidence-based practitioners and one that helps to focus scarce learning time on evidence that is highly relevant to patient needs.[1] Focusing clinical uncertainty into an answerable question will enable you to search for research in a systematic way. This should help to reduce the volume of search results to a manageable amount.

Where do questions come from?

Uncertainty and questions arise from many clinical and management situations. For example, a question that arose during my work in palliative care related to the development and use of pain diaries for patients with advanced cancer. I realized that I didn't actually know whether completing pain diaries was useful in the palliative care of patients with cancer. Was time being spent developing something that had previously been shown to be useless or even harmful? After all, it is conceivable that monitoring one's pain in a diary actually heightens one's awareness and experience of pain. I needed to search the literature to find out if any research had been done on this topic. To focus my search, I developed the following question: *Does the use of pain diaries in the palliative care of patients with cancer lead to improved pain control?*

Elements of a question

Generally, there are four elements to a question: *Population, Intervention, Comparison*, and *Outcome*. These elements have become known as PICO,[1, 2] and this format has proved successful in helping clinicians to learn how to formulate searchable, answerable questions.[3] Recently, a fifth element of question development – the *Time frame* in which the question occurs – has been proposed, and PICO becomes PICOT.[2]

Focusing attention on each of these elements ensures that all aspects of the clinical uncertainty you are trying to address are included in your question. This is particularly helpful when communicating the uncertainty to colleagues and also guides effective search strategies.[1] Each of the elements of a question will be described in turn.

Population

The *population* is the client group or clinical scenario of interest. This can be a single patient or group of patients with a particular condition or health care problem. In my example, the population is 'people with cancer receiving palliative care'. The population may also consist of individuals with similar demographic characteristics. Alternatively, if you are a manager, the scope of the population may be a wider aspect of delivering or organizing health services, such as nurse-led care for people with chronic conditions.

Other examples of populations include:

- A person with a grade two pressure sore (an individual)
- People with hypertension (a group of people with a particular condition)
- Children under 10 years of age (a population with similar demographic characteristics)
- Primary health care for the elderly (an aspect of health care delivery)
- Organization of an outpatient department (aspects of organizing health care for a particular population)

Intervention of interest

The *intervention* is the aspect of health care of interest. In my example, the question was whether the use of pain diaries to record pain was a useful treatment for the palliative care of people with cancer, i.e. 'pain diaries' are the intervention. Interventions come in many guises, and recognizing these can help you to develop a strategy for searching for the evidence. Interventions can be:[4]

- Therapeutic (e.g. different wound dressings)
- Preventive (e.g. influenza vaccination)
- Diagnostic (e.g. measurement of blood pressure)
- Organizational (e.g. implementation of a computerized appointments system)

If your clinical uncertainty is about people's experiences or the meaning of a complex phenomenon to those involved, then your question may be more concerned with a situation than in intervention. These types of questions, which are usually addressed by qualitative research evidence (see Chapter 8), may just require a population component and a *situation*. For example, if you were interested in improving mammography services, you might wish to focus on how women are given the results of mammography. It would be important to understand women's experiences of receiving the results of mammography in order to learn from their good and bad experiences. As well, dissatisfaction with the experience of mammography may also reduce adherence to the screening programme. In this example, the population of interest is 'women' and the situation is 'routine mammography screening for early breast cancer'. Your clinical question might be *What are women's experiences of receiving the results of mammography screening?* Questions that are addressed by qualitative research typically do not fit the PICOT format, and a much simpler structure of the population and situation components will usually suffice.[5]

Comparison interventions

Clinical decisions by definition involve choosing between alternative courses of action (or no action), and thus focused clinical questions (particularly intervention and diagnostic questions) often include an element of comparison. Examples are whether paracetamol (acetaminophen) is better than ibuprofen for the relief of pyrexia in children, or whether temperature taking in children is more accurate using glass-mercury rectal thermometers or tympanic membrane thermometry. Careful thought about useful comparisons for your clinical questions will help you to get more useful answers to your questions.

For questions about interventions (and we know that these are the questions most commonly raised by nurses[6]), the relevant comparison may be standard care or no intervention at all. The pain diaries example could be phrased as *Does the use of pain diaries in the palliative care of patients with cancer lead to improved pain control compared with not using diaries?* The comparison here is 'not using diaries'. Another example incorporating a comparison intervention might be *Do people receiving treatment for venous leg ulcers in community leg ulcer clinics have improved healing rates compared with those receiving care at home?* This question involves a comparison of two treatment settings: specialized community clinics and home care.

Outcome of interest

The *outcome*, or the effect we are hoping to achieve by using the intervention, is an area of question development that often gets missed if not using a structured format such as PICOT. Thinking about outcomes during question formulation is important because knowing what you hope to achieve by using the intervention helps to narrow the focus of your search to studies that report the outcome of interest. When you start thinking about outcomes, you may identify more than one outcome that is important to your question. In the pain diary example, we would be interested in whether 'pain control' improved as a result of visual recording of pain levels. However, we might also be interested in people's 'perceptions' of using a pain diary as part of their care. Both outcomes are important but would likely require separate search strategies given that different types of research would be needed to address these different questions (see Chapters 7 and 8). Therefore, it is helpful to list all of the outcomes of interest and then prioritize your searching accordingly.

In the example comparing use of paracetamol and ibuprofen in children, the outcome of interest would be 'reduction in pyrexia'; another outcome of interest might be 'reduction of pain'. In the example comparing community leg ulcer clinics with care at home, the outcome of interest would be 'leg ulcer healing', although one also might be interested in the outcomes of 'quality of life' and 'cost-effectiveness'.

Time frame

This element focuses on the period of time over which the question occurs. It might not always be relevant, but including it in the structure reduces the chance that it might be forgotten in situations where it might be a useful.[2] All three of our examples could include time as an element. That is, it would be helpful to know over what period of time it is useful to get people to record their pain in diaries – perhaps for 48 hours before a review of their pain control. A shorter time frame of 1 hour would be appropriate for the comparison of the effectiveness of paracetamol with ibuprofen for children with pyrexia. The time frame would be much longer in our comparison of community clinics and care at home for leg ulcers since leg ulcers can take months to heal. In this example, 6 months would be an appropriate time frame to specify.

Putting it all together

The individual elements of a question are crucial when it comes to searching for evidence. One of the easiest ways to do this is to use a table (see Table 3.1).

Putting each part of the question into its appropriate column eases the task of developing a searchable question. It is important to remember that the order of the elements

Table 3.1 The PICOT table

Population	Intervention	Comparison	Outcome	Time frame

Table 3.2 Component parts of a question

Population	Intervention	Comparison	Outcome	Time frame
Children with pyrexia	Paracetamol	Ibuprofen	Apyrexia	1 hour

within a question does not have to follow the order of the columns (i.e. population, intervention, comparison intervention, outcome, and time frame). It is also worth remembering that not all questions will require an entry in every column of the table.

The example of comparing paracetamol with ibuprofen to reduce fever in children is broken down into its component parts in Table 3.2. This leads to the formulation of the following question: *In children with pyrexia, is paracetamol more effective than ibuprofen in achieving apyrexia within 1 hour of administration?*

Different types of questions

Several other types of important questions can arise out of clinical uncertainty (Table 3.3). It is important to be able to identify what type of question you are asking because this will help in your search for the best type of research to answer the question. Chapters 7 and 8 focus on the process of identifying the best research design to answer these different types of questions; there is no overall 'best' research design. Examples of different types of clinical question are shown in Table 3.3.

Finding answers

Thinking about all the elements of the clinical uncertainty you are trying to address using the PICOT format provides you with terms you can use to begin your search for answers. Chapters 4, 5 and 6 describe various aspects of effective searching. Developing a focused question can save a great deal of searching time, with the key words of the question becoming the key terms for a search. Perhaps of all health care professionals, nurses spend most time at the bedside and have little or no protected time to find evidence for practice.[7] By developing focused questions, nurses can make efficient use of their time searching for research evidence and, given the right resources, can increasingly base their practice on evidence.

Table 3.3 Different types of clinical questions[6]

Type of question	Example
Health care interventions. *What are the health outcomes of different interventions?*	Does compression bandaging increase the healing of venous leg ulcers compared with no compression?
Causation and harm. *What might be causing disease/ill health/adverse effects?*	Does the combined measles, mumps and rubella childhood immunization lead to an increased risk of autism compared with separate vaccines given at different times?
Prognosis. *What are potential future outcomes of a condition?*	Does having a stroke increase risk of dementia in older people?
Diagnosis or assessment. *Does a diagnostic test differentiate between people with and without a condition?*	Is audiometry more accurate than the whispered voice test for detecting hearing impairment in older people?
Meaning. *Describing, exploring and explaining aspects of health and illness*	What are the experiences of using pain diaries of people with cancer receiving palliative care?
Economics. *Studying the economic efficiency of health care interventions and programmes*	Are four-layer elastic bandages more cost-effective than multilayer inelastic bandages for healing venous leg ulcers?

LEARNING EXERCISE

Identify areas of your practice where there is uncertainty – it's even better if you can do this with a colleague! It might help to reflect on the *Why do we do it this way?* types of questions that student nurses and new members of staff ask when they visit your practice area for the first time. Practise focusing these uncertainties into searchable questions using the PICOT format. For each question that you focus, try to identify what type of question it is (i.e. intervention, causation, prognosis, etc., as outlined in Table 3.3).

References

1 Strauss SE, Richardson WS, Glasziou P, Haynes RB. *Evidence-Based Medicine: How to Practice and Teach EBM*. Third edition. Edinburgh: Elsevier Churchill Livingstone, 2005.
2 Fineout-Overholt E, Johnston L. Teaching EBP: asking searchable, answerable clinical questions. *Worldviews Evid Based Nurs* 2005;2:157–60.
3 Nollan R, Fineout-Overholt E, Stephenson P. Asking compelling clinical questions. In Melnyk BM, Fineout-Overholt E (editors). *Evidence-Based Practice in Nursing and Health Care: A Guide to Best Practice*. Philadelphia: Lippincott Williams & Wilkins, 2005:25–38.
4 Richardson WS, Wilson MC, Nishikawa J, Hayward RS. The well-built clinical question: a key to evidence-based decisions. *ACP J Club* 1995;**123**(3):A12–13.
5 Collins S, Voth T, DiCenso A, Guyatt G. Finding the evidence. In: DiCenso A, Guyatt G, Ciliska D (editors). *Evidence-Based Nursing. A Guide to Clinical Practice*. St Louis: Elsevier Mosby, 2005:20–43.
6 McCaughan D, Thompson C, Cullum N, Sheldon T, Raynor P. Nurse practitioner and practice nurses' use of research information in clinical decision making: findings from an exploratory study. *Fam Pract* 2005;**22**:490–7.
7 Blythe J, Royle JA. Assessing nurses' information needs in the work environment. *Bull Med Libr Assoc* 1993;**81**:433–5.

Chapter 4

OF STUDIES, SUMMARIES, SYNOPSES, AND SYSTEMS: THE '4S' EVOLUTION OF SERVICES FOR FINDING CURRENT BEST EVIDENCE

R. Brian Haynes

Practical resources to support evidence-based health care decisions are rapidly evolving. New and better services are being created through the combined forces of increasing numbers of clinically important studies, increasingly robust evidence synthesis and synopsis services, and better information technology and systems. The need for these resources is being spurred by demands for higher quality at lower cost from health services, but the impact of better information resources is being blunted by noisy pretenders promising 'the Earth' but yielding just the dirt. Providers and consumers of evidence-based health care can help themselves to identify current best evidence by recognizing and using the most 'evolved' information services for the topic areas of concern to them.

Figure 4.1 provides a '4S' hierarchical structure, with original *studies* at the base, *syntheses* (systematic reviews) of evidence just atop the base, then *synopses* of studies and syntheses next up, and the most evolved, evidence-based information *systems* at the top. Information seekers should begin looking at the highest level resource available for the problem that prompted their search.

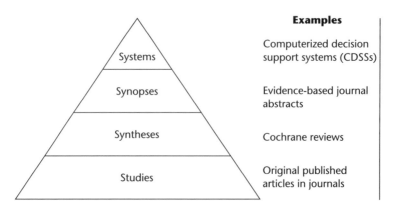

Figure 4.1 '4S' levels of organization of evidence from research. Reproduced with permission from Haynes RB. Of studies, syntheses, synopses, and systems: the '4S' evolution of services for finding current best evidence. *ACP J Club* 2001;**134**:A11–13.

Systems

A perfect evidence-based clinical information system would integrate and concisely summarize all relevant and important research evidence about a clinical problem and would automatically link, through an electronic medical record, a specific patient's circumstances to the relevant information. The user would then consult the system – indeed, be reminded by the system – whenever the patient's record was reviewed. The information contained in the system would be based on an explicit review process for finding and evaluating new evidence as it is published and then reliably updated whenever important new research evidence became available. Thus, clinicians and patients could always have the benefit of the current best evidence. The system would not tell decision makers what to do – those judgements would require integration of the system's evidence with the patient's circumstances and wishes, the skills of the nurse, and the resources available.[1] Rather, the system would ensure that the cumulative research evidence about a patient's problem was immediately at hand, potentially with important features related specifically to the patient highlighted. Furthermore, to maximize speed of use, a short synopsis would be the user's first point of interaction, although there would be links to summaries and then to original studies so that the user could delve as deeply as needed to verify the accuracy, currency and details of the synopsis.

Current systems don't reach this level of perfection as yet, but production models exist for parts of such systems. Electronic medical record systems with computerized decision support rules have been shown in randomized trials to improve the process, and sometimes the outcome,[2] of care, but these cover a limited range of clinical problems, are not necessarily based on current best evidence, and are mainly 'homebuilt' and thus not easily disseminated to most practice settings.

Given that we have some way to go before current best evidence is integrated into electronic medical records, some excellent, but less developed systems are now readily available. For example, some electronic textbooks, such as UpToDate (http://www.uptodate.com), integrate evidence-based information about specific clinical problems and provide regular updating. Although the evidence is cited with this resource, it falls short with respect to being explicit about how evidence is selected. *Clinical Evidence* (www.clinicalevidence.com) does have an explicit review process and integration of evidence about prevention and intervention for a broad and expanding array of clinical problems as diverse as changing smoking behaviour and treating venous leg ulcers and ear wax. It provides a model for the 4S approach to building information systems that are firmly based on underpinning studies, syntheses, and synopses, but it is not comprehensive in its topic coverage. *Clinical Evidence* is also available on Ovid (http://www.ovid.com) as a separate title.

Although these systems are not integrated with electronic medical records, they can be accessed through the same computers that run electronic records, so that one need not go to a remote location to find them. Unfortunately, connecting the right information to a specific patient's problems requires that clinicians understand evidence-based care principles and that they apply some effort and skill in using the resources. Fortunately, emerging information systems reduce these burdens considerably.

Table 4.1 A prototype for evidence synopsis for hand-held computers

Question	Study groups	Outcome	EER	CER	RRR (95% CI)	NNT (CI)
Are antibiotics effective for treatment of women with symptoms of urinary tract infection but negative results on urine dipstick testing?	Experimental: 26 women were allocated to trimethoprim, 300 mg, for 3 days. Control: 33 women were allocated to placebo	Dysuria at 7 days	10%	41%	77% (20 to 94)	4 (2 to 16)

Conclusion: In women with symptoms of urinary tract infection but negative urine dipstick results for both nitrites and leucocytes, trimethoprim for 3 days reduced dysuria at 7 days.

Based on: Trimethoprim reduced dysuria in women with symptoms of urinary tract infection but negative urine dipstick test results. *Evidence-Based Nursing* 2006;**1**:17. Abstract of: Richards D, Toop L, Chambers S, Fletcher L. Response to antibiotics of women with symptoms of urinary tract infection but negative dipstick urine test results: double blind randomised controlled trial. *BMJ* 2005;**331**:143.

EER = experimental event rate, CER = control event rate, RRR = relative risk reduction, CI = confidence interval, NNT = number needed to treat; RRR, NNT and CIs calculated from data in article.

Synopses

When no evidence-based information system exists for a clinical problem, then synopses of individual studies and reviews are the next best source. What busy practitioner has time to use evidence-based resources if the evidence is presented in its original form or even as detailed systematic reviews? Although these detailed articles and reviews are essential building blocks, they are often indigestible if consumed on the run. The perfect synopsis would provide exactly enough information to support a clinical action. The declarative title for each abstract that appears in *Evidence-Based Nursing*, *Evidence-Based Medicine*, and *ACP Journal Club* represents an attempt at this (e.g. 'Trimethoprim reduced dysuria in women with symptoms of urinary tract infection but negative urine dipstick test results'). In some circumstances, this can be enough information to allow a decision-maker to proceed, assuming familiarity with the nature of the intervention and its alternatives, or to look further for the details, which, for an ideal synopsis, would be immediately at hand. The full abstract related to the above declarative title, as well as the related clinical commentary, can be found in *Evidence-Based Nursing*.[3] The synopsis in Table 4.1 contains the essential information on the effects in a format that could be adopted to wireless palmtop Internet devices.

Syntheses

If more detail is needed or no synopsis is at hand, then databases of systematic reviews (syntheses) are available, notably the *Cochrane Library* (http://www3.

interscience.wiley.com/cgi-bin/mrwhome/106568753/HOME). Users in the United Kingdom enter via the National Library for Health (http://www.library.nhs.uk) and Ovid's Evidence-Based Medicine Reviews (EBMR) service (http://www.ovid.com). These summaries are based on a rigorous search for evidence, explicit scientific review of studies uncovered in the search, and systematic assembly of the evidence to provide as clear a signal about the effects of a health care intervention as the evidence will allow. Stimulated by the success of the Cochrane Collaboration, the number of systematic reviews in the literature has grown tremendously over the past few years. If *Evidence-Based Nursing* (http://ebn.bmjjournals.com) doesn't have a review on the topic you are interested in, it may be worthwhile to look in MEDLINE, using the Clinical Queries 'Find Systematic Reviews' service (http://www.ncbi.nlm.nih.gov/entrez/query/static/clinical.shtml). Clinical Queries are also available for both MEDLINE and CINAHL through Ovid: check with your local library to see if they have implemented this feature for either or both MEDLINE and CINAHL. Better still, Ovid's EBMR provides one-stop shopping for both Cochrane and non-Cochrane systematic reviews. Details of searching these and other resources for high quality syntheses are provided in Chapters 5 and 6.

Studies

If all of the preceding 'Ss' fail (i.e. no systems, synopses or syntheses), then it's time to look for original studies. These can be retrieved on the web in several ways. If you don't know which database is best suited to your question, search engines that are tuned for health care content can assemble access across a number of web-based services. At least two of these search engines are attentive to issues of quality of evidence, namely TRIP (Turning Research into Practice, http://www.tripdatabase.com and SUMSearch (http://sumsearch.uthscsa.edu). These both do basic sorting of articles retrieved from a range of databases, but users must appraise the individual items retrieved to determine which fall within the schema presented here. Many will not, especially when convenience of access is favoured over quality. If the search is for an intervention, then the *Cochrane Library* and Ovid's EBMR also include the Cochrane Controlled Trials Register. If none of these services provides a satisfying result, it is time to go to the main search screen of any of the single databases, such as CINAHL, EMBASE/Excerpta Medica, PsycInfo, or MEDLINE's PubMed (http://www.ncbi.nlm.nih.gov/entrez/query.fcgi). The Clinical Queries screen in PubMed (http://www.ncbi.nlm.nih.gov/entrez/query/static/clinical.shtml) and Ovid limits for MEDLINE and CINAHL provide detailed search strategies that home in on clinical content for diagnosis, prognosis, therapy and aetiology. If you still have no luck and the topic is, say, a new intervention (that someone has asked about but you don't yet know about), then try Google (http://www.google.com). It is incredibly fast and can get you to a product monograph in a few milliseconds. At least you will find what the manufacturer of the intervention claims it can do, as well as detailed information on adverse effects, contraindications and prescribing. The Google homepage allows you to add a Google search window to your web browser's home page. Unless you are a very slow typist, this is the fastest way to get to almost any service on the Internet, including all of the ones named in this chapter that are accessible on the web. You can also use Google to find independently prepared product monographs in MEDLINEPlus, provided free by the United States National Library of Medicine: just type MEDLINEPlus 'xxx' in the Google search window, where 'xxx' is the name of the intervention (e.g. type 'MEDLINEPlus trimethoprim' for the example discussed in this chapter). More details on search strategies are found in Chapters 5 and 6.

It's worth emphasizing that almost all of the resources just reviewed are available on the Internet. The added value of accessing these services on the web is considerable, including links to full text journal articles, consumer information, and complementary texts.

Is it time to change how you seek best evidence?

Compare the 4S approach with how you usually seek evidence-based information. Is it time to revise your tactics? If, for example, it surprises you that CINAHL and MEDLINE are so low on the 4S list of resources for finding current best evidence, then this communication will have served a purpose: resources for finding evidence have evolved over the past few years, and searches can be much quicker and more satisfying for answering clinical questions if the features of your quest match those of one of the evolved services. This is in no way a knock against single databases such as CINAHL or MEDLINE. They provide premier access routes to the studies and reviews that form the foundation for all of the other more specialized databases reviewed above. There are big rewards from becoming familiar with these new resources and using them whenever the right clinical question presents itself.

LEARNING EXERCISE

Update your knowledge of the management of uncomplicated urinary tract infections in women by searching for information in at least one of each of the following types of publications: a system, a synopsis, a synthesis and an original study. Keep track of your time at each step. Reviewing your success with all of these types of services, how far down the 'pyramid' of services did you need to travel before you found an accurate representation of current best management? How long did it take you to get there? Repeat each of the steps as you learn more about searching for evidence in Chapters 5 and 6. Once you have yourself organized, you should be able to check resources at each level in less than 10 minutes – and you should find the current best answer in *Clinical Evidence* within the first 5 minutes.

Conflict of interest statement

Brian Haynes has direct or indirect connections with many of the evidence-based resources used as examples above, including *ACP Journal Club* (Editor), *Evidence-Based Medicine* (Co-editor), *Cochrane Library* (Reviewer and former Board Member and Cochrane Centre Director), *Clinical Evidence* (Advisory Board), and PubMed and Ovid Clinical Queries (Developer). These resources are used to illustrate the concepts in the paper; there are other, and perhaps better, examples.

Note

This text was originally published in *ACP J Club* 2001;**134**:A11–13 and is republished here with permission.

References

1 DiCenso A, Cullum N, Ciliska D. Implementing evidence-based nursing: some misconceptions. *Evidence-Based Nursing* 1998;1:38–9.
2 Hunt DL, Haynes RB, Hanna SE, Smith K. Effects of computer-based clinical decision support systems on physician performance and patient outcomes: a systematic review. *JAMA* 1998;280:1339–46.
3 Trimethoprim reduced dysuria in women with symptoms of urinary tract infection but negative urine dipstick test results. *Evidence-Based Nursing* 2006;1:17. Abstract of: Richards D, Toop L, Chambers S, Fletcher L. Response to antibiotics of women with symptoms of urinary tract infection but negative dipstick urine test results: double blind randomised controlled trial. *BMJ* 2005;331:143.

Chapter 5

SEARCHING FOR THE BEST EVIDENCE. PART 1: WHERE TO LOOK

K. Ann McKibbon and Susan Marks

Clinicians are continually challenged to keep up with the rapidly growing and changing information base relevant to their areas of practice. They must not only locate relevant information but must also assess its quality, asking themselves *Do I, or should I, believe this information?* Increasingly, they must deal with conflicting information. For example, one study may report that treatment A (e.g. compression stockings) was better than treatment B (e.g. taking aspirin and walking around) for reducing the incidence of venous thromboembolism during air travel, but another study may report just the opposite. Nurses need to know how to search for the best available evidence and to evaluate what they find so that they can ensure that their professional practice is current. As well, more and more people are searching the Internet for health-related information and using this information to make decisions.[1] Nurses have a role in assessing the information that people bring to health care encounters and, if appropriate, supplying better or more relevant evidence.

This is the first of two chapters on practical searching for the best evidence. In Chapter 4, Haynes described a multi-level categorization of information sources that nurses can use to meet their information needs. This chapter will provide examples of searching in some resources from the first three of the 4S levels introduced by Haynes (i.e. systems, synopses and syntheses); the final S, studies, will be addressed in Chapter 6. We will also describe other types of information resources, including accessing statistical data and being alerted to new advances in your areas of expertise and interest. Chapter 6 will focus on techniques for the efficient retrieval of high-quality information from an important information source for nurses: electronic bibliographic databases, specifically CINAHL and MEDLINE. As suggested by Haynes in Chapter 4, we urge you to use CINAHL and MEDLINE only if other 'higher level' resources that synthesize or summarize information are not available, and you must find original studies, critically appraise them, and apply the results to your specific clinical question. We start with textbook-like resources or systems that distil or consolidate research.

Textbook-like resources: systems

Textbooks provide information for two types of needs. Whether texts are traditional, paper-based products or available online, books are invaluable for addressing specific 'stable' information needs, that is, facts that seldom change, such as gross anatomy, basic principles and mechanisms, and specific disease characteristics. If the texts are up to date and based on current best clinical evidence, they can also provide summaries of new or complex topics or discuss issues in the context of other related areas of knowledge. The following are examples of the types of questions that can be answered using textbooks:

- What are the developmental milestones for 2-year-old children?
- What is the incubation period for chickenpox?
- What does the literature say about using hip protectors to prevent injuries in older adults who are prone to falling?

Many health professionals feel that they need access to one or two standard general textbooks and several specialty texts to cover their specific areas of expertise (e.g. neurology or paediatrics). With the substantial costs of producing clinically useful textbooks or systems and the move towards interdisciplinary care, many of the newer health-related resources include content appropriate for both nurses and physicians. *Clinical Evidence*, published by the BMJ Publishing Group (http://www.clinicalevidence.com/ceweb/conditions/index.jsp), and PIER (Physicians' Information and Education Project), produced by the American College of Physicians (http://pier.acponline.org/index.html), are two online systems that include much information that is relevant to nurses. Both focus their content on giving direction to primary care practitioners and emphasize evidence for making treatment decisions; very little content deals with assessment (screening or diagnosis), prognosis, or causation. Each system describes and provides links to the evidence that underpins their recommendations. They differ in terms of the information they provide. *Clinical Evidence* provides evidence for both the benefits and harms of an intervention, and readers decide how to apply the evidence in clinical practice. PIER prescribes actions based on the evidence (e.g. instructs caregivers to use education and behavioural modification to improve sleep quality in people with dementia[2]). Both resources are readily available through hospital or library access systems. Individuals not affiliated with a major health sciences library must pay subscription costs to access these systems. They are easy to search using either a simple search term box or selecting from a list of specified conditions and diseases. What follows is advice from *Clinical Evidence* and PIER on the use of hip protectors to prevent injuries in elderly people prone to falling.

Clinical Evidence **searching term:** hip protectors
Clinical Evidence **clinical advice summary:** 'One systematic review found that hip protectors reduced hip fractures compared with no hip protectors in nursing home residents, although the result was of borderline significance. There was no significant difference between hip protectors and no hip protectors in any other fracture.'[3]
PIER searching term: hip protectors
PIER advice: 'Target interventions at reducing or eliminating risk factors, recognizing that exercise, avoiding polypharmacy, and hip protectors (in institutionalized patients) are effective. (A level of evidence.)'[4]

Synopses: distilled information sources

Despite the peer review process, not all research studies published in journals are methodologically sound, and some are more sound than others. Before you apply the results of a study, you need to assess the strength of the study, determine what the results were, and decide whether the results are appropriate and applicable to your clinical situation. These three steps take time and skill. Some information resources have already done the work of assessing the strength of individual studies or reviews and provide a summary of the results: that is, they have done the work of critically appraising the study. If this work, or distillation, is done accurately and appropriately, clinicians simply need to decide if they can use the information in their decision-making: that is, to match the information to the specific clinical question or need. Haynes (Chapter 4) classifies these resources as *synopses*.

The evidence-based journal series (*Evidence-Based Nursing, Evidence-Based Medicine*, and *Evidence-Based Mental Health*) and *ACP Journal Club* are examples of distilled information sources or synopses. Primary research studies or systematic reviews that meet specific methodological criteria are identified from the current international health care literature. Studies or reviews that are clinically relevant and have results that warrant attention (up to 25 studies or reviews/issue) are selected and summarized in structured abstracts; each abstract is accompanied by a commentary that is written by a clinician and links the study findings to clinical practice. Each abstract and accompanying commentary fits on a single printed page.

Whereas *Evidence-Based Nursing* focuses on nursing-related research, *ACP Journal Club* is directed at internists, and *Evidence-Based Medicine* is for general practitioners and others interested in broad coverage of important advances in medicine. Other examples of such synopsizing journals in various areas of health care can be found at http://www.ebmny.org/journal.html.

Regular reading of evidence-based abstract journals is a quick and efficient way for clinicians to keep up to date. When issues of journals like *Evidence-Based Nursing* are collated, they provide small concentrated databases of high-quality studies, with the key information for each study presented in a concise and consistent format. Readers of these synopses save time in two ways: they do not have to do the work of separating the 'wheat' from the 'chaff', and they do not have to read the sometimes lengthy full-text articles to find the 'bottom line' of the study. Examples of collections of synopses of original studies and systematic reviews are the OVID Evidence-Based Medicine Reviews database of *ACP Journal Club* (http://www.ovid.com/site/catalog/DataBase/904.jsp?top=2&mid=3&bottom=7&subsection=10) and InfoPOEMs Information Retriever (http://www.infopoems.com/). Another synthesized resource that can be used by nurses is the Database of Reviews of Effects or DARE (http://www.york.ac.uk/inst/crd/crddatabases.htm#DARE). DARE is an online collection of synopses of systematic reviews. In the health care context, a *systematic review* article is defined as an article that poses a clinical question, uses predefined methods to search for studies that provide evidence to answer the question, chooses articles for data extraction and analysis using predefined inclusion and exclusion criteria, and combines the evidence across the included studies using appropriate statistical and clinical methods and understandings. If studies are judged to be sufficiently similar, the results of multiple studies may be combined using statistical methods. This type of systematic review is called a *meta-analysis*.[5]

Haynes includes systematic reviews as a third category in his hierarchy of information resources (see Chapter 4). DARE reviews include expert direction on application of the evidence from each systematic review, making DARE a synthesized information resource based on systematic reviews. Each DARE review provides an assessment of the strength of the review methods, a summary of the results, clinical implications, and author contact information. DARE is available free on the Internet, although access to the full text of reviews can be problematic, expensive, or both.

A search of DARE in mid-2007 identified 2510 synopses of systematic reviews that included the terms 'nursing' or 'nurses'.

Consolidated information sources

When searching for information on a specific topic, you will often find conflicting data from different studies on the same topic. Differences in individual study results may occur because studies use different designs, methods or outcomes. Systematic reviews, as described in the previous section on syntheses, attempt to reconcile these differences by synthesizing or amalgamating the findings of multiple primary studies on the same topic.

The Cochrane Collaboration is an international network of health care professionals, scientists and lay people committed to producing and maintaining systematic reviews of the effects of health care interventions. The collected systematic reviews and citations of controlled trials and randomized controlled trials are published in the *Cochrane Library* (available on the Internet at http://www.cochrane.co.uk/en/clibintro.htm for a fee, through various commercial providers, or free of charge under a national agreement). The *Library* includes four databases:

- The Cochrane Database of Systematic Reviews is updated quarterly. Issue 2, 2007, contains the full text of 3094 systematic reviews and protocols for 1707 planned or ongoing systematic reviews. The database includes systematic reviews on many nursing-related topics, such as adherence to medications, support during childbirth, breast feeding, caregiver support and postpartum depression, doctor–nurse collaboration, effects of limited asthma education, stroke units, and treating scabies.
- The DARE database described above.
- The Cochrane Review Methodology Database comprises references to articles on the theory and methods of systematic reviews and on critical appraisal.
- The Cochrane Controlled Trials Register is a database of citations of controlled trials and has >495 000 entries. Note that because the entries are controlled trials, most information included in the *Cochrane Library* relates to interventions.

Many other systematic reviews can be found in the large bibliographic databases, such as MEDLINE and CINAHL, and in professional journals.

The Internet

The Internet has brought both blessings and curses for nurses, as for others. It has given health professionals and patients access to many valuable information sources. Unfortunately, because of the speed at which the Internet is expanding and the lack

of quality control of information that is published, the high-quality and clinically important sources are often hidden in a morass of information that is of questionable, or
at least uncertain, quality. Research on assessing the quality of information found on
Internet sites is in its early stages. A systematic review by Gagliardi and Jadad[6] identified
98 rating schemes for evaluating the quality of Internet sites that provide health information, and almost all were incompletely developed and gave little information on test
reliability and validity. Given this, it is important for nurses to judge the quality of
information found on a given Internet site by using common sense (e.g. consider the
source), checking it out with a colleague, and applying the principles of critical appraisal
and evidence-based practice that are discussed in subsequent chapters of this book.
These assessment skills become even more important given the number of patients
using information found on the Internet as a basis for health-related decisions.[1]

Nurses can search the Internet to address various information needs. For example,
they can help patients with newly diagnosed cancer to identify Internet sites that provide accurate disease-specific information from a professional perspective, in a form
that is understandable from a patient perspective, as well as online support groups
and electronic mailing lists.[6] Access to the Internet provides an excellent opportunity for patients to become more knowledgeable about their conditions and treatments and more involved in decision-making related to their own health care. Nurses
can access some of the information resources discussed in previous sections of this
chapter on the Internet at no cost. They can also learn about new topics by accessing Internet tutorial sites published by reputable universities and organizations.
Professional associations offer access to many online continuing education courses
(e.g. American Nursing Association at http://www.nursingworld.org/ and UK Royal
College of Nursing at http://www.rcn.org.uk/). MEDLINEPlus from the US National
Library of Medicine (http://medlineplus.gov/), the UK National Library for Health
(http://www.library.nhs.uk/), and UK NHS Direct Online (http://www.nhsdirect.
nhs.uk/) provide high-quality, readily available information for practitioners and
patients. Many of these sites include health videos explaining conditions, interventions, diagnostic tests, and other patient education issues. Many nurses use
Google to search the Internet, although other useful search engines are available
(http://searchenginewatch.com/showPage.html?page=2156221).

Some services allow you to search across multiple sources. For example, the TRIP
(Turning Research into Practice) database is a free Internet resource designed to retrieve
evidence from >150 sources (http://www.tripdatabase.com). The search results are
organized into categories based on the 4S approach described by Haynes in Chapter
4 and include evidence-based synopses (e.g. from *Evidence-Based Nursing* abstracts,
Clinical Evidence), clinical answers (i.e. services that match the best available
evidence to the question), systematic reviews, guidelines (by country/area of origin),
etextbooks, clinical calculators, medical images, patient information leaflets, and
MEDLINE (automatic searches of PubMed using the validated search filters that are
described further in Chapter 6).

Keeping up to date

E-mail can help you keep abreast of evidence in newly published studies and systematic reviews. One can easily receive the tables of contents of journals or newly
published articles on specific topics or subscribe to services that notify advances across

many journals. PubMed, through their My NCBI service (http://www.ncbi.nlm.nih.gov/books/bv.fcgi?rid=helppubmed.section.pubmedhelp.My_NCBI), allows you to establish a search that will automatically e-mail you citations of newly published articles based on specific content (e.g. asthma in adolescents or patient education in diabetes care) or journal titles. The Chinese University of Hong Kong maintains a website with links to sign up for e-mail alerts from all major journal publishers (http://www.lib.cuhk.edu.hk/information/publisher.htm). bmjupdates+ is a free service alerting users to newly published studies and systematic reviews in more than 110 journals (http://bmjupdates.mcmaster.ca/index.asp). You choose the frequency with which you want to receive email notifications, state the disciplines in which you are interested, and set the score level on clinical relevance and newsworthiness as determined by peer raters in multiple disciplines. The content is currently being expanded to include alerts to content rated by nurses.

Searching for statistical data

Nurses sometimes need to access health-related statistics. The web pages of the University of Michigan (http://www.lib.umich.edu/govdocs/stats.html) and the US National Library of Medicine (http://www.nlm.nih.gov/services/statistics.html) are good places to start to look for international, national, and local statistics on mortality, morbidity, utilization, and manpower needs.

In Chapter 6, we will describe searching for original or primary studies using the CINAHL and MEDLINE databases. Although these large databases are sometimes difficult to search, they both provide access to evidence important to nursing care and practice.

Summary

Nurses need information as they conduct their daily activities. Different information needs are best met by using specific sources or combinations of sources. Textbooks, journals, bibliographic databases, products that distil or consolidate research, and the Internet each have a place in addressing information needs. A proactive approach to these sources, a decent computer, an Internet connection, and a small personal library can provide practising nurses with adequate information access at a reasonable cost in terms of money, time and energy.

LEARNING EXERCISES

1. As community nurse, you facilitate a support group for new mothers. During the sessions, mothers have raised the following questions:
   (a) What are the developmental milestones that I should be looking for as my child approaches 6 months of age? One year of age?
   (b) Our family is planning a trip to visit my parents in East Africa. Will we need to get any vaccinations? Which ones? Will my baby need to get vaccinated as well?
   (c) Does mumps–measles–rubella vaccination cause autism?
   For each question, identify the type of resource that would be most appropriate and conduct the search.

2. Use the TRIP database (http://www.tripdatabase.com/) to find out what evidence exists on the benefits of antioxidants.
3. Can you identify specific guidelines for providing nutritional advice to people with diabetes? (Hint: see 'Filter by' box in TRIP.)

Solutions to learning exercises
1a. Information on developmental milestones is likely to be fairly stable (facts that seldom change). Try a paediatric textbook.
1b. Information on vaccinations required by specific countries is likely to be changing often because of changing incidences of infectious diseases. Try the Internet. In Google, entering the terms 'East Africa travel vaccination' identifies a US Centers for Disease Control and Prevention website on Health Information for Travellers to Countries in East Africa (http://www.cdc.gov/travel/eafrica.htm).
1c. This is a question of treatment harm. Try searching for a systematic review in the Cochrane Library. There is indeed a Cochrane review by Demicheli V, Jefferson T, Rivetti A, Price D. Vaccines for measles, mumps and rubella in children. Cochrane Database of Systematic Reviews 2005, *Issue 4: CD004407.*

References

1 Wainstein BK, Sterling-Levis K, Baker SA, Taitz J, Brydon M. Use of the Internet by parents of paediatric patients. *J Paediatr Child Health* 2006;**42**:528–32.
2 McCurry SM, Gibbons LE, Logsdon RG, Vitiello M, Teri L. Training caregivers to change the sleep hygiene practices of patients with dementia: the NITE-AD project. *J Am Geriatr Soc* 2003;**51**:1455–60.
3 Mosekilde L, Vestergaard P, Langdahl B. Fracture prevention in postmenopausal women. Clinical Evidence [online] 2005. http://www.clinicalevidence.com/ceweb/conditions/msd/1109/1109_contribdetails.jsp (accessed 17 April 2006).
4 Christmas C. Hip fracture. In: PIER [online database]. Philadelphia: American College of Physicians, 2006. http://pier.acponline.org (accessed 17 April 2006).
5 Mulrow C, Cook D, editors. *Systematic Reviews: Synthesis of Best Evidence for Health Care Decisions.* Philadelphia: American College of Physicians, 1998.
6 Gagliardi A, Jadad AR. Examination of instruments used to rate quality of health information on the internet: chronicle of a voyage with an unclear destination. *BMJ* 2002;**324**:569–73.

Chapter 6

SEARCHING FOR THE BEST EVIDENCE. PART 2: SEARCHING CINAHL AND MEDLINE

K. Ann McKibbon and Susan Marks

Chapter 5 described several types of information resources (systems, synopses, and syntheses) that nurses can use to support clinical practice and other professional activities. This chapter will focus on another type of information resource: large bibliographic databases, which provide access to primary studies and systematic reviews related to nursing practice and research. We will describe how to harness the full potential of two databases (CINAHL and MEDLINE) for use in clinical decision-making. We will show you some fast and efficient ways to locate citations of high-quality studies with findings that are ready for clinical application. Speed and efficiency are important to nurses: McKnight[1] reported that patient care duties and time demands often stand in the way of accessing information for decision-making.

In Chapter 5, we suggested that nurses with clinical questions should start seeking answers using textbook-like resources (systems), synopses such as those included in *Evidence-Based Nursing*, and systematic reviews (syntheses). These resources should constitute a first-line information-seeking approach – three of the '4 Ss' described by Haynes in Chapter 4. This chapter focuses on searching two large bibliographic databases (CINAHL and MEDLINE) to address questions that cannot be answered using the more refined summarized resources or when comprehensive coverage of a topic is needed: the fourth S (*studies*) in the information resources pyramid.

Proverbially speaking, looking for clinically useful and high-quality reports of original studies is like looking for a needle in a haystack. The health care literature contains an abundance of reports and papers that are in the early stages of development. Relatively few items in large databases like MEDLINE and CINAHL are studies with findings that are appropriate for clinical application. One estimate is that for every 5000 ideas that are initially postulated as improvements in health care, only one is fully evaluated and proved to be effective for changing health care practice.[2] Thus, effective and efficient literature searching is critical.

Many articles abound on nurses' use of electronic resources such as CINAHL and the Internet. A survey by Griffiths and Riddington[3] showed that nurses at a hospital in the United Kingdom used online resources, specifically CINAHL, MEDLINE, and full-text journals. Twenty-seven per cent reported regular use of CINAHL, and 18% reported regular use of MEDLINE. In 2005, Pravikoff *et al.*[4] surveyed more than 1000 nurses in the United States, who reported reliance on peers and the Internet as well as use of MEDLINE and CINAHL. Both studies showed that nurses felt they needed more skills and training on how best to use electronic information tools such as CINAHL and MEDLINE.

What is CINAHL, why should I use it, and how do I access it?

CINAHL (Cumulated Index to Nursing and Allied Health Literature) is considered to be the premier database for nurses and allied health professionals. It includes material from 1982 and is growing at a rate of 10% per year. It is smaller than MEDLINE (800 000 vs 15 million records) but includes a wider variety of resources and a higher proportion of articles important to nurses. In addition to journal articles, CINAHL also includes citations to books, book chapters, pamphlets, audiovisuals, dissertations, educational software, conference proceedings, standards of professional practice, nurse practice acts, critical paths, and research instruments. Many citations also include bibliographies and links to the full text of articles, features that enhance the usual searching methods.

CINAHL is available from many vendors (http://www.cinahl.com/prodsvcs/prodsvcs.htm), and access is a membership benefit of the American Nurses Association, American Association of Colleges of Nursing, and some other organizations. In this chapter, we will focus on the Ovid Technologies platform for CINAHL and CINAHL direct. Most nurses associated with large institutions, hospitals, or educational organizations will have online access to Ovid CINAHL through their libraries.

What is MEDLINE, why should I use it, and how do I access it?

MEDLINE, produced by the United States National Library of Medicine, is the largest and probably most frequently used health care database worldwide. With citations dating back to 1966, it includes more than 15 million citations from more than 5164 health care journals as of 2007 (http://www.nlm.nih.gov/bsd/index_stats_comp.html and http://www.nlm.nih.gov/bsd/bsd_key.html). Although many of the journals are medical in nature, several nursing journals are also indexed in MEDLINE. It is also important to note that much of the research relevant to nursing practice, especially research related to teams and multidisciplinary care, is published in non-nursing journals.

Many options exist for online access to MEDLINE (http://www.diabetesmonitor.com/database.htm). Most health sciences or hospital libraries provide access via Ovid Technologies. Nurses can also access MEDLINE using PubMed, a free online version of MEDLINE designed for health professionals (http://www.ncbi.nlm.nih.gov/entrez/query.fcgi). Many patients and families also use PubMed: over 2 million searches are done each day.

The remainder of this chapter will focus on Ovid MEDLINE and PubMed, the MEDLINE platforms that are available to most nurses.

Searching for clinically useful articles made easy

Clinically useful articles (similar to those abstracted in *Evidence-Based Nursing*) can be difficult to identify quickly and easily in CINAHL and MEDLINE. Searching for such clinically relevant articles is challenging because so few of them exist and because they are mixed in with thousands of other articles and reports that, although possibly important, do not include the type of evidence on which practice changes should be based. The ability to limit online search results to articles that are clinically relevant and important would no doubt be helpful to busy nurses, physicians, and other health professionals. The articles we have just described can be identified because they use distinct methododological and research techniques (e.g. a randomized controlled design to identify the effectiveness of interventions, or ethnographic methods to address questions related to different cultural understandings of death and dying). Textwords and phrases related to research methods can be harnessed to retrieve only studies with these specific characteristics and leave behind articles that are less likely to contain information ready for clinical application.

Using terms and phrases unique to the research methods of studies, the Health Information Research Unit at McMaster University, Canada (http://hiru.mcmaster.ca/hedges) has developed sets of predefined search strategies that can be used to retrieve studies in CINAHL and MEDLINE related to the following categories of clinical care questions:

- Intervention/treatment
- Screening and diagnosis
- Prognosis
- Causation/aetiology/harm
- Clinical prediction guides
- Economics
- Qualitative studies
- Systematic reviews

The strategy sets described above are referred to as *clinical queries*. They are built into Ovid CINAHL and MEDLINE and PubMed. Each clinical query for the above categories is available at three levels so that you can choose the relative size of your retrieval result for a given topic:

- A *high specificity (narrow or specific) strategy* maximizes the retrieval of high-quality, clinically relevant articles while keeping to a minimum the number of non-relevant citations retrieved. This strategy is most useful for those interested in 'a few good studies' without having to go through a large retrieval set.
- A *high sensitivity (broad or sensitive) strategy* maximises the number of relevant citations without worrying about the retrieval of non-relevant citations. More relevant citations are returned as well as more non-relevant citations. People who want to obtain the maximum number of relevant citations (e.g. researchers or people working on a systematic review who need to identify all relevant literature on a topic) should use this level of strategy sets.
- An *optimizing (minimal difference) search strategy* balances the difference in the scope of highly sensitive and highly specific search results. Such an optimized search strategy set is for people interested in a more 'middle of the road' approach to

citation retrieval, ensuring a relatively high proportion of relevant articles, without too many non-relevant ones.

Experimentation with the three levels of clinical queries will help you to understand which level of search strategy is best for you in a specific situation.

Not all clinical care categories and search strategy levels are available in Ovid CINAHL or MEDLINE or PubMed. The strategies, however, work in a similar manner in all databases and platforms. In the following sections, we provide examples to show the application of strategies in each database.

How to apply clinical queries in CINAHL

Ovid CINAHL provides access to search strategies for identifying treatment, prognosis, causation, and qualitative studies, as well as systematic reviews. Ovid uses *limits* to filter search results after searches for content are completed. Traditional limits in Ovid searching include limiting to articles written in English and to those that include human participants. You 'collect' your content in a search session and then 'limit' your initial retrieval down to a more manageable size. An example will make this description clearer. Suppose that you are interested in understanding whether the grief process is different for the families and close friends of people who commit suicide. The search has two components: grief and suicide. Because the question relates to the subjective experiences of the participants, it would likely be best addressed by a qualitative study (see Chapter 8).

Signing on to Ovid CINAHL, you first ask for all articles that are indexed as being about grief (Figure 6.1). The first 'grief' in the figure (GRIEF/) retrieves articles to which indexers have assigned the term 'grief'. The second 'grief' (grief.tw.) retrieves articles that have the word grief in the title or abstract. The third 'grief' (grief.mp.) retrieves all articles that have grief anywhere in the record (title, abstract or indexing), which in this case is 3209 articles. Doing the same retrieval for 'suicide', the system tells us that 5475 articles include the word suicide in the title, abstract, or indexing. Putting the two ideas (grief and suicide) together (using the Boolean AND) indicates that 100 articles deal with both concepts. One hundred articles are still too many for a busy clinician to review, so the next step is to move on to the limit function of Ovid. See the arrow in Figure 6.1 to show how limiting is accomplished.

To apply limits, click on the 'More Limits' button. You will see the screen shown in Figure 6.2. We have asked for articles that

- are written in English
- have abstracts
- were published from 2000 on
- are qualitative studies

You then hit the 'Limit a search' button, and we now have only seven citations, rather than 100, to review. One citation in the retrieval result is a phenomenology study designed to explore and interpret the lived experience of six people who had lost a family member to suicide.[5]

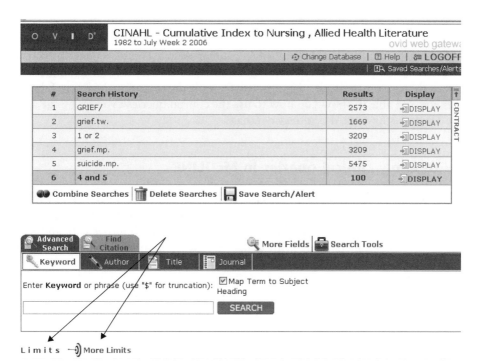

Figure 6.1 Searching for articles on both grief and suicide. Printed with permission of Wolters Kluwer.

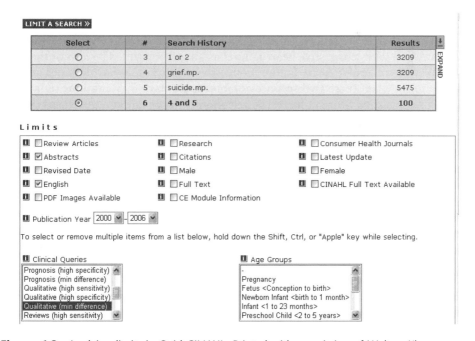

Figure 6.2 Applying limits in Ovid CINAHL. Printed with permission of Wolters Kluwer.

CINAHL online direct does not yet have the clinical queries embedded within their service, although they are considering implementation. You can, however, enter the search strategies as you would any other content terms. The web page (http://hiru. mcmaster.ca/hedges) includes the clinical queries for CINAHL searching to limit retrievals to those articles with a high probability of being clinically important. Librarians are willing and able to show you how to use the clinical queries by entering the appropriate terms in the CINAHL direct database.

How to apply clinical queries in MEDLINE

The use of clinical queries in Ovid MEDLINE is almost identical to the Ovid CINAHL implementation. As an example, we describe a search designed to retrieve evidence that nurses who use telephone or e-mail communication can improve care and reduce hospital admissions in patients with congestive heart failure. This question is best addressed by a quantitative study. Because so many more quantitative studies exist, searching for them is sometimes more difficult than searching for qualitative studies. One method that helps with both the formulation of questions and the translation of the concepts into search strategies is to phrase the question using the PICO format (see Chapter 3), whereby

P(atient) = patients with congestive heart failure
I(ntervention) = nurses using telephone or email
C(omparison) = without nurses using telephone or e-mail (terms not added to search)
O(utcome) = any outcome (term was not added to the search as we hope that hospital admission is included with other reported outcomes)

The 'content' search in Ovid MEDLINE (see Figure 6.3) found 20 articles on nursing care in congestive heart failure ('nursing care' as an index term combined (using the Boolean AND) with 'congestive heart failure' as an index term). The idea of the nursing aspects of congestive heart failure (congestive heart failure/nu) provides another 367 citations. When these two sets are combined, we have 375 citations on nursing aspects of congestive heart failure. The telephone and e-mail concept yields 16 464 citations. Combining our retrieval sets for nursing aspects of congestive heart failure and telephone and e-mail communication (again, using the Boolean AND), we now have 29 citations. Limiting these 29 citations to treatment studies (using the sensitive clinical query identified above) published in English that have abstracts and include human participants brings the retrieval set down to 16 citations. The first three are shown in Figure 6.4. The first, a study by Sisk et al.[6] of 406 patients with heart failure, found that those who received a nurse-led intervention (including regular telephone follow-up) had fewer hospital admissions at 12 months than those who received usual care (143 vs. 180 hospital admissions or 0.13 fewer hospital admissions/person/year).

PubMed's implementation of the clinical queries uses the same sets of strategies but provides a slightly different approach to searching. Strategies to identify articles on treatment, diagnosis, prognosis, clinical practice guides, and causation are available for use at http://www.ncbi.nlm.nih.gov/entrez/query/static/clinical.shtml. The clinical query for qualitative studies is included as a special (not clinical) query at the Health Services Research page http://www.nlm.nih.gov/nichsr/hedges/search.html.

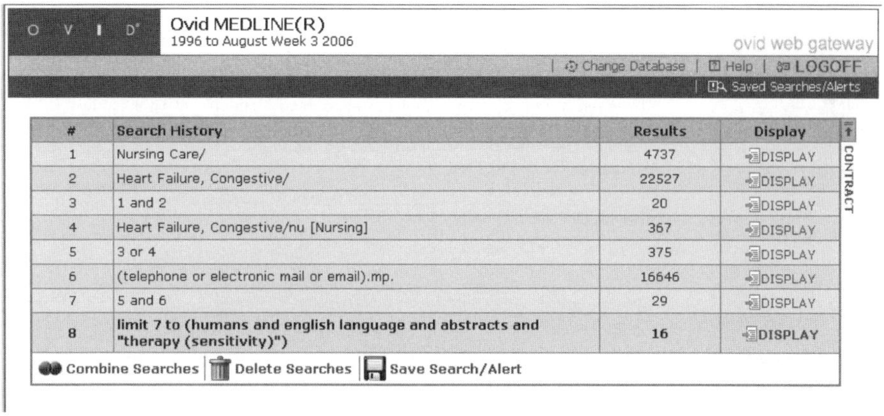

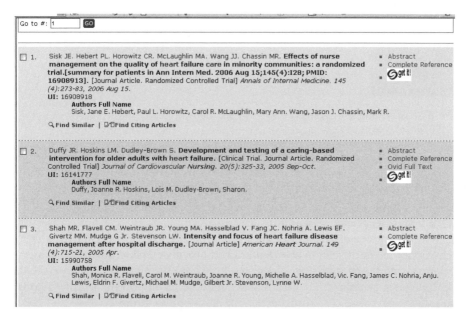

Figure 6.3 Searching with limits in Ovid MEDLINE (1996–2006 database subset). Printed with permission of Wolters Kluwer.

Figure 6.4 First three citations retrieved from search for studies on congestive heart failure and telephone follow-up. Printed with permission of Wolters Kluwer.

Use of the clinical queries in PubMed starts before you enter your content terms. Consider a search to identify tools that will help you to predict which residents will have fractures in a nursing home setting. The search in PICO format is

P(atient) = patients in nursing homes
I(ntervention) = prediction guide
C(omparison) = no prediction guide
O(utcome) = fractures (or prediction of fractures)

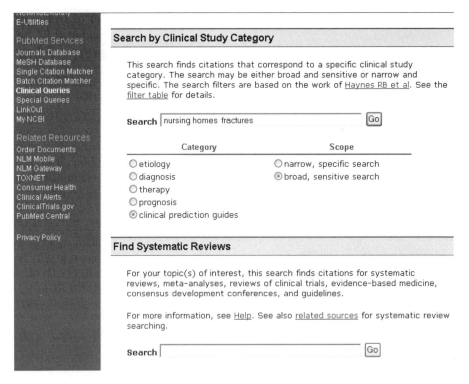

Figure 6.5 Searching using clinical queries in PubMed.

Your search content is entered into the box (nursing homes – the PICO 'P', and fractures – the PICO 'O'). Your search strategy choice is clinical prediction guide (the PICO 'I'), and the complete search is done once you click the Go button (see Figure 6.5). Note that you only have a choice of a broad (sensitive) or a narrow (specific) search but not the optimization choice that Ovid provides. The sensitive search identifies 92 citations, and the specific search identifies five citations. A study by Montero-Odasso et al.[7] includes evidence that gait velocity may be an important factor to consider when estimating risk of fractures in nursing home populations.

Additional search tips and information – CINAHL

Many online sites exist to help you learn searching skills for CINAHL. For example, here is one from Ovid: http://www.ovid.com/site/products/ovidguide/nursing.htm. To find others, use Google and the term 'CINAHL tutorials'. Choose one with which you are comfortable and that is published by an institution or organization you trust.

- CINAHL provides information on scales and questionnaires, as well as a variety of non-study-type literature.
- Librarians who work in your institution are often willing to spend time providing training in group or one-on-one training sessions.

Additional search tips and information – PubMed

- The 'see-related' button helps you to find other studies related to a specific article.
- A good tutorial on how to search in PubMed is available at http://www.nlm.nih.gov/bsd/disted/pubmed.html. You can find others using a Google search.
- Although you can limit your searching to 'nursing journals', be aware that this limit does not help you to find evidence important to nursing but limits the retrieval to those articles published in nursing journals. Note that approximately 75% of high-quality studies selected for abstraction in *Evidence-Based Nursing* are published in non-nursing journals.[8]

Summary

The large bibliographic databases CINAHL and MEDLINE can provide valuable information support for nurses. The databases provide access to citations of studies and systematic reviews. [Other sources such as the *Cochrane Library* and Database of Abstracts of Reviews of Effects (DARE) are better resources to identify systematic reviews.] Use of predefined search strategies (clinical queries) that filter retrieval results to identify high-quality, clinically appropriate studies of treatment, assessment, prognosis, causation and clinical prediction, as well as qualitative studies and systematic reviews, can make searching faster and easier. Nurses need to learn how best to use CINAHL and MEDLINE, and we encourage you to seek this training from practice, peers, librarians, or tutorials.

LEARNING EXERCISES

1. Conduct a search in both PubMed and CINAHL to identify studies comparing the benefits of using nurse practitioners versus physicians in family practice settings. Hint: an RCT on this topic was published in *JAMA* 2000. See if you can get this study to appear in your list of results.
2. Conduct a PubMed search to determine the health benefits and risks of being tall (or short). Hint: use Clinical Queries. From your retrieval result, select a citation of interest and click on the 'Related articles and links' button.

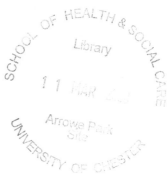

Solutions to learning exercises
1. *Mundinger MO, Kane RL, Lenz ER, Totten AM, Tsai WY, Cleary PD, Friedwald WT, Siu AL, Shelanski ML. Primary care outcomes in patients treated by nurse practitioners or physicians: a randomized trial. JAMA 2000;**283**:59–68.*
2. *Search Clinical Queries using the aetiology category. Three examples of studies that your search might identify are listed below:*
   (a) *Nettle D. Women's height, reproductive success and the evolution of sexual dimorphism in modern humans. Proc Biol Sci 2002;**269**:1919–23. (Nettle states that tall men and short women have the greatest 'reproductive success'.)*
   (b) *Forsen T, Eriksson J, Qiao Q, Tervahauta M, Nissinen A, Tuomilehto J. Short stature and coronary heart disease: a 35-year follow-up of the Finnish cohorts of the Seven Countries Study. J Intern Med 2000;**248**:326–32. (Forsen et al. state that tall men have a 19% decrease in coronary artery disease mortality in Finland).*
   (c) *Palmer JR, Rosenberg L, Harlap S, Strom BL, Warshauer ME, Zauber AG, Shapiro S. Adult height and risk of breast cancer among US black women. Am J Epidemiol 1995;**141**:845–9. (Palmer et al. assessed the incidence of breast cancer in black women using case-control methods and concluded, 'After control for multiple confounders, the relative risk estimate for women <61 inches (<154.9 cm) tall was 0.5 (95% confidence interval (CI) 0.3–0.7) relative to the median height of 64–65 inches (162.6–165.1 cm). Among women > or = 61 inches (> or = 154.9 cm) tall, there was little indication of any variation in risk with increasing height. The findings suggest that short stature is associated with a decreased risk of breast cancer in US black women.')*

References

1 McKnight M. The information seeking of on-duty critical care nurses: evidence from participant observation and in-context interviews. *J Med Libr Assoc* 2006;**94**:145–51.

2 Matson E. Speed kills (the competition). *Fast Company* 1996 Aug/Sep:84–91.

3 Griffiths P, Riddington L. Nurses' use of computer databases to identify evidence for practice – a cross-sectional questionnaire survey in a UK hospital. *Health Info Libr J* 2001;**18**:2–9.

4 Pravikoff DS, Tanner AB, Pierce ST. Readiness of US nurses for evidence-based practice. *Am J Nurs* 2005;**105**:40–51.

5 Fielden JM. Grief as a transformative experience: weaving through different lifeworlds after a loved one has completed suicide. *Int J Ment Health Nurs* 2003;**12**:74–85.

6 Sisk JE, Herbert PL, Horowitz CR, McLaughlin MA, Wang JJ, Chassin MR. Effects of nurse management on the quality of heart failure care in minority communities: a randomized trial. *Ann Intern Med* 2006;**145**:273–83.

7 Montero-Odasso M, Schapira M, Soriano ER, Varela M, Kaplan R, Camera LA, Mayorga LM. Gait velocity as a single predictor of adverse events in health seniors aged 75 years and older. *J Gerontol A Biol Sci Med Sci* 2005;**60**:1304–9.

8 McKibbon KA, Wilczynski NL, Haynes RB. What do evidence-based secondary journals tell us about the publication of clinically important articles in primary healthcare journals? *BMC Med* 2004;**2**:33.

Chapter 7

IDENTIFYING THE BEST RESEARCH DESIGN TO FIT THE QUESTION. PART 1: QUANTITATIVE RESEARCH

Jackie Roberts and Alba DiCenso

Evidence-based nursing is about applying the best available evidence to a specific clinical uncertainty or question. Different types of clinical questions require evidence from different research designs. No single design has precedence over another. Instead, the design chosen must fit the particular research question.[1] Questions focused on the cause, prognosis (course), diagnosis, prevention, treatment or economics of health problems are best answered using research designs that gather quantitative data, whereas questions about the meaning or experience of illness are best answered using designs that gather qualitative data. Many different quantitative and qualitative research methods exist, each with a specific purpose and with strengths and limitations. In this chapter, the most rigorous research designs that use quantitative data to address questions of prevention or treatment, causation and prognosis will be outlined. Chapter 8 will describe the use of research designs to address questions of meaning or experience, which are based on qualitative data.

Questions about the effectiveness of prevention and interventions

The *randomized controlled trial (RCT)* is the strongest design for questions of whether health care interventions are beneficial (i.e. do more good than harm). An RCT is a true experiment in which people are randomly allocated to receive a new intervention (*experimental group*) or a conventional intervention (*comparison group*) or no intervention at all (*control group*). Because the play of chance alone determines the allocation of participants to study groups, the only systematic difference between groups should be the intervention. Investigators follow participants forward in time (*follow-up*), and then assess whether they have experienced a specific outcome (Figure 7.1). The two most important strengths of RCTs are (1) the random allocation of participants to groups, which helps to ensure that groups are similar in all respects except exposure to the intervention, and (2) the longitudinal nature of the study, whereby exposure to the intervention precedes the development of the outcome. These two features help to ensure that any differences in outcome can be attributed to the intervention. Disadvantages of this design include the cost of conducting a trial, the long period of follow-up before patients experience the outcome,

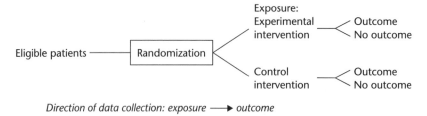

Direction of data collection: exposure ⟶ outcome

Figure 7.1 Randomized controlled trial design.

and the possibility that patients who agree to participate in a trial may differ from those to whom the results would be applied (*generalizability*).

If you are a school nurse who wants to find an effective intervention to prevent initiation of smoking among adolescents, you should look for evidence from RCTs. An example is a trial in which schools are randomly allocated to an experimental group or a control group. Those allocated to the experimental group receive an innovative intervention that is taught in small groups and provides opportunities for adolescents to practise smoking avoidance behaviours, whereas those allocated to the control group receive traditional lectures about the ill effects of smoking. The students are followed up for several years, and data are collected and compared on the number of students in each group who begin to smoke. In most RCTs, individuals are randomly allocated to groups. In this study, schools are the *unit of randomization* to reduce the likelihood of students discussing their experiences of the intervention with students in the control group. To avoid such *contamination*, investigators often randomize units such as classrooms, schools, or communities rather than individuals; this method of randomization is called *cluster randomization*.

If you are a primary care nurse practitioner and are wondering whether you should suggest nicotine gum to help smokers to stop smoking, again you should look for evidence from RCTs. In such trials, smokers are randomly allocated to nicotine gum (experimental group) or placebo gum, which looks and tastes like nicotine gum but contains no active ingredients (control group). Participants are then followed up, and data are collected and compared on the number in each group who stopped smoking.

There are occasions, however, when evaluating an intervention using an RCT may not be ethical or feasible. In such instances, we must rely on a less rigorous design, such as a *cohort analytic study* (also known as a *longitudinal or prospective study*). This study design is similar to the RCT in that two or more comparison groups receive different interventions, or no intervention, and are followed up to determine who experiences the outcome of interest. The important difference between cohort analytic and randomized controlled designs is the absence of random allocation to study groups in the former. In cohort analytic studies, participants often select themselves or are selected by a clinician to receive the intervention (Figure 7.2). This is an important limitation because groups may differ in ways other than exposure to the intervention (*selection bias*). Group differences in outcomes at the end of the study may be because of differences in the groups that existed before the intervention began (*baseline differences*). The intervention therefore may appear to have had an effect on an outcome when, in fact, initial differences in the groups influenced the outcome. Thus,

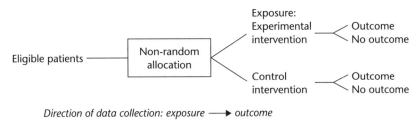

Direction of data collection: exposure ⟶ outcome

Figure 7.2 Cohort analytic study design.

examining characteristics of groups at baseline and comparing them for differences is important. However, there may be differences in factors that cannot be measured, and such differences would remain unknown.

Continuing with the example of a school-based smoking prevention programme, if school administrators were unhappy about random allocation of schools to groups, a cohort analytic study might be done rather than an RCT. In such a study, several schools are approached and asked if they would like to receive the innovative intervention (intervention group) or traditional lectures (control group). Without random allocation to groups, it may be that schools that choose the innovative intervention differ from those that choose not to receive it in ways that may influence the outcome (e.g. socioeconomic status or parental smoking habits). The study findings may show that students who received the innovative intervention were less likely to start smoking, but this outcome may have been influenced by the baseline characteristics of the group rather than, or as well as, the intervention. In other words, this group may not have been as likely to smoke even if they did not receive the innovative intervention. Even if investigators document group differences in baseline characteristics or use statistical techniques to adjust for differences, other factors that were not considered may be responsible for differences in outcome.

Using a cohort analytic design for the nicotine gum example, smokers who want to stop smoking are offered nicotine gum, and those who choose to take it (intervention group) are compared over time with those who choose not to take it (control group). Again, the major limitation of this design is that smokers who choose to take nicotine gum may differ from those who choose not to take it with respect to known and unknown baseline characteristics that may influence the outcome. Nicotine gum may appear to increase quit rates when, in fact, the increase may be because of variables such as higher motivation to stop smoking, younger age, or fewer years of smoking.

Questions about the cause of a health problem or disease

The RCT is the most rigorous design to determine whether some factor (*exposure*) causes an outcome. Using this design, participants are randomly allocated to be or not to be exposed to a potential causative agent and then followed up to compare the number in each group who experience the outcome. In questions of causation, however, it may not be ethical or feasible to randomly allocate people to exposure to the causative agent. The next best evidence comes from cohort analytic studies.

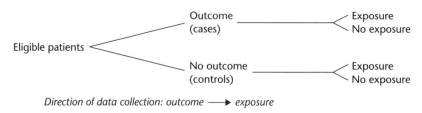

Direction of data collection: outcome ⟶ exposure

Figure 7.3 Case–control study design.

In this design, investigators follow up people who are exposed to and not exposed to a causative agent. The major strength of RCTs and cohort analytic studies is that those entering the study have not yet experienced the outcome. Investigators are certain, therefore, that exposure to the causative agent (smoking) precedes the development of the outcome (lung cancer). This issue of *temporality* – that is, that the causative agent precedes the development of the outcome – is crucial for establishing a causal relationship.[2]

When the outcome of interest is rare or takes a long time to develop, neither RCTs nor cohort analytic studies may be feasible. In these circumstances, a case-control design is often used. In a *case-control design*, patients with the outcome of interest (cases) and those without the outcome of interest (controls) are identified. The investigators then look back in time to determine whether participants had previous exposure to the causative agent (Figure 7.3). Investigators may be able to match the case and control patients on important variables that may influence the outcome (e.g. age, sex and other health conditions). In this way, the groups are as similar as possible, and the specific effect of the causative agent on the outcome can be examined more confidently. Strengths of this design are that it allows the assessment of causation when an outcome is rare or takes a long time to develop and that it includes a control group. Limitations are the difficulties in establishing that the exposure actually occurred before the outcome (temporality); obtaining accurate information about exposure to a causative agent that has occurred in the past (relies on accuracy of people's memory or on completeness and accuracy of medical records); and identifying a control group that is similar in all other factors that may have influenced the outcome, especially when some of these factors are unknown.

When considering whether smoking causes lung cancer, it is unethical to randomize participants to smoke or to not smoke and then follow them over time to determine who develops lung cancer. An RCT is therefore not possible. Cohort analytic studies have been done in which investigators followed up a group of smokers and a group of non-smokers, who were matched on as many other explanatory variables as possible. However, given that lung cancer develops over a long period of time, these studies took many years to complete. Case-control studies are often a more feasible option when the disease in question is rare and when a cohort analytic study would need to be extremely large and costly to identify a sufficient number of people who develop the disease. Using a case-control design for the smoking and lung cancer example, people with lung cancer are matched to people without lung cancer on several important variables. All participants are asked about their past smoking behaviour, and the groups are compared to see whether those with lung cancer were more likely to have smoked.

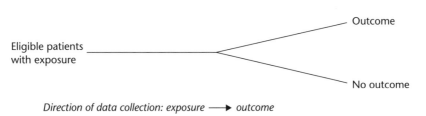

Direction of data collection: exposure ⟶ outcome

Figure 7.4 Cohort study design.

Questions about the course of a condition or disease (prognosis)

When we are interested in the likelihood that people will experience or develop an outcome given their exposure to a disease or condition, the best design is a *cohort study*. An example of a prognosis question is whether infants who are preterm and small for gestational age are likely to have cognitive and motor delays during early childhood.[3] In this example, the conditions are being preterm and small for gestational age. An example of a prognosis question related to a disease is *How likely are patients with ulcerative colitis to develop bowel cancer?* In a cohort study, a group of patients who are at a uniform point in the development of or exposure to the disease or condition (e.g. at first onset or initial diagnosis) (*inception cohort*) and are free of the outcome of interest are followed up to determine who develops the outcome (Figure 7.4).

In the case of lung cancer, an example of a prognosis study is to assemble a group of patients who have just been diagnosed with lung cancer and follow them over time to determine when, or if, certain symptoms appear or how long patients survive.

The longitudinal nature of the cohort study design ensures that the disease or condition precedes the outcome. The disadvantages of this design are the expense and time required to follow up large numbers of participants until some develop the outcome and the differential care and treatment patients may receive over the follow-up period.

Single studies versus systematic reviews

Questions about the cause, course, prevention or treatment of disease or about diagnostic tests have usually been addressed by more than one study. To help practitioners and health policy makers keep up with the literature related to specific topics, systematic reviews of the literature are conducted. In a *systematic review*, eligible research studies are viewed as a population to be systematically sampled and surveyed. Individual study characteristics and results are then abstracted, quantified, coded, and assembled into a database that, if appropriate, is statistically analysed much like other quantitative data. The statistical combination of the results of more than one study, or *meta-analysis*, effectively increases the sample size and results in a more precise estimate of effect than can be obtained from any of the individual studies used in the meta-analysis. Rigorous systematic reviews provide a summary of all methodologically sound studies related to a specific topic. This is much more powerful than the results of any one single study and avoids the potential bias of reading only some of the existing studies on a particular question. However, if the studies under review are not methodologically sound, then the results of the meta-analysis will also be biased.[1]

Summary

Several research designs can be used to gather quantitative data. The designs described in this chapter are the most rigorous for addressing questions of treatment, causation, and prognosis. When looking for studies related to these questions, awareness of these designs will help nurses to identify those studies and systematic reviews that are worth reading and have the potential to inform practice. In addition, researchers often collect both quantitative and qualitative data within a single study. Such mixed methods and approaches can illuminate diverse, but related, concepts such as the frequency of a particular health state and the meaning of it to those who experience it.

LEARNING EXERCISES

Identify two or three recurring clinical uncertainties that you have (it would be particularly good to do this with a colleague). Write them down in PICO format (see Chapter 3). For each, think carefully about the ideal study design to conduct research that might help to reduce your uncertainty.

References

1 DiCenso A, Cullum N, Ciliska D. Implementing evidence-based nursing: some misconceptions. *Evidence-Based Nursing* 1998;1:38–40.
2 Hill AB. *Principles of Medical Statistics*. London: Lancet, 1971:313.
3 Hutton JL, Pharoah PO, Cooke RW, Stevenson RC. Differential effects of preterm birth and small gestational age on cognitive and motor development. *Arch Dis Child Fetal Neonatal Ed* 1997;76:F75–81.

IDENTIFYING THE BEST RESEARCH DESIGN TO FIT THE QUESTION. PART 2: QUALITATIVE RESEARCH

Jenny Ploeg

Qualitative research methods have become increasingly important as ways of developing nursing knowledge for evidence-based nursing practice. Qualitative research answers a variety of questions related to nursing's concern with human responses to actual or potential health problems. The purpose of qualitative research is to describe, explore, and explain the phenomena being studied.[1] Qualitative research questions often take the form of *What is this?* or *What is happening here?* and are more concerned with the process than the outcome.[2] This chapter provides an overview of qualitative research, describes three common types of qualitative research, and gives examples of their use in nursing.

Sampling, data collection and data analysis

Sampling refers to the process used to select a portion of the population for study. Qualitative research is generally based on non-probability and purposive sampling rather than probability or random approaches.[3] Sampling decisions are made for the explicit purpose of obtaining the richest possible source of information to answer the research question. Purposive sampling decisions influence not only the selection of participants, but also settings, incidents, events, and activities for data collection. Some of the sampling strategies used in qualitative research are maximum variation sampling, homogeneous sampling, and snowball sampling.[4] Qualitative research usually involves smaller sample sizes than quantitative research.[5] Sampling in qualitative research is flexible and often continues until no new themes emerge from the data, a point called *data saturation*.

Many data collection techniques are used in qualitative research, but the most common are interviewing and participant observation.[6] Unstructured interviews are used when the researcher knows little about the topic, whereas semi-structured interviews are used when the researcher has some idea of the questions to ask about a topic. Participant observation is used to observe research participants in as natural a setting as possible. Participant observation techniques differ in the extent to which the researcher is visible and involved in the setting.[6] To learn more about the topic being studied, qualitative researchers may also use other data sources such as journals, newspapers, letters, books, photographs, and video tapes. Collection of qualitative data is also common in experimental and epidemiological studies (e.g. randomized controlled trials) that use mixed-methods approaches.[7]

Qualitative data

Whereas analysis of quantitative data focuses on statistics, analysis of qualitative data focuses on codes, themes and patterns in the data.[8] Increasingly, qualitative researchers use computer software programs to assist with coding and analysis of data.[9] The product of qualitative research varies with the approach used. Qualitative research may produce a rich, deep description of the phenomenon being studied or a theory about the phenomenon. Qualitative research reports often contain direct quotes from participants that provide rich illustrations of the study themes. Qualitative research, unlike its quantitative counterpart, does not lend itself to empirical inference to a population as a whole; rather it allows researchers to generalize to a theoretical understanding of the phenomenon being examined.

In the current context of pressure towards evidence-based health care, there is new enthusiasm for qualitative meta-synthesis, or meta-study.[10, 11] *Meta-study* involves the analysis and synthesis of qualitative findings, methods, and theories or frameworks from different studies to develop overarching or more conclusive ways of thinking about phenomena.[11] More details about the analysis of qualitative data are provided in Chapter 13.

Types of qualitative research

There are many different types of qualitative research, such as ethnography, phenomenology, grounded theory, life history, and case study.[8] As in quantitative research, it is important for nurse researchers to select the qualitative research approach best suited to the research question. Three of the most commonly used approaches to qualitative research in nursing are phenomenology, ethnography and grounded theory.[6] The goals and methods associated with each approach will be described briefly in the following sections. Examples of studies that use each approach are summarized to illustrate some of the similarities and differences among approaches. More complete descriptions and comparisons of these approaches and their use in nursing are available.[2, 5, 12]

Phenomenology

The aim of a phenomenological approach to qualitative research is to describe accurately the lived experiences of people and not to generate theories or models of the phenomena being studied.[13] The origins of phenomenology are in philosophy, particularly the works of Husserl, Heidegger and Merleau-Ponty.[13] Because the primary source of data is the life world of the individual being studied, in-depth interviews are the most common means of data collection. Furthermore, emerging themes are often validated with participants because their (i.e. participants') meanings of that lived experience are central in phenomenological study.

Phenomenology was used to answer the following research question: *What is the lived experience of adults who are integrating a hearing loss into their lives?*[14] The convenience sample consisted of 32 adults with mild to profound hearing loss. Data were collected through semistructured, audiotaped interviews with participants. Analysis involved identification of core and major themes in the data and validation of the findings with selected participants. The core theme of 'dancing with' eloquently captured participants' perceptions of moving, gracefully or awkwardly, with the changes required by hearing loss, never sure of the next steps. The major themes of 'dancing with' loss and fear, fluctuating feelings, courage amidst change, and an altered life perspective provide readers with a rich description of participants' perceptions of what it was like to live with hearing loss. These findings offer nurses a deep understanding of the phenomenon that can be applied in their interactions with people living with hearing loss. The phenomenological approach was key to uncovering participants' meanings of the complex and dynamic process of integrating hearing loss into their lives.

Ethnography

The goal of ethnography is to learn about a culture from the people who actually live in that culture.[15] A culture can be defined not only as an ethnic population but also as a society, a community, an organization, a spatial location, or a social world.[16] Ethnography has its roots in cultural anthropology, which aims to describe the values, beliefs and practices of cultural groups.[15] The process of ethnography is characterized by intensive, ongoing, face-to-face involvement with participants of the culture being studied and by participating in their settings and social worlds during a period of fieldwork. The essential data collection methods of participant observation and in-depth interviewing permit researchers to learn about the meanings that informants attach to their knowledge, behaviours and activities.[17] The social, political and economic contexts of a culture are important parts of an ethnographic study, unlike a phenomenological study.

An ethnographic approach was used to answer the following research question: *What is it like to be a young urban African-American who has at least one AIDS-afflicted family member?*[18] Stories of six young people are described in the article. There was an extensive four-year period of in-depth fieldwork that included telephone and in-person interviews and participant observation. The stories powerfully illustrated how the culture in which the youths had to survive was so alienating that they deliberately sought exposure to HIV. The findings provide an important understanding for nurses working with adolescents in either preventive or acute care roles. The ethnographic approach was uniquely suited to bringing attention to the important influence of the contexts of marginalization, insensitive social policies, and demanding caretaking responsibilities on the lives of these youths.

Grounded theory

The purpose of a grounded theory approach to qualitative research is to discover social-psychological processes.[19] Grounded theory was developed by Glaser and Strauss in the 1960s and is founded philosophically on symbolic interactionism.[20] Distinct features of grounded theory include theoretical sampling and the constant comparative method. *Theoretical sampling* refers to sampling decisions made throughout the entire research process, in which participants are selected based on their knowledge of the topic and on emerging study findings. In data analysis, the researcher constantly compares incidents, categories and constructs to determine similarities and differences and to develop a theory that accounts for behavioural variation. Both observation and interviewing are commonly used for data collection.

Grounded theory was used to answer the following research question: *What is the process of reimaging after an alteration in body appearance or function?*[21] The theoretical sample consisted of 28 participants who had experienced body image disruptions such as significant weight change, amputation or paralysis of body parts, and scars from burns, surgery or trauma. Participants were interviewed at 3, 6, 12 and 18 months after the physical alteration. The constant comparative method of concurrent data collection and analysis was used to develop a three-phase theory of the process of reimaging: (1) body image disruption, (2) wishing for restoration, and (3) reimaging the self. Nurses can use this understanding of the phases of reimaging to assist clients through the process by anticipating potential needs or problems, providing information and support, and exploring alternative problem-solving strategies. The grounded theory approach was ideally suited to discovering the social-psychological process of reimaging.

Summary

The examples of nursing research studies using three different approaches exemplify the value of qualitative research in answering important nursing questions. The studies also provide rich illustrations of the differences and similarities between the disparate approaches that are captured by the term 'qualitative research'. The examples differ in the type of research question asked, philosophical underpinnings, methods used, and, to some extent, the final product. Each study, however, resulted in important new information about the phenomena studied. This new information facilitates deeper understanding of participants' experiences by nurse readers and, as long as nurses remain aware of the theoretical rather than empirical basis for generalizing from qualitative findings, has the potential for influencing nursing practice in similar situations.

LEARNING EXERCISES

Identify a knowledge gap in your practice that could be addressed by a qualitative research study. With a colleague,

1. Identify which of the three qualitative approaches (phenomenology, ethnography or grounded theory) would best answer your research question, and discuss why.
2. Identify the qualitative research question for your issue.
3. Discuss the data collection techniques you could use to answer your research question.
4. Discuss how you might use findings from qualitative studies in your practice.

References

1 Marshall C, Rossman GB. *Designing Qualitative Research*. Fourth edition. Thousand Oaks: Sage, 2006.
2 Munhall PL. *Nursing Research: A Qualitative Perspective*. Third edition. Sudbury: Jones and Bartlett Publishers and National League for Nursing Press, 2001.

3 Kuzel AJ. Sampling in qualitative inquiry. In: Crabtree BF, Miller WL, editors. *Doing Qualitative Research*. Second edition. Thousand Oaks: Sage, 1999:33–45.

4 Meadows LM, Morse JM. Constructing evidence within the qualitative project. In Morse JM, Swanson JM, Kuzel AJ, editors. *The Nature of Qualitative Evidence*. Thousand Oaks: Sage, 2001:187–200.

5 Morse JM. Designing funded qualitative research. In: Denzin NK, Lincoln YS, editors. *Handbook of Qualitative Research*. Thousand Oaks: Sage, 1994:220–35.

6 Morse JM, Richards L. *README FIRST for a User's Guide to Qualitative Methods*. Thousand Oaks: Sage, 2002.

7 Tashakkori A, Teddlie CB, editors. *Handbook of Mixed Methods in Social and Behavioral Research*. Thousand Oaks: Sage, 2002.

8 Tesch R. *Qualitative Research: Analysis Types and Software Tools*. New York: Falmer, 1990.

9 Weitzman EA. Software and qualitative research. In Denzin NK, Lincoln YS, editors. *Handbook of Qualitative Research*. Second edition. Thousand Oaks: Sage, 2000:803–29.

10 Paterson BL, Thorne SE, Canam C, Jillings C. *Meta-study of Qualitative Health Research: A Practical Guide to Meta-analysis and Meta-synthesis*. Thousand Oaks: Sage, 2001.

11 Thorne S, Jensen L, Kearney MH, Noblit G, Sandelowski M. Qualitative meta-synthesis: reflections on methodological orientation and ideological agenda. *Qual Health Res* 2004;**14**:1342–65.

12 Streubert Speziale HJ, Carpenter DR. *Qualitative Research in Nursing: Advancing the Humanistic Imperative*. Fourth edition. Philadelphia: Lippincott Williams and Wilkins, 2006.

13 Van Manen M. *Researching Lived Experience: Human Science for an Action Sensitive Pedagogy*. Second edition. London, Ontario: Althouse Press, 1997.

14 Herth K. Integrating hearing loss into one's life. *Qual Health Res* 1998;**8**:207–23.

15 Spradley JP. *The Ethnographic Interview*. New York: Harcourt Brace Jovanovich College Publishers, 1979.

16 Hammersley M. *What's Wrong with Ethnography? Methodological Explorations*. New York: Routledge, 1992.

17 Germain CP. Ethnography: the method. In: Munhall PL editor. *Nursing Research: A Qualitative Perspective*. Third edition. Sudbury, MA: Jones and Bartlett Publishers and National League for Nursing Press, 2001:277–306.

18 Tourigny SC. Some new dying trick: African American youths 'choosing' HIV/AIDS. *Qual Health Res* 1998;**8**:149–67.

19 Strauss A, Corbin JM. *Basics of Qualitative Research: Techniques and Procedures for Developing Grounded Theory*. Second edition. Thousand Oaks: Sage, 1998.

20 Glaser B, Strauss A. *The Discovery of Grounded Theory: Strategies for Qualitative Research*. Chicago: Aldine Transaction, 1967.

21 Norris J, Kunes-Connell M, Spelic SS. A grounded theory of reimaging. *ANS Adv Nurs Sci* 1998;**20**:1–12.

Additional resources

Creswell JW. *Qualitative Inquiry and Research Design: Choosing among Five Approaches*. Second edition. Thousand Oaks: Sage, 2007.

Creswell JW. *Research Design: Qualitative, Quantitative and Mixed Methods Approaches*. Second edition. Thousand Oaks: Sage, 2003.

International Institute for Qualitative Methodology. University of Alberta. http://www.uofaweb.ualberta.ca/iiqm/Links.cfm

Qualitative Health Research journal, Sage (monthly).

The Qualitative Report (online journal). Nova Southeastern University. http://www.nova.edu/ssss/QR/index.html

Chapter 9

IF YOU COULD JUST PROVIDE ME WITH A SAMPLE: EXAMINING SAMPLING IN QUANTITATIVE AND QUALITATIVE RESEARCH PAPERS

Carl Thompson

When undertaking any research study, researchers must choose their sample carefully to minimize bias. This chapter highlights why practitioners need to pay attention to issues of sampling when appraising research, and discusses sampling characteristics that readers should look for in quantitative and qualitative studies. The chapter focuses on the randomized controlled trial (RCT) as an example of quantitative research, and on grounded theory as an example of qualitative research. Although these two designs are used as examples, the general principles outlined can be applied to all quantitative and qualitative research designs.

What is sampling?

Research studies usually focus on a defined group of people, such as patients receiving mechanical ventilation or the parents of chronically ill children. The group of people in a study is referred to as the *sample*. Because it is too expensive and impractical to include the total population in a research study, the ideal study sample represents the total population from which the sample was drawn (e.g. all patients receiving mechanical ventilation or all parents of chronically ill children). This point – that studying an entire population is, in most cases, unnecessary – is the key to the theory of sampling. *Sampling* means studying a proportion of the population rather than the whole population. The results of a study that has assembled its sample appropriately can be more confidently applied to the population from which the sample was drawn. Using the examples provided earlier, we can say that the authors of one study 'sampled' 54 patients from a 'population' of patients who required mechanical ventilation in order to test out the effects of music therapy on anxiety,[1] and in another study, researchers 'sampled' 50 children (and their parents) from a 'population' of all children admitted to hospital for chronic health conditions in order to test out a stress-relieving intervention.[2] In both studies, the researchers examined a small portion of the populations of interest so that they could say something that would apply to the entire populations.

When reading a paper that sets out to say something about a population by studying a sample, readers need to assess the external validity. *External validity* is the degree to which the findings of a study can be generalized beyond the sample used in the study. The ability to generalize is almost totally dependent on the adequacy of the sampling process. Nurses should consider several possible threats to external validity when appraising a paper and deciding whether the results could be applied to patients in their care:

- *Unusual sample selection*: Study findings may be applicable only to the group studied. For example, the findings of a study of a telephone support programme for caregivers of people with Alzheimer's disease that recruited a sample from local Alzheimer's Association branches would not necessarily apply to the population of caregivers as a whole because most caregivers do not belong to such local groups and, therefore, are different from the sample.
- *Distinctive research settings*: The particular context in which a study takes place can greatly affect the external validity of the findings. For example, Tourigny[3] sampled six African-American youths to learn about deliberate exposure to HIV. The study took place in the context of extreme poverty in a uniquely deprived urban setting in the United States (US). The opportunity for a suburban community nurse in the United Kingdom (UK) to apply the theory generated by this study may be limited by the very different social settings involved.
- *History*: The passage of time can affect the findings. For example, studies of mechanisms for implementing research findings within health care organizations might be affected by the organizational and structural changes that occur at local and national levels over time. Examples of such reorganization include the effects of separating health care provision from purchasing through the National Health Service (NHS) 'internal market' of the late 1980s and the creation of health maintenance organizations in the US.
- *Population-specific research constructs*: The particular constructs, concepts, or phenomena studied may be specific to the group sampled. For example, researchers evaluating the concept of 'quality' in health care should recognize that professionals and consumers may differ in their perceptions of the concept and should be explicit about how they actually measured it.

Sampling in quantitative research

Quantitative research is most often used when researchers wish to make a statement about the chance (or probability) of something happening in a population. For example, a person is 65% less likely to die a cardiac-related death if she eats a Mediterranean-type diet compared with the recommended Step 1 diet of the American Heart Association.[4] Quantitative studies usually use sampling techniques based on probability theory. *Probability sampling*, as it is known, has two central features: (1) The researcher has (in theory) access to all members of a population, and (2) every member of the population has an equal and non-zero chance of being selected for the study sample. In other words, they cannot have 'no chance' of being sampled.

Three concepts relevant to probability samples are sampling error, random sampling, and sampling bias. Each of these will be described below.

Sampling error

Probability samples allow researchers to minimize sampling error in that they provide the highest chance of the sample being representative of the total population. Sampling error occurs in all probability samples and is unavoidable because no sample can ever totally represent the population. There will always be a gap between a sample's representativeness and the population's known or unknown characteristics: the *sampling error*. Readers of quantitative studies should look for evidence that the researchers tried to combat sampling error. Specifically, the authors should have identified the study sample using a random selection process and provided a statistical justification for the sample size. The size of the sampling error generally decreases as the size of the sample increases.

Random sampling

Random selection works because, as individuals enter a sample, their characteristics, which differ from those of the population, balance the characteristics of other individuals. For example, in a randomly selected sample of users of mental health services, some users will be from upper socioeconomic groups, and these will be balanced by others who are from lower socioeconomic groups.

Successful random sampling requires a sufficiently large sample. If a sample is large enough, then differences in outcomes that exist between groups will be detected statistically, whereas, if it is too small, important differences may be missed. One of the clues that can alert readers to a study that is not large enough is the confidence interval around a study finding. Although not all studies report confidence intervals, these are becoming increasingly popular in the reporting of quantitative studies. A *confidence interval* provides a statement of the level of confidence that the true value for a population lies within a specified range of values. A *95% confidence interval* can be described as follows: if sampling is repeated indefinitely, with each sample leading to a new confidence interval, then in 95% of the samples, the interval will cover the true population value.[5] The larger the sample size, the more narrow the confidence interval and, therefore, the more precise the estimate.

Sampling bias

Unlike sampling error, which cannot be avoided completely, sampling bias is usually the result of a flaw in the research process, and increasing the size of the sample just increases the effect of the bias. *Sampling bias* occurs when a sample is not representative of the population. An example of sampling bias has already been highlighted in the section on external validity: sampling only caregivers from Alzheimer's Association groups introduces a sampling bias if the study aim is to generalize to the whole population of caregivers of people with Alzheimer's disease. *Bias*, in the context of RCTs, can be thought of as '. . . any factor or process that tends to deviate the results or conclusions of a trial away from the truth'.[6] Two important biases related to sampling that could affect the generalizability of study findings are referral filter bias and volunteer bias. In *referral filter bias*, the selection that occurs at each stage in the referral process from primary to secondary to tertiary care can generate patient samples that are very different from one another.[7] For example, the results of a study of people with asthma under the care of specialists are not likely to be generalizable to individuals with asthma in primary care settings. In *volunteer bias*, people who volunteer to participate in a study may have exposures or outcomes (e.g. they tend to be healthier) that differ from those of non-volunteers.[8]

When appraising a research report, readers can ask a simple set of questions to assess whether sampling bias exists:

- Who was included in the sample?
- What was the source of recruitment into the study? (Community or hospital? Specialized centres or general hospitals?)
- How were subjects recruited? (Approached by health care professionals or study researchers? Paid or unpaid?)
- Which people were approached to be in the study? (Consecutive individuals? Volunteers or only people the researcher believed would be useful candidates?)
- What were the inclusion *and* exclusion criteria for the sample? What were the demographics (e.g. age and sex) of the sample? Did they have any medical conditions or a history of previous interventions that could affect the results of the study?

Some research designs – specifically RCTs – use probability theory slightly differently. In these studies, individuals might be initially sampled on a non-probability basis (e.g. all people attending an asthma clinic in one year) and then randomly allocated to an experimental or control group (e.g. self-management education or usual care). It is in the process of allocation that probability theory comes into play. Through random allocation, and provided that the sample is large enough, all factors that influence outcomes (both known and unknown) are evenly distributed between the groups and therefore, at the end of the study, any differences among the groups can be attributed to the intervention. Randomization alone, however, does not allow researchers to generalize to a population. Questions of sample size and the representativeness of the sample as a whole are still important. Readers should look for evidence that the sample was large enough and that there were no baseline differences between the experimental and control groups. If they are satisfied on these two counts, they can go on to consider the similarities between the study sample and the individuals for whom they provide care. If they are similar, then the study sample can be said to be representative, and readers can feel confident in applying the study findings in practice.

Sampling in qualitative research

Not all research designs are concerned with generalizing from a sample to a population of people. Qualitative studies use rich and deep description to inform our understanding of concepts and contribute to broader theoretical understanding. For example, a study of the experiences of older adults making the transition to life in a nursing home says nothing about the amount of experience or the probability of 'adjustment' to a nursing home; instead, the author simply describes what that experience might be like.[9] On the basis of this rich description, the author proposed a three-stage theory about the process of adjustment to a nursing home placement. What this means is that nurses should consider the possibility that these stages might need to be addressed in patients undergoing this transition. Good qualitative enquiry leads to theoretical generalizability rather than statistical inference. Because we want to generalize about the shape or content of a concept or contribute to a theoretical understanding of an aspect of health care, sampling in qualitative research is driven by a set of concerns very different from those that drive quantitative designs. 'The purpose [of sampling in qualitative research] is not to establish a random or representative sample drawn from a population but rather to identify specific groups of people who either possess characteristics or live in circumstances relevant to the social phenomenon being studied. Informants are identified because they will enable exploration of a particular aspect of behaviour relevant to the research. This allows the researcher to include a wide range of types of informants and also to select key informants with access to important sources of knowledge.'[10]

Qualitative researchers use non-probability sampling techniques as the basis for their studies. For example, if a researcher wants to know more about the content of unpleasant experiences among people receiving primary health care, it would be of no value to ask a random sample of the population because most people have relatively little experience of receiving primary care. It would be far more advantageous to interview people who were unhappy with the care they received (perhaps identified from complainant records). If we wanted to know the extent of unhappy experiences among consumers, the sampling strategies would be reversed, and we might randomly select individuals from the whole population and attempt to measure the amount of dissatisfaction.

Non-probability sampling

Just as various approaches to sampling are used in quantitative studies, several approaches to non-probability sampling are used in qualitative research. The same questions asked of probability samples can be asked of non-probability samples. Questions of sample size, however, are not as important here. Rather, it is the 'fitness for purpose', or quality, of the sample that should be described in the paper. This is difficult to judge in qualitative studies because the adequacy of the sample often can only be judged by the quality of the analysis of the data generated. In some qualitative studies, sampling continues until no new themes emerge from the data, a point called *data saturation*. However, as with quantitative findings, various terms exist to describe qualitative non-probability sampling:

- *Convenience or opportunistic sampling*: as with quantitative studies, this involves choosing individuals who are closest to hand or easiest to access.
- *Homogeneous sampling*: researchers decide at the outset to select participants who can provide similar stories or narratives on a phenomenon; often, selection is based on shared demographic or theoretical characteristics.
- *Heterogeneous or maximum variation sampling*: this is the opposite of homogeneous sampling: researchers decide at the outset to select participants who can provide different narratives or accounts of experiencing a phenomenon; often, selection is based on different demographic or theoretical characteristics.
- *Snowball sampling*: this approach is used when no sampling frame exists or access to individuals in a frame might be difficult because of cultural or social reasons. Often this approach is used with powerful or elite groups (e.g. police officers, physicians, or criminals), where access to the closed parts of networks depends on referral from a member of the social group. Usually, an initial respondent is asked if

they know of any other potential participants who might be willing to speak with the researcher. Sometimes informants are asked if they would be willing to approach other potential informants on behalf of researchers.

- *Theoretical sampling*: this approach, associated with the grounded theory approach to qualitative research,[11] aims to seek out data that challenge, and therefore develop, emerging ideas and hypotheses revealed by previous data collection. Initial cases are sampled based on shared characteristics to gain a broad understanding of the phenomenon under investigation. Then, individuals are sought who may prove exceptions to the arguments being developed. When it is no longer possible to advance the arguments further (i.e. theoretical avenues of inquiry are exhausted), a state of *theoretical saturation* is said to have been achieved.

Regardless of the specific technique used, the earlier questions remain useful as a way of focusing your scrutiny:

- Who was included in the sample? That is, are participants able to adequately contribute to knowledge and understanding?
- What was the source of recruitment into the study? Is this context likely to influence the shape of the analysis presented?
- How were subjects recruited? (Approached by health care professionals or study researchers? Paid or unpaid?) Are these factors likely to alter the stories, accounts, or behaviours presented and, if so, how did the researcher account for this?
- Which individuals were approached to be in the study? (Consecutive individuals? Volunteers or only people the researcher believed would be useful candidates?)
- What were the inclusion and exclusion criteria for the sample? What were the demographics (e.g. age and sex) of the study sample? Did informants have any medical conditions or a history of previous interventions that might affect the study findings? In qualitative research, the findings are usually the accounts that people provide or the behaviours presented.

All of these questions remain relevant, but clues that should help readers to assess the adequacy of a qualitative sample include the believability of the final product and the sense of completeness of the analysis presented. A solid qualitative paper should generate a theory or description that encompasses a range of experiences or values and makes explicit the limitations of qualitative research in regard to conventional generalizability.

Quantitative and qualitative and sampling: a final word of caution

This chapter has used the quantitative–qualitative distinction to highlight the primary differences between probability and non-probability sampling strategies. In reality, however, this distinction is often blurred, and many studies use a combination of two or more approaches. This is not a criticism: sampling is an integral part of the application of research methodology and, because of this, it should be guided by the research question. Like so much in evidence-based health care, the key questions to ask about the sampling strategy of a study relate to the 'fitness for purpose'. Three questions capture the quality of any sample:

1. Are the study participants similar enough to the people for whom I provide care? In quantitative terms, this enables you to judge whether the results of the study can be applied to your population. In qualitative terms, the similarity of individuals enables you to judge whether the concepts or experiences being explored would be meaningful to your practice.
2. Was the sample selected in such a way that it could introduce bias into the research? This concept is applicable to both quantitative and qualitative research. In qualitative research, however, the boundaries or limitations of theoretical generalizability are usually encompassed in the description of the participants.
3. Was the sample large enough? In quantitative research, this means *Was the sample large enough to detect a difference between groups if a difference existed?* In qualitative research, this means *Were there enough people (or was sufficient time spent with a few people) to provide rich meaningful description and convincing analysis?*

Summary

An understanding of how participants are assembled for a study, plus additional information on their characteristics (e.g. age, sex and disease severity), will help readers to decide whether a study sample is sufficiently similar to their own patients and they can apply the results to their own practice.[7]

LEARNING EXERCISES

1. Which of the following use simple random sampling? Provide a brief example of the sampling method used in each.
   (a) A lottery game (such as the UK national lottery)
   (b) The UK, Canadian, or American general election (but not the Australian)
   (c) A census of all patients detained under the UK Mental Health Act
2. Table 9.1 represents the Modified Early Warning risk assessment scores (MEWS) for patients in the Springfield Medical Admissions Unit (MAU) for a 6-month period.
   (a) What is the total population of the MAU?
   (b) The nurse wants to sample 50% of the individuals. How many patients would this be?
   (c) The nurse wants to keep the correct proportion of men to women in the sample. Using the following formula, calculate the number of men that should be included in the sample.

   $$\frac{\text{number of males}}{\text{number of total patients}} \times \text{size of sample survey}$$

   (d) What type of sampling technique has been used here?
   (e) If the nurse wishes to sample 180 patients, how many men and women per MEWS category should be surveyed? Put your answers in a table. (Results should be rounded to the nearest whole number.)
3. Suppose you wish to conduct a grounded theory study of individuals who abuse alcohol. Who would you start with and why? How might your sampling strategy go next as a result of talking with your first subsample?

Table 9.1 Modified Early Warning risk assessment scores (MEWS)* for patients in the Springfield Medical Admissions Unit (MAU) for a 6-month period

	MEWS	1	2	3	4	5	6	7	8	9	10	11	12
Men	9	8	9	9	13	20	23	28	78	74	69	71	60
Women	6	8	11	10	13	18	35	34	63	62	61	88	70
Total	**15**	**16**	**20**	**19**	**26**	**38**	**58**	**62**	**141**	**136**	**130**	**159**	**130**

* Scores ≥5 are indicative of heightened risk of a critical event such as cardiac arrest.

Table 9.2 Modified Early Warning risk assessment scores (MEWS)* for patients in the Springfield Medical Admissions Unit (MAU) for a 6-month period, proportionate to sex by MEWS score

	MEWS	1	2	3	4	5	6	7	8	9	10	11	12
Men	2	2	2	2	2	4	4	5	15	14	13	13	11
Women	1	2	2	2	2	3	7	6	12	12	12	17	13
Total	**3**	**4**	**4**	**4**	**4**	**7**	**11**	**11**	**27**	**26**	**25**	**30**	**24**

* Scores ≥5 are indicative of heightened risk of a critical event such as cardiac arrest.

Solutions to learning exercises

1a. *A lottery uses the simple random sampling method. All of the numbers (total population) are put into a barrel, and the required number (sample) is drawn at random. Each item has an equal chance of selection.*

1b. *An election is an example of non-random sampling (volunteer sampling) because each member of the population (18 years or older) can participate if they decide to do so. Australia is different; because voting is compulsory, it is, in effect, a census (although, of course there is a form of sampling error because some people still will not vote).*

1c. *A census does not use simple random sampling because every member of the target population must be included.*

2a. *The total patient population of the MAU is 950.*

2b. *A sample of 50% of the MAU's population would equal 475 individuals.*

2c. *In order to keep the sample proportionate to the number of men and women in the MAU, roughly 236 men and 240 women should be included in the sample.*

2d. *The sampling method used here is stratified sampling.*

2e. *Table 9.2 features the breakdown of the sample of 180 patients so that it is proportionate to sex by MEWS score.*

3. *There is no correct answer here but you might like to consider that not all individuals who abuse alcohol are easily identifiable. You could use people who score above a certain point in validated screening tools, such as the CAGE questionnaire (http://pubs.niaaa.nih.gov/publications/Assesing%20Alcohol/ InstrumentPDFs/16_CAGE.pdf) or you could sample people who attend self-help clinics (although probably not Alcoholics Anonymous as it's anonymous!). Remember, though, that it is the phenomenon of alcohol abuse that you are seeking to illuminate. Whomsoever you use, they should be able to recount an important dimension of the phenomenon of abusing alcohol.*

References

1 Chlan L. Effectiveness of a music therapy intervention on relaxation and anxiety for patients receiving ventilatory assistance. *Heart Lung* 1998;**27**:169–76.

2 Burke SO, Handley-Derry MH, Costello EA, Kauffmann E, Dillon MC. Stress-point intervention for parents of repeatedly hospitalized children with chronic conditions. *Res Nurs Health* 1997;**20**:475–85.

3 Tourigny SC. Some new dying trick: African American youths 'choosing' HIV/AIDS. *Qual Health Res* 1998;**8**:149–67.

4 de Lorgeril M, Salen P, Martin JL, Monjaud I, Boucher P, Mamelle N. Mediterranean dietary pattern in a randomized trial: prolonged survival and possible reduced cancer rate. *Arch Intern Med* 1998;**158**:1181–7.

5 Satin A, Shastry W. *Survey Sampling: A Non-mathematical Guide.* Ottawa: Statistics Canada, 1985:7–32.

6 Jadad AR. *Randomised Controlled Trials: A Users' Guide.* London: BMJ Books, 1998:28.

7 Sackett DL, Haynes RB, Guyatt GH, Tugwell P. *Clinical Epidemiology: A Basic Science for Clinical Medicine.* Second edition. Boston: Little, Brown and Company, 1991.

8 Sackett DL. Bias in analytic research. *J Chronic Dis* 1979;**32**:51–63.

9 Wilson SA. The transition to nursing home life: a comparison of planned and unplanned admissions. *J Adv Nurs* 1997;**26**:864–71.

10 Mays N, Pope C, editors. *Qualitative Research in Health Care.* London: BMJ Books, 1996:12–13.

11 Glaser BG and Strauss AL. *The Discovery of Grounded Theory: Strategies for Qualitative Research.* New York: Aldine Publishing Company, 1967.

Additional resource

http://informationr.net/rm/RMeth22.html Not always health related but an excellent set of resources and workbooks.

Chapter 10

THE FUNDAMENTALS OF QUANTITATIVE MEASUREMENT

Donna Ciliska, Nicky Cullum and Alba DiCenso

In this chapter we provide a basic introduction to the quantitative measurement of health outcomes (e.g. blood pressure, quality of life, patient satisfaction, costs) of the type that will frequently be encountered in studies of treatment, causation, prognosis, diagnosis and economic evaluations.

Health can be measured in many different ways. The various aspects of health that can be measured are referred to as *variables*.[1] For example, in a study exploring the effects of exercise and structured exercise programmes on health, the interventions (known as the *independent* variables) are lifestyle and structured exercise programmes, and the outcomes (known as the *dependent* variables) are physical activity and cardiorespiratory fitness.[2] In a treatment study, the independent variables are those that are under the control of investigators, and the dependent variables are those that may be influenced by the independent variable. In a causation study, investigators rely on natural variation between both variables and look for a relation between the independent and dependent variables. For example, when considering whether smoking causes lung cancer, smoking is the independent variable and lung cancer is the dependent variable.

Types of variables

Variables can be classified as nominal, ordinal, interval, or ratio variables depending on the type of data they represent. *Nominal (categorical) variables* are simply names of categories. Nominal variables that have only two possible values are referred to as *dichotomous variables*; examples include handedness (right or left), survival (dead or alive), or the presence or absence of a specific feature (e.g. depressed or not depressed, diabetes or no diabetes). Other nominal variables may have several possible values (e.g. race can include white, black, Hispanic, and others). The actual number of categories can be determined by the researcher; for example, race can be defined as having two values (black or non-black) or as having several possible values, as indicated above. No hierarchy is presumed with nominal data – that is, being right-handed is not twice as good as being left-handed (although, historically, there was considerable prejudice against those with left-hand dominance). In contrast, *ordinal variables* are sets of 'ordered' categories.[1] For example, patients are often asked to rate the severity of their pain on a scale of 0–10, where 0 is no pain and 10 is unbearable, excruciating pain. Although we can safely say that a pain rating of 8 is worse than a pain rating of 5, we do not really know how much these two ratings differ because we do not know the size of the intervals between each rating.[1] Ordinal scales have also been used to grade pressure ulcer severity and to classify the staging of various cancers (e.g. stage I, II or III). *Interval variables* consist of an ordered set of categories, with the additional requirement that the categories form a series of intervals that are all exactly the same size. Thus, the difference between a temperature of 37°C and 38°C is 1 degree, as is the difference between 38°C and 39°C, and so on. However, an interval scale does not have an absolute zero point that indicates complete absence of the variable being measured. Because there is no absolute zero point on an interval scale, ratios of values are not meaningful – that is, two values cannot be compared by claiming that one is 'twice as large' as another. A *ratio variable* has all of the features of an interval variable but adds an absolute zero point, which indicates the complete absence (none) of the variable being measured. The advantage of an absolute zero is that ratios of numbers on the scale reflect ratios of magnitude for the variable being measured.[3] To illustrate, 100°C is not twice as hot as 50°C (interval data), but 100 cm is twice as long as 50 cm, and a pulse of 80 beats/min is twice a pulse rate of 40 beats/min (ratio data).

The reason for stressing the differences between types of variables is that the type of variable dictates, to a large extent, the method of statistical analysis used by the researcher. It is meaningless to discuss the average or mean value of nominal or ordinal data because they are categories. Thus, the notion of a 'mean' or 'average' sex or race makes no sense; counts or frequencies of the number of individuals in each category, however, are useful. Conversely, the mean blood pressure (ratio variable) in a sample of patients is more meaningful than a count of the number of patients with each blood pressure measurement. In Chapters 11, 12 and 17, we will explore different ways to describe and analyse quantitative data.

Issues in measurement

It is important to remember that most measurements in health care research encapsulate several things: the 'real' or true value of the variable being measured, the variability of the measure, the accuracy of the instrument with which we are measuring, and perhaps the position of the patient or the skills and expectations of the person doing the measurement. Some of these elements are within the control of the measurer (e.g. ensuring that a scale is at 0 before we weigh someone), whereas other elements are not (e.g. a patient's blood pressure varies by time of day, and therefore researchers should try to assess blood pressure at the same time each day).

Some measures are more *objective* than others and are less likely to be influenced by human error or bias. A few examples of objective measures include all-cause mortality (i.e. whether one is 'dead' or 'alive') and serum cholesterol concentrations. In contrast, *subjective measures* may be influenced by the perception of the individual doing the measuring (e.g. patient-reported pain ratings). Most paper-and-pencil questionnaires are subjective measures. The Beck Depression Inventory is an example of a subjective paper-and-pencil questionnaire.

Frequency counts, such as incidence or prevalence, are often used when we want to know the extent of a disease or condition in a population. Others may be more interested in the beneficial and harmful effects of an intervention, such as differences in the rates of sexually transmitted diseases after a behavioural intervention provided to minority women.

What measurement issues should I consider when reading an article?

Are the measures reliable and valid?

These are two critically important properties of measurement. *Reliability* refers to the degree to which a measure gives the same result twice (or more) under similar circumstances, and it may relate to the measure being used or the people using it. For example, if a patient's blood pressure is measured every 4 minutes on the same arm, by the same nurse, and the patient is not subject to any intervention such as activity or medication, you would expect to get similar sphygmomanometer readings each time. The extent to which repeated readings are similar is called *reliability*. Assessment of the similarity of repeated readings taken by the same nurse provides a measure of *intra-rater* or *within-rater reliability*. You would also hope that two different nurses measuring the same patient's blood pressure under the same circumstances would get similar readings. The extent to which the readings from two different nurses are similar is known as *inter-rater* or *between-rater reliability*.

Validity is the ability of a measurement tool to accurately measure what it is intended to measure. There are many different types of validity, but one of the most important is *criterion-related validity*, which requires comparison of a given measure with a *gold standard*, or the best existing measure of the variable.[4] In a study by Steer *et al.*,[5] the results obtained using the Beck Depression Inventory for Primary Care were compared with the results of a standardized interview conducted by a physician using *DSM-IV* criteria. The interview results were considered to be the gold standard. Other examples of commonly used alternatives to the gold standard include sphygmomanometer measures of blood pressure instead of direct central venous pressure readings and a simple urine hormone test instead of serum hormone concentrations as a test for pregnancy.

Is the measure subject to bias?

There are several potential sources of bias. It is not important to remember what they are called, but you should be able to recognize sources of bias in a study. One way that bias can occur in a study is when the health care providers, patients and data collectors participating in an intervention study are not *blinded* or *masked* to the treatment allocation. In an ideal world, health care providers delivering the intervention, patients, and the research staff measuring the outcomes would not know which treatment the patient was receiving. Although this level of blinding is possible in randomized trials evaluating new drugs, it is far more difficult to achieve in evaluations of most nursing interventions. Often, neither the nurses delivering an intervention nor the patients receiving the intervention can be masked (e.g. nurses know that they are providing a patient education intervention, and patients know that they are receiving it). In such studies, it is often possible, however, to 'mask' the person measuring the outcome. By ensuring that the person measuring the outcome is unaware of a patient's group allocation, researchers try to minimize the bias that could be introduced by the unconscious adjustments assessors might make if they were aware of a patient's group allocation. For example, in a study by Dunn et al.,[2] which compared two interventions to increase physical activity, the people who assessed blood pressure, pulse rate and body fat did not know which intervention participants had received. If they had known, this might have influenced their perceptions when they were doing the measurements, particularly if they had a clear opinion about which intervention was most effective. Similarly, participants reporting their own levels of activity might alter their reporting of actual behaviour depending on whether they enjoyed the intervention or wished they had been allocated to a different group. When describing the study design, authors should specify whether the study was blinded and explicitly state which groups were blinded. For more on blinding, see Chapter 18.

Another common type of bias is *social desirability bias*, in which people's responses to questions may reflect their desire to under-report their socially unfavourable habits, such as the number of cigarettes smoked, illicit drug use, or unsafe sexual practices. Conversely, people may overestimate what they perceive to be socially desirable practices, such as exercise participation or daily intake of fruits and vegetables.

A third type of bias is *recall bias*, which acknowledges that human memory is fallible. Reports of seat-belt use 5 years ago or fibre intake last month, for example, are not as accurate as concurrent or prospective measurements, where seat-belt use or dietary intake are recorded on a daily basis.

Investigators often use strategies to try to overcome these potential biases. These strategies include having outcome assessors who do not know the purpose of a study or which intervention a patient received; having study participants complete self-report questionnaires in a private area to ensure that their responses to sensitive or potentially embarrassing questions are confidential; and collecting information prospectively (i.e. as it happens), rather than retrospectively (historically).

Summary

Readers of research reports need to consider the types of measures used, the reliability and validity of the measures, and the methods used to minimize bias in the measurement of outcomes. These are some of the elements to be considered when assessing the quality of studies.

LEARNING EXERCISES

1. Working with a colleague, think of a few examples of nominal, ordinal, interval and ratio variables. Explain to each other why each is an example of a specific type (e.g. nominal).
2. Explain to a colleague why it is important to know the difference between nominal, ordinal, interval and ratio data.
3. Identify a trial (using any bibliographic database). Read the article to determine which variables are dependent and which are independent. Then, determine whether the variables are nominal, ordinal, interval or ratio data.

References

1 Norman GR, Streiner DL. *PDQ Statistics*. Toronto: BC Decker Inc, 1986.
2 Dunn AL, Marcus BH, Kampert JB, Garcia ME, Khol HW 3rd, Blair SN. Comparison of lifestyle and structured interventions to increase physical activity and cardiorespiratory fitness: a randomized trial. *JAMA* 1999;**281**:327–34.
3 Gravetter FJ, Wallnau LB. *Essentials of Statistics for the Behavioral Sciences*. California: Brooks/Cole Publishing Company, 1998.
4 Anthony D. *Understanding Advanced Statistics. A Guide for Nurses and Health Care Researchers*. Volume 4. Edinburgh: Churchill Livingstone, 1999.
5 Steer RA, Cavalieri TA, Leonard DM, Beck AT. Use of the Beck Depression Inventory for Primary Care to screen for major depression disorders. *Gen Hosp Psychiatry* 1999;**21**:106–11.

Chapter 11

SUMMARIZING AND PRESENTING THE EFFECTS OF TREATMENTS

Trevor A. Sheldon

Health care professionals and policy makers are increasingly aware of the need for their decisions to be informed by the best available research evidence. Practitioners need enough knowledge and skills to identify and interpret methodologically sound research. This chapter aims to help you to do this by looking at how the results of intervention, or treatment, studies are summarized and presented for different types of health outcomes. Chapter 12 explains how statistical techniques are used to assess the probability that an observed treatment effect occurred by chance and what is meant by a 'statistically significant' result.

Measures of health and disease

Many measures are used to assess the health outcomes of an intervention, ranging from those trying to capture an effect on people's general health (e.g. Short Form-36) to measures of a specific dimension relevant to a particular disease (e.g. Beck Depression Inventory).[1,2] Some are measures of patients' perceptions of their health; more often, however, they are measures that clinicians or researchers believe to be important. Regardless, these measures are generally either continuous or discrete, a distinction that is important because the type of measure used determines the way in which the results are presented and analysed.

Continuous measures

When the outcomes of a study are continuous (e.g. temperature, blood pressure, urine output, or cholesterol concentrations), researchers are usually interested in the extent to which these values change after exposure to an intervention. Studies that use continuous outcome measures may compare the average values of the variable (e.g. mean or median) after treatment. In a study of treatment for arthritis, researchers may measure changes in levels of pain or mobility on one or more pain or mobility scales. In conditions that are life threatening, studies may assess outcomes such as length of survival.

Recently, emphasis has shifted to more patient-centred measures of health. These measures assess patient ratings of health along several dimensions, such as physical functioning, social functioning, mental health and pain, and either score these separately in the form of a health profile (e.g. Nottingham Health Profile or the SF-36) or combine the ratings of different dimensions into a single number or index [e.g. Euroqol (EQ5D) or General Health Questionnaire].[1,2] All of these use continuous scales.

Once the change in score has been determined for each individual patient, the overall change in score for the group that received the intervention is compared with the overall change in score for the control group. How is this done? Many biological phenomena, such as height, are distributed 'normally' in the population. The term *normal* in this context refers to the symmetrical bell-shaped curve when the values for a large sample are plotted (Figure 11.1). Most values cluster around the middle value, with fewer at either end of the scale. The scores for a group of people are usually summarized using an average – either the mean or the median. The *mean* is calculated by adding all the values together and dividing by the number of observations. The *median* is the value of the middle observation when all observations are put in order; 50% of observations lie above the median and 50% lie below. When data are normally distributed, the mean and median are equal, and the mean value is used to summarize the data. However, when data deviate significantly from a normal distribution, also known as a *skewed distribution* (Figure 11.2), it is more informative to use the median rather than the mean value to summarize the data.

Not everyone in a group responds to an intervention in the same way or to the same degree, so not only are we interested in the average effect, but also we should know something about the extent to which the values are spread out or are dispersed or vary. This can be done by describing the *range* of values in a group (i.e. minimum and maximum values recorded). Other methods of recording this dispersion include the *interquartile range*, between which 50% of all the observations lie (Figure 11.1), or the *standard deviation (SD)*, which is a measure of the average amount individual values differ from the mean of the group; the lower the SD, the smaller the spread of values.

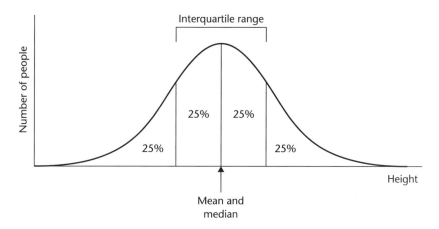

Figure 11.1 A normal distribution curve: variables such as height are distributed like this in the population.

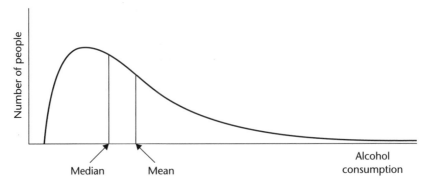

Figure 11.2 A skewed distribution curve: variables such as alcohol consumption are distributed like this in the population.

Discrete measures

Instead of measuring health outcomes on a continuous scale, studies often focus on discrete health events, such as the occurrence of a disease, death, or hospital discharge. What these outcomes have in common is that the event either occurs or does not; they are *discrete*, or *dichotomous, measures*.

For a group of people, discrete outcomes can be summarized as the percentage or proportion of people who experience an event during the follow-up period. For example, in a study of patients admitted to hospital with acute stroke, 61 out of 110 patients (55%) on general medical wards died within 7 years.[3] In a study of pressure bandages after coronary angioplasty,[4] 3.5% of patients allocated to pressure bandages experienced bleeding compared with 6.7% of those allocated to no bandages. These proportions express the probability or *risk* that a person in the group of interest experienced the event at some point during the follow-up period. This summary measure can be extended to take into account not only whether people experienced the event, but also the rate or speed at which they did so. For example, if 20% of study participants are dead after 2 years, the risk of them dying by 2 years would be 20%, regardless of whether they all died by 1 year or 2 years. The *rate*, however, measures the number of people experiencing the event per unit of time (*incidence*). If all deaths occurred by 1 year, the rate would be 20 per 100 person years (20 deaths for each 100 people followed up for 1 year), whereas if they all died by 2 years, the incidence would be halved, or 10 per 100 person years.

Continuous measures are often recast as discrete measures in evaluative studies, especially if there is a threshold above or below which there is a clinical difference. In the area of acute and critical care, the Glasgow Coma Scale is a continuous measure that includes 15 points. However, cut-off levels can be used to signify different levels of impairment: scores of 3–8 could signify severe impairment, scores of 9–12 could signify moderate impairment, and scores ≥13 could signify mild impairment. Studies may focus on changes in scores or the percentage of patients with severe impairment. For example, in studies of depression, one can measure the extent of depression using a depression scale or one can assign a threshold value to the scale, above which people receive a diagnosis of depression and below which people are classified as not depressed. In other words, the first approach measures how depressed people were before and after treatment, whereas the second uses a threshold measure, which can determine whether more or fewer people were depressed at the end of treatment compared with baseline. An example of the second approach is found in a review of St John's Wort for depression,[5] in which patients were classified as 'responders' or 'non-responders' to treatment.

Measures of effect and association

The previous section described different ways of measuring health outcomes. In this section, we examine how these measures are used to determine whether an intervention has an effect on an outcome and the size and direction of this effect. As before, the approach depends on whether the outcome is measured as a continuous or discrete variable. Remember that differences in the outcomes of patients who receive different interventions are not necessarily caused by the interventions. Changes in a health measure over time or between groups do not necessarily imply causation. It may be that patients in different groups were different to begin with or were managed differently in other respects, or that the outcomes were assessed differently. These are important criteria by which treatment studies should be appraised and are discussed in Chapter 15. It could also be that differences occurred by chance. One of the purposes of statistical analysis is to determine whether this is likely to be the case (see Chapter 12).

Continuous measures

Studies that use continuous outcome measures often compare the mean (or median) values of the outcome at the end of the follow-up period or the average change in outcome for the intervention and control groups from the baseline to the end of follow-up. If the average values (or changes) differ between the groups, it suggests that there may be differences in effect between the intervention and the control conditions. For example, a study evaluating the effect of oral contraceptives on dysmenorrhoea in adolescent girls used the pain subscale of the modified Moos Menstrual Distress Questionnaire (MMDQ).[6] The mean MMDQ score for the oral contraceptive group was 3.1 and for the placebo group it was 5.8; the difference in mean pain scores of 2.7 suggested a reduction in pain due to oral contraceptive use (see Chapter 12). In another example,[7] researchers assessed the effects of bereavement support for homosexual men, using a composite score for grief and distress before and after bereavement support in the treatment group and before and after standard care in the control group. They then compared the mean change (in this case, a decrease) in the distress–grief composite score in each group and found a greater reduction in the group that received bereavement support (1.09) than in the control group (0.47).

Another way of expressing differences in outcome for continuous measures is to put the average difference in the context of the amount of dispersion or variation (by dividing the difference in means by the SD). This is called the *standardized difference* and has no units. It simply expresses the effect of an intervention in terms of the number of SDs between the averages of the two groups. In a systematic review of self-management education for adults with asthma, one outcome measure was mean forced expiratory volume in 1 second (FEV_1).[8] Patients who received self-management education had a higher standardized mean FEV_1 (by 0.1) compared with those who

Intervention (exposure)	Event		Total
	Yes	**No**	
Yes	a	b	**a + b**
No	c	d	**c + d**

Figure 11.3 Numbers of people who receive (don't receive) an intervention and who experience (don't experience) an event.

received regular medical review. This means that the mean FEV$_1$ was 0.1 standard deviation higher in one group than in the other.[8] This is a very small difference and so is unlikely to be clinically important (see Chapter 12).

Standardized means also allow for comparison of the size of the treatment effect when different outcome measures are used and are therefore used in meta-analyses, which attempt to compare and combine the results of several studies measuring difference outcomes. You will often encounter reporting of standardized differences in systematic reviews in the *Cochrane Library*. Because standardized differences have no units, they have no direct clinical meaning and so are more difficult to interpret. In studies of effectiveness, a rule of thumb is that standardized mean differences > 0.5 indicate interventions that are very effective, and differences between 0.25 and 0.5 indicate interventions that are moderately effective.

Discrete measures

The measure of effect when using discrete outcomes (e.g. dead or alive) compares the risk of (i.e. proportion) experiencing an event in the intervention and control groups (see Figure 11.3).

The risk of an event in the intervention group (R^i) is simply the proportion of people in that group who experience the event (e.g. having a heart attack),

$$R^i = \frac{a}{a + b}$$

The corresponding risk in the control group is

$$R^c = \frac{c}{c + d}$$

There are two ways in which the outcome, or event rates, can be compared in participants who receive and do not receive the intervention. The *relative risk (RR)*, or *risk ratio*, is the risk of patients in the intervention group experiencing the outcome divided by the risk of patients in the control group experiencing the outcome:

$$RR = \frac{R^i}{R^c} = \frac{a/(a + b)}{c/(c + d)}$$

Table 11.1 Results of the Trondheim Stroke Unit trial. Table created using data from Indredavik *et al.* 1999[3]

Treatment group	Outcome after 7 years		
	Dead	**Alive**	**Total**
Stroke unit (treatment)	41	69	110
General ward (control)	61	49	110

If the intervention and control conditions have the same effect, then, assuming that the groups are comparable in all other respects, the risk of the event (e.g. death) will be the same in both groups; i.e. the top and bottom of the fraction will be the same, and the RR will be 1.0. If the risk of death is reduced in the intervention group compared with the control group, then the RR will be <1.0. If, however, the intervention is harmful, then the RR will be >1.0. The further the RR is from 1.0, the greater the strength of association between the intervention and the outcome.

The study of acute stroke care previously mentioned can help to illustrate this point. Table 11.1 shows the results of the Trondheim Stroke Unit trial for 220 patients, half of whom were admitted to a general medical ward and half to a specialized stroke unit.[3]

The risk of death in the stroke unit group was 41/110 = 0.37 or 37%. The risk of death in the control group was 61/110 = 0.55 or 55%. We can see that the risk of death was lower in the stroke unit group and can summarize this using the risk ratio:

$$RR = \frac{\text{risk of death in the treatment group}}{\text{risk of death in the control group}} = \frac{0.37}{0.55} = 0.67$$

Thus, over 7 years, the risk of dying after admission to a stroke unit was 0.67 or 67% of the risk of dying after admission to a medical ward. In other words, for every 100 people who die after admission to a general medical ward for stroke, only 67 would die if admitted to a stroke unit. This could also be expressed as a relative risk reduction (RRR) of 33% (i.e. 33 out of 100 patients would not die if admitted to a stroke unit).

Seeing this estimate of the effect, or the risk reduction, would likely prompt health professionals to consider urging a review of stroke care if their hospital did not have a stroke unit. However, they first might want to be sure that the effect was real (see Chapter 12), that the study was well conducted, and that other studies confirmed the apparently beneficial effects (see Chapters 15 and 19).

For various statistical reasons, some studies express the outcome as the odds of the event (*a/b*) rather than the risk of the event [*a/(a+b)*]. The *odds ratio (OR)* is the odds of the event in the intervention group (*a/b*) divided by the odds of the event in the control group (*c/d*):

$$OR = \frac{a/b}{c/d} = \frac{ad}{bc}$$

As with the RR, an OR of 1.0 means there is no difference between groups, and an OR <1.0 means that the event is less likely in the intervention group than the control group. When the event being measured is quite rare, the OR and RR are numerically similar because the values of a and c are insignificantly small.

The use of the OR can be illustrated with results of the Trondheim Stroke Unit trial (Table 11.1). The effect of stroke unit care can be summarized using the OR:

$$\frac{\text{odds of death in the treatment group}}{\text{odds of death in the control group}} = \frac{41/69}{61/49} = \frac{0.59}{1.24} = 0.48$$

Thus, the odds of dying in the treatment group are 48% of the odds of dying in the control group.

Clinical importance and impact

ORs and RRs are measures of the strength of association between an intervention and an outcome. However, they do not tell us much about the impact or clinical significance of the intervention and whether the intervention is worth considering.

It is important to remember that the RR indicates the 'relative' benefit of a treatment, not the 'actual' benefit; in other words, it does not take into account the number of people who would have developed the outcome anyway. The impact of a treatment is captured by the *absolute risk difference* or, when the risk is reduced, the *absolute risk reduction (ARR)*. The ARR can be calculated by simply subtracting the proportion of people experiencing the outcome in the intervention group from the proportion experiencing the outcome in the control group. The absolute difference in risk tells us how much the reduction is a result of the intervention itself.

For example, in a study of depression, if 2% of participants in the control group are depressed (i.e. $R^c = 0.02$) and a treatment halves the risk of depression to 1% (i.e. $R^i = 0.01$), then the RR is

$$\frac{R^i}{R^c} = \frac{0.01}{0.02} = 0.5$$

Although an RR of 0.5, or a halving of the risk, looks like a large effect, the absolute difference in risk is

$$R^c - R^i = 0.02 - 0.01 = 0.01 \text{ or } 1\%$$

This is a risk reduction of only one event per 100 people. This sounds a lot less impressive than a statement that a treatment halves the risk of depression. So, when reading a report of an intervention study, we need to interpret the RR or OR within the context of how frequently the outcome occurs in the population.

Another approach to expressing the effect of an intervention is the *number needed to treat (NNT)* (see Chapter 17), which conveniently expresses the absolute effect of the intervention. This is simply 1 divided by the absolute risk difference:

$$\frac{1}{(R^c - R^i)} = \frac{1}{0.01} = 100$$

In other words, one would need to treat 100 patients to prevent one additional case of depression. The NNT represents the number of patients who would need to be treated to prevent one additional event and is a useful way of expressing clinical effectiveness – i.e. the more effective an intervention, the lower the NNT.

To illustrate this, consider the impact of the same intervention, which still halves the risk of depression in the treatment group compared with the control group, but this time in a population at higher risk (e.g. people who have had a previous episode of depression). If the risk of the event in the control group (R^c) is now 0.2, or 20%, then the risk in the intervention group (R^i) will be half that: 0.1, or 10%. Now the absolute risk difference is 0.2 – 0.1 = 0.1, and the NNT is 1/0.1 = 10. In other words, only 10 people would need to be treated to prevent one additional case of depression. The effectiveness of the treatment as measured by the OR or RR is the same, but the impact is much greater because the intervention is being applied to a population with a much higher risk of depression.

An example of how the difference between relative and absolute differences can affect the interpretation of the study results is provided by epidemiological studies that compared the risk of death in women using third- and second-generation oral contraceptives.[9] These studies found that the OR for death in third- versus second-generation pills was 1.5 (an approximate 50% increase in the risk of death). This sounds like a lot. However, the risk of death in women who take either type of pill is very low. The absolute increase in risk for third-generation pills compared with second-generation pills is only six deaths per million women. In other words, there would be one extra death for every 166 666 women taking the third-generation pill! As you can see, it is important to be aware of the absolute risk of an event when trying to assess the importance of a finding expressed as an RR or RRR.

Relative and absolute differences in risk can each be expressed in four different ways, depending on the outcome measured (i.e. a 'good' event such as a healed wound or a 'bad' event such as a heart attack) and the direction of effect. A risk reduction occurs when the risk of a bad event decreases. A benefit increase occurs when the risk of a good event increases. A risk increase occurs when the risk of a bad event increases, and a benefit reduction occurs when the risk of a good event decreases.

Summary

Measures of health and disease are usually either discrete or continuous, and the form they take influences the way results of health-related studies are presented and analysed. Researchers typically measure how health interventions shift the average (mean or median) values of continuous measures. Apart from the average, it is extremely informative to know about the spread of continuous data using measures such as the range and the standard deviation. Discrete measures of health are often summarized as the percentage of people experiencing that outcome, e.g. the percentage of wounds healed. Researchers frequently want to determine whether there seems to be an association between exposure (e.g. to an intervention) and an outcome, and what the strength of that association is, and measures such as relative risk and odds ratios (for discrete measures) and standardized difference (for continuous measures) are used for this. Absolute differences in risk and the number needed to treat (NNT) give readers of research an indication of the *clinical* importance of a treatment effect.

LEARNING EXERCISES

1. A large trial of one of the statins (Simvastatin) compared coronary heart disease mortality rates in 4444 patients, half of whom received the drug and half placebo.[10] The 4S study was a secondary prevention trial, carried out with patients after a heart attack or symptoms of heart disease (angina) – in other words, those at high risk of a fatal event. The results are shown in Table 11.2.

   Answer the following questions using the spaces provided as prompts:

   (a) Calculate the risk of death and odds of death in the statin and no statin groups.

   Risk of death in statin group   ... / ... =
   Risk of death in control group   ... / ... =
   Odds of death in statin group   ... / ... =
   Odds of death in control group ... / ... =

   (b) Use your results to calculate the risk ratio and odds ratio (two measures of effect). What do they show about the association between the use of statins and death?

   $$\text{Risk ratio} = \frac{\text{risk of death in statin group}}{\text{risk of death in control group}} = ...$$

   Thus the risk death for those receiving statins was ... % of the risk for those not receiving statins.

   $$\text{Odds ratio} = \frac{\text{odds of death in statin group}}{\text{odds of death in control group}} = ...$$

   Thus the odds of death for those receiving statins was ... % of the odds for those not receiving statins.

   How might you interpret these results, and how would you explain the difference between the risk ratio and odds ratio?

   (c) Calculate the absolute reduction in risk associated with use of statins in this study.
   (d) In a population of 10 000 people with the risk shown in the control group of this study, how many deaths would be averted? Calculate the number needed to treat (NNT).

2. Repeat the same calculations as above using data from another statin trial (WOSCOPS), which evaluated the effect of Pravastatin on people with no evidence of heart disease but increased

Table 11.2 Results of the 4S study.[10] Table created using data from Scandinavian Simvastatin Survival Study Group 1994[10]

Intervention	5-year outcome		
	Dead	Alive	Total
Statin (treatment)	182	2039	2221
No statin (control)	256	1967	2223

Table 11.3 Results of WOSCOPS[11]. Table created using data from Shepherd 1995[11]

Intervention	5-year outcome		
	Dead	Alive	Total
Statin (treatment)	106	3196	3302
No statin (control)	135	3158	3293

cholesterol concentrations (a primary prevention trial).[11] The results of the WOSCOPS trial are summarized in Table 11.3.

Compare the number of lives saved per 10 000 people treated and the NNT in the WOSCOPS and 4S studies. Can you explain the differences?

Solutions to learning exercises
1a.

Risk of death in statin group	182/2221 = 0.082
Risk of death in control group	256/2223 = 0.115
Odds of death in statin group	182/2039 = 0.089
Odds of death in control group	256/1967 = 0.130

1b. Risk ratio = 0.71
Risk of death for those receiving statins was 71% of the risk for those not receiving statins.
Odds ratio = 0.68
Odds of death for those receiving statins was 68% of the odds for those not receiving statins. The results suggest that statins reduce the risk of death so that, when used, only about one-third of those who would previously have died now die over a 5-year period. The risk ratio and the odds ratio are very similar, the odds ratio being slightly lower (implying a slightly larger treatment effect) because, when calculating the odds of an event, we take the number not experiencing the event to be the denominator rather than the total number at risk of the event.[12]

1c. The absolute reduction in risk associated with using statins is 0.115 − 0.082 = 0.033 or 3.3%.

1d. In a population of 10 000 people, the number of deaths averted would be the absolute reduction in risk × 10 000 = 0.033 × 10 000 = 330 deaths averted. The NNT is 1/0.033 = 30.3, which rounded up to the next whole number is 31. Thus, you would need to treat 31 people with statins to save one life over 5 years.

2. Using the data from the WOSCOPS trial:

Risk of death in statin group:	106/3302 = 0.032
Risk of death in control group:	135/3293 = 0.041
Odds of death in statin group:	106/3196 = 0.033
Odds of death in control group:	135/3158 = 0.043
Risk ratio:	0.032/0.041 = 0.78
Odds ratio:	0.033/0.043 = 0.77
Absolute risk reduction is 0.041 − 0.032 = 0.009	

In a population of 10 000, the number of lives saved would be 0.009 × 10 000 = 90. The NNT is 1/0.009 = 111. Thus, fewer lives were saved by statins in the WOSCOPS study than in the 4S study. This is because the WOSCOPS study was concerned with primary prevention, and so the participants were at lower risk of death from coronary heart disease. The 4S study was concerned with secondary prevention (participants had already had a heart attack). The difference in the nature of the participants in the two studies is best seen by comparing the death rates in the control groups: 11.5% in the 4S (secondary prevention) study and 4% in the WOSCOPS (primary prevention) study. Therefore, even though the relative risk of death with statin treatment was similar for both trials (0.71 for 4S and 0.78 for WOSCOPS), the impact of the treatment in the lower risk patient group is less than in the high risk group. This difference in treatment effects is further illustrated by the difference in the NNTs from the two trials.

References

1 Bowling A. *Measuring Disease*. Second edition. Milton Keynes: Open University Press, 2001.

2 Bowling A. *Measuring Health: A Review of Quality of Life Measurement*. Third edition. Milton Keynes: Open University Press, 2005.

3 Indredavik B, Bakke F, Slørdahl SA, Rokseth R, Haheim LL. Stroke unit treatment. 10-year follow-up. *Stroke* 1999;**30**:1524–7.

4 Botti M, Williamson B, Steen K, McTaggart J, Reid E. The effect of pressure bandaging on complications and comfort in patients undergoing coronary angiography: a multicenter randomized trial. *Heart Lung* 1998;**27**:360–73.

5 Linde K, Mulrow CD, Berner M, Egger M. St John's wort for depression. *Cochrane Database Syst Rev* 2005;(2):CD000448.

6 Davis AR, Westhoff C, O'Connell K, Gallagher N. Oral contraceptives for dysmenorrhea in adolescent girls: a randomized trial. *Obstet Gynecol* 2005;**106**:97–104.

7 Goodkin K, Blaney NT, Feaster DJ, Baldewicz T, Burkhalter JE, Leeds B. A randomized controlled clinical trial of a bereavement support group intervention in human immunodeficiency virus type 1-seropositive and -seronegative homosexual men. *Arch Gen Psychiatry* 1999;**56**:52–9.

8 Powell H, Gibson PG. Options for self-management education for adults with asthma. *Cochrane Database Syst Rev* 2003;(1):CD004107.

9 Spitzer W, Lewis MA, Heinemann LA, Thorogood M, MacRae KD. Third generation oral contraceptives and risk of venous thromboembolic disorders: an international case-control study. Transnational Research Group on Oral Contraceptives and the Health of Young Women. *BMJ* 1996;**312**:83–8.

10 Scandinavian Simvastatin Survival Study Group. Randomised trial of cholesterol lowering in 4444 patients with coronary heart disease: the Scandinavian Survival Study (4S). *Lancet* 1994;**344**:1383–9.

11 Shepherd J, Cobbe SM, Ford I, Isles CG, Lorimer AR, MacFarlane PW, McKillop JH, Packard CJ. Prevention of coronary heart disease with pravastatin in men with hypercholesterolemia. West of Scotland Coronary Prevention Study Group. *N Engl J Med* 1995;**333**:1301–7.

12 Davies HT, Crombie IK, Tavakoli M. When can odds ratios mislead? *BMJ* 1998;**316**:989–91.

Chapter 12

ESTIMATING TREATMENT EFFECTS: REAL OR THE RESULT OF CHANCE?

Trevor A. Sheldon

Chapter 11 described how the outcomes of clinical trials are measured and summarized before analysis. One of the things we are interested in when critically reading a report of a clinical trial that assesses the effects of an intervention is whether the results provide an accurate estimate of the true treatment effect in the type of patients included in the study. In this chapter, we will discuss how to determine, through the use and interpretation of statistical tests, whether a treatment has a real effect on health outcomes or if the differences in outcomes are likely to be due to chance.

Sampling error

Even if a study has been conducted in a methodologically sound (unbiased) way, a study result such as '5% more wounds healed in the treatment group compared with the control group' does not necessarily mean that this is a *true treatment effect*. The finding could be a chance occurrence even when there is no true effect. To illustrate this point, imagine that you are playing a game with dice. We know that, on average, each of the numbers 1 to 6 should come up an equal number of times in unbiased dice. However, when your friend throws two or even three sixes in a row, you are unlikely (depending on the friend) to infer that the dice are loaded (biased) or that he is cheating. Instead, you would probably conclude that this was just luck. This example shows us that even if there is no true effect (i.e. the dice are not loaded), we can observe events that look as though there is an effect, simply because of chance (*sampling error*). This is particularly the case when there are small numbers of observations. For example, if the number six came up in two out of four throws (i.e. 50% of the time), we would assume it was because of chance. However, if it occurred in 100 out of 200 throws, then we would tend to reject the idea that this was just a result of chance and instead accept an explanation that the dice were loaded (and that you would need to choose your friends better).

Exactly the same logic can be applied to the results of evaluations of clinical interventions. It is possible that the result of a study showing that one treatment is associated with better (or worse) outcomes is only because of chance. This is particularly likely to be the case if the study is small. Therefore, when we examine the results of a study, we want to see the extent to which they are likely to have occurred

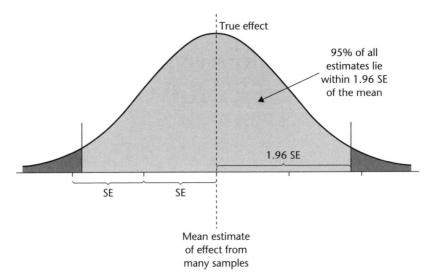

True effect

95% of all
estimates lie
within 1.96 SE
of the mean

1.96 SE

SE   SE

Mean estimate
of effect from
many samples

Figure 12.1 Sampling distribution of study results – not all studies give the same results due to sampling error. SE = standard error.

by chance. If the results are highly unlikely to have occurred by chance, we accept that the findings reflect a real treatment effect.

Unlike the dice, which we can check by throwing them repeatedly to see if our run of sixes was a chance finding or because of some bias, we can't easily repeat every clinical trial many times to check if the findings are real. We have to make do with our one study. Of course, replication of the results of studies is an important part of the scientific process, and we would be more confident if the results were confirmed by subsequent studies.

Statistical theory tells us that if we could repeat the same evaluation several hundred times with different samples of the same number of patients, the result (e.g. the mean difference or relative risk reduction) would not always be the same. If we plotted the results of these trials on a graph, the shape of the curve (i.e. the distribution of the results) would be approximately normal, or bell shaped (Figure 12.1). On average, the results of the studies would give us a correct estimate of the true treatment effect. However, any one study result could vary from this 'true' effect by chance. The amount of chance variation from the 'true' effect is given by the measure of spread or standard deviation of this distribution, which, because it indicates the amount of random sampling error that is likely, is called the *standard error* (SE). The larger the SE, the more individual study results will vary away from the true effect.

Confidence intervals

The discussion above shows that we cannot assume that a single study estimate of the effect of an intervention is the true effect because considerable random variation can exist. Therefore, any one study cannot give us a certain true value of the effect because it may vary from the true value by chance. However, because of the normal shape of the sampling distribution (Figure 12.1), we know (from statistical theory that we do not need to explore here) that 95% of all possible studies give an estimate of the effect of the intervention being evaluated that lies 1.96 SEs on either side of the true value. This leads to the important observation that *in 95% of evaluations, the true value of the treatment effect will lie within 1.96 SEs on either side of the estimate of effect found in our single study.* In other words, there is a 95% probability that this range (1.96 SEs on either side of a single study effect size) includes the true value. This is called a 95% *confidence interval (CI)*, and it provides a plausible range within which we are 95% confident the true value of the treatment effect will lie (Figure 12.1).

If we want to be more confident that our interval includes the true value, we can use a wider interval, such as a 99% CI, which lies 2.58 SEs on either side of the estimate. In this case, there is only a 1 in 100 chance that the true value falls outside of this range.

The wider the CI, the less *precise* is our estimate of the treatment effect. This precision depends on the spread of the sampling distribution (Figure 12.1) measured by the SE. This in turn depends on the sample size and the variability of what is being measured. The smaller the number of patients in a trial or number of events observed (e.g. deaths), the greater will be the sampling error or the spread of the sampling distribution (Figure 12.2). The greater the sampling error, the more likely it is that any one experiment will differ by chance from the true or average value, and so the wider will be the 95% CI. On the other hand, if we increase the number of participants in a study or the number of people who are likely to experience an event such that the distribution becomes less spread out, individual study results will fall much closer to the true or average result, and the SE and the width of the CI will be reduced (Table 12.1). This is similar to saying that we are more confident in using the results of throwing dice many times to assess whether they are biased than when we throw them only a few times.

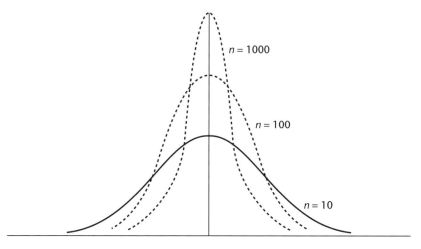

Figure 12.2 The larger the sample (*n*), the smaller the sampling error and the narrower the confidence interval will be and so the more precise the estimate of the effect size.

Table 12.1 Larger sample sizes give more precise confidence intervals

Sample size (each group)	Estimated reduction in blood pressure	95% confidence interval
50	6 mmHg	−1.0 to 13.0 mmHg
100	6 mmHg	1.1 to 10.9 mmHg
200	6 mmHg	2.5 to 9.5 mmHg
1000	6 mmHg	5.2 to 6.8 mmHg

Presenting uncertainty about a treatment effect using CIs is now the method preferred by many good health care journals. In addition to giving the plausible range of the size and direction of the treatment effect, CIs can also be used to give an idea of whether or not a treatment has any effect. If the CI around a difference in mean blood pressure reduction or a difference in the proportion of wounds healed includes the value zero (i.e. no difference in average or proportions), then we cannot be confident that the treatment is better than the control condition. Similarly, if the CI of an odds ratio or relative risk includes the value 1 (i.e. same odds or risk in treated and untreated groups; see Chapter 11), then we cannot be confident that a difference exists between the intervention and control conditions. This is equivalent to carrying out a hypothesis test (see below).

To illustrate the interpretation of a 95% CI, let us consider some examples. Murchie et al.[1] assessed whether nurse-led clinics in primary care improved secondary prevention of heart disease at four years after the intervention. They reported a 25% relative reduction in the risk of dying, with a 95% CI of 2 to 42. This means that we are 95% certain that nurse-led clinics reduce the risk of mortality somewhere between 2% and 42% when compared with usual care. We infer that if the study was well conducted, these clinics were effective. If the CI had included no reduction in risk (i.e. zero), then we would not have been 95% confident of its effectiveness.

To give another example, a systematic review of breast screening (either by self examination or clinical examination)[2] reported that the relative risk increase for biopsies with benign results was 88%. The 95% CI around this estimate was 77% to 99%; in other words, we are 95% confident that there is an increased risk of benign biopsies of between 77% and 99%. The 95% CI around the estimated increase in the relative risk of breast cancer mortality of 5% was −10% to 24%. Since this range includes an increase of zero, we cannot be confident that breast self-examination is either harmful or beneficial in terms of breast cancer mortality.

A third example illustrates the use of CIs when the measure of effect is the difference in the average of a continuous variable. In Chapter 11, we reported the estimate of the effect of low-dose oral contraceptives for dysmenorrhoea in adolescent girls as a difference in means (between oral contraceptive and placebo groups) of 2.7 on Moos Menstrual Distress Questionnaire scores at 3 months.[3] The 95% CI around this estimate was 0.88 to 4.53. Because the entire interval lies above zero, we can be 95% confident that this treatment reduces dysmenorrhoea.

By contrast, Chapter 11 also reported a standardized mean difference of 0.1 when comparing self-management with regular medical review of patients with asthma.[4] The 95% CI around this estimate was −0.14 to 0.15, and because this includes zero, we are not confident that there is a true difference.

Hypothesis testing and p-values

Instead of trying to estimate a plausible range of values within which the true treatment effect is likely to lie (i.e. a CI), researchers often begin with a formal assumption that no effect exists (the *null hypothesis*). This is a bit like the situation in a court of law where a person charged with an offence is assumed to be innocent. The aim of the evaluation is similar to that of the prosecution: to gather enough evidence to convince a neutral observer to reject the null hypothesis and to accept, instead, the alternative hypothesis that the treatment does have an effect (or that the defendant is guilty). The greater the quantity and quality of evidence that is not compatible with the null hypothesis, the more likely we are to reject it and accept the alternative. In a court case, the more evidence there is against the defendant, the more likely it is they are guilty and will be convicted.

In a clinical evaluation, the greater the treatment effect (expressed as the number of SEs away from zero), the more likely it is that the null hypothesis of zero effect is not supported and that we will accept the alternative that a true difference exists between the treatment and control groups. In other words, the number of SEs that a study result varies from the null value is equivalent, in our court case analogy, to the amount of evidence against the innocence of the defendant. The SE is regarded as the unit that measures the likelihood that the result is not because of chance. The more SEs the result is from the null, the less likely it is to have arisen by chance and the more likely it is to be a true effect.

For example, if a study shows a mean difference in blood pressure of 5 mmHg when the SE is 5 mmHg, then the result is only 1 SE above or below the null of no difference. We know that 68% of study results are likely to lie within 1 SE of zero even when there is no treatment difference, simply by chance. In this case, there is insufficient evidence from the study to make us reject the null hypothesis; the result is compatible with chance. However, if the study result is a treatment difference of 15.1 mmHg (i.e. more than 3 SEs above or below zero), then we are more likely to reject the null hypothesis because we know that, when no real treatment effect exists, 99.7% of studies will have a result that is within 3 SEs of zero (15 mmHg). The probability of an experiment giving a result of a 15 mmHg reduction in blood pressure by chance when no real treatment effect exists is less than 0.3% (3 out of 1000).

The question then becomes *What is the burden of proof required to accept that a treatment is effective?* In other words, how unlikely must it be that a result is due to chance (i.e. how many SEs must a result be from the null) for us to accept the alternative that a treatment difference really exists? We need to use some rule or criterion to decide when a result will be regarded as compatible with the null hypothesis and when it is so unlikely to be due to chance that we reject the null hypothesis and accept instead that the treatment makes a difference (or, in the courtroom example, that the defendant is guilty). Traditionally, researchers have used probabilities less than 5% (1.96 SE) or less than 1% (2.56 SE) as cut-offs. In other words, if the estimate of treatment effect is more than 1.96 SE above or below the null value, then the probability of this or a more extreme result occurring by chance when the null is, in fact, true is less than 5% or 1 in 20; we say it is statistically significant at the 5% level or $p < 0.05$. Similarly, if the result is more than 2.58 SE above or below zero, then it is regarded as statistically significant at the 1% level ($p < 0.01$). For example, in the study of nurse-led coronary heart disease secondary prevention clinics,[1] the mean change in the overall score for six health status domains in the

SF-36 questionnaire over one year of follow-up was 0.59 in patients allocated to nurse clinics and 0.06 in the control group. The difference between the groups of 0.53 was highly statistically significant at $p < 0.001$; that is, the probability that this result was due to chance was less than 1 in 1000. Therefore, nurse-led clinics are likely to be effective at improving key aspects of health in patients with coronary heart disease.

Type I error: the risk of a false-positive result

By now it should be clear that, because of the play of chance, we cannot know the true treatment effect with complete certainty, even when no study bias exists. All we can do is make probabilistic statements that indicate how likely it is that the true value lies within a range (i.e. the CI) and how likely it is that the result or one greater is a result of chance (p-value). This means that there is always the possibility of being wrong. Because of this uncertainty, we can make two main types of errors. One type of error is to reject the null hypothesis falsely (i.e. to say that a treatment effect exists when, in fact, the null is true or, in our court case example, to falsely convict the defendant). This false positive is called a *type I error*. The risk or probability of this type of error is given by the p-value or statistical significance of the treatment effect. If a treatment difference in blood pressure is 11 mmHg ($p = 0.04$), and we infer that a real treatment effect exists, then we have a 4 in 100 risk of being wrong (because 4% of all experiments of the same type would have reported this or a larger difference by chance). So, the type I error or p-value is 4%. The lower the p-value, the less likely it is that the result is a false positive and the lower the risk of a type I error. This is the same as saying that the more evidence we have to support the guilt of a defendant, the less likely it is that an innocent person will be falsely convicted. To some extent, the level of type I error that one accepts depends on the costs and consequences of making an incorrect inference and saying that a treatment works when, in fact, it does not. Because this will vary according to what is evaluated, use of a single cut-off for all research studies is not very sensible, and guidance has been published.[5]

In addition, this approach to considering research results is being challenged by a different school of statistics: Bayesian statistics. This method suggests an approach to understanding how the results of research studies can be considered in light of previous knowledge, including expert views (valued in professional practice), in order to inform clinical decision-making.[6,7]

Type II error: risk of a false-negative result

The uncertainty, of course, works the other way as well. Even if insufficient evidence is presented in a trial to convict a defendant, this doesn't necessarily mean that she is innocent: it could be that a guilty person was wrongly acquitted. Similarly, even if we cannot exclude chance as the explanation of the result of a study, it does not necessarily mean that the treatment is ineffective. This type of error – a false-negative result – where we wrongly accept the null hypothesis of no treatment effect is called a *type II error*.

This is a particular problem of small studies because they have more sampling error and so larger SEs. The larger the SE, the harder it is to exclude chance and, therefore, the greater the probability of falsely accepting the null hypothesis of no treatment effect. In small studies, even large estimates of treatment effect do not provide sufficient evidence of a true effect (i.e. they are not statistically significant) because the SE is so large. We say that the study has low *power* to detect a treatment effect as statistically significant when such an effect really does exist.

If a study is too small, the CIs can be so wide that they cannot really exclude a value indicating no effect. For example, several studies of debriding agents for the treatment of chronic wounds are so small that their estimates have large CIs. A study of cadexomer iodine, for example, reported an odds ratio for healed wounds of 5.5 favouring cadexomer iodine compared with dextranomer.[8] However, because only 27 patients were included in the trial, the 95% CI was wide, ranging from 0.88 to 34.48. Thus, the study was too small to be able to exclude an odds ratio of 1 (no treatment difference). If the study had been larger, a statistically significant treatment effect might have been found.

One of the problems in clinical research is the plethora of studies that are too small and so have insufficient power. In these cases, one cannot interpret a statistically non-significant result to mean that no treatment effect exists. Because so many studies are too small and have low power, it is possible that important clinical effects are being missed (type II error). One approach for dealing with this problem is to pool or combine the results of similar studies to get an overall and more precise estimate of treatment effect. This approach is called meta-analysis and is discussed in Chapter 19.

When a study is undertaken, the sample size should be sufficiently large to ensure that the study will have enough power to reject the null hypothesis if a clinically important treatment effect exists. Researchers should, therefore, carry out a power or sample size calculation when designing a study to ensure that it has a reasonable chance of correctly rejecting the null hypothesis. This *a priori* power calculation should be reported in the paper.

Tests for different types of outcome measures

In Chapter 11, we described different ways of expressing treatment effects based on the type of outcome measure used. Type of outcome measure also affects the type of statistical test used to determine the extent to which an estimate of treatment effect is due to chance.

Continuous measures

When a trial uses a continuous measure such as blood pressure, the treatment effect is often calculated by measuring the difference in mean improvement in blood pressure between groups (see Chapter 11). In these cases (if the data are normally distributed), a *t*-test is commonly used. If, however, the data are highly skewed, it is better to test for differences in the median, using non-parametric tests such as the Mann–Whitney U test.

Categorical variables

When a study measures categorical variables and expresses results as proportions (e.g. numbers infected or wounds healed), then a χ^2 (chi-squared) test is used. A χ^2 test assesses the extent to which the observed proportion in the treatment group differs from what would have been expected by chance if no real difference existed between the treatment and control groups. Alternatively, if an odds ratio is used, the SE of the odds ratio can be calculated and, assuming a normal distribution, 95% CIs can be calculated, and hypothesis tests can be conducted.

Paired analysis

The tests described in the previous section apply to situations where independent groups of patients are being compared; that is, the people in one treatment group are different from those in the comparison group. There are, however, situations where patients in the groups are matched with each other, or where patients are used as their own 'controls'. In these 'paired' comparisons, it is not appropriate to use the tests outlined above, and paired analyses are needed. For normally distributed continuous measures, one can use the paired *t*-test. For skewed continuous paired data, the Wilcoxon signed-rank test is available. In the case of categorical outcomes, several alternative tests are available, such as McNemar's test. The important thing to remember is that, if the design of the comparison is paired or matched, the analysis must also be paired.

Statistical significance is not clinical significance

Thus far, we have focused on ways of testing whether an estimate of treatment effect found in a trial is likely to be an accurate reflection of the true effect or whether it is likely to have arisen by chance. Researchers and readers of research often focus excessively on whether a result is statistically significant (i.e. unlikely to be the result of chance). However, just because a test shows that a treatment effect is statistically significant, it does not mean that the result is *clinically* important. For example, if a study is very large (and therefore has a small SE), it is easier to find small and clinically unimportant treatment effects to be statistically significant. Consider, for example, a very large randomized controlled trial comparing hospital readmission rates in patients receiving a new heart drug with patients receiving usual care. A 1% reduction in readmissions is reported in the treatment group (49% readmissions versus 50% in the usual care group). This is highly statistically significant ($p < 0.0001$) mainly because this is a large trial. However, it is unlikely that clinical practice would be changed on the basis of such a small reduction in readmissions.

Summary

When reading reports of clinical trials, it is important to remember that apparent differences in the outcomes of patients in different treatment groups may be chance occurrences and not necessarily true treatment effects. Ideally, the results of clinical trials (presented as risk differences, odds ratios, or differences in means) are presented with CIs around them. CIs represent the degree of uncertainty around a result: the narrower the CI, the more precise the result. When a statistically significant difference is present, it is also important to consider whether the difference is clinically important and whether it is large enough to warrant a change in practice.

LEARNING EXERCISES

1. A study found that group-based education for people with type II diabetes was associated with a reduction in fasting blood glucose concentrations compared with a control group. The mean difference in fasting blood glucose concentrations was −1.17 mmol/l. The 95% CI is −1.63 to −0.72 mmol/l. What do you conclude about the effect of the educational intervention on blood glucose concentrations?

2. An evaluation examined the effect of nurse home visits to low-income, first-time mothers.[9] The outcomes included birth weight, number of hospitalizations, number of days in hospital, and an emotional/cognitive stimulation score. The means, mean differences, and 95% CIs around the mean differences are shown in Table 12.2. What do you conclude about the effect of nurse home visits on birth weight and the degree to which the home environment was cognitively and emotionally stimulating?

3. A systematic review of nine RCTs examined the effect of graduated compression stockings in preventing deep venous thrombosis in people who went on long flights.[10] What do the results in Table 12.3 tell us about the effect on deep and superficial venous thromboses?

Solutions to learning exercises

1. *The study shows an estimated reduction in fasting blood glucose of 1.17 mmol/l. Because any value within the 95% CI would mean a reduction in blood glucose concentrations (i.e. the 95% CI does not include zero or any increase in blood glucose), it is reasonable to infer that the result represents a real reduction in fasting blood glucose concentrations, and not a chance reduction. Assuming that we are content that the study design and conduct were rigorous, we can conclude that group-based education was effective in reducing fasting blood glucose concentrations.*

2. *The mean difference in the emotional/cognitive stimulation score is positive (1.3), and the 95% CI included only positive values (0.4 to 0.22); thus, we are 95% confident that nurse home visits did improve this aspect of development. Initially, it appears that home visits were also associated with a reduction in birth weight (mean difference was −18.2 g, the negative sign indicating a reduction), but because the 95% CI (−98.7 to 62.4 g) includes both decreases and increases in birth weight, we cannot be confident that there is a true effect on birth weight as a consequence of nurse home visits.*

3. *The results show a large reduction in deep venous thrombosis risk with stocking use, and that this difference is not likely to be due to chance because the 95% CI excludes no effect or an increase in risk. On the other hand, the small estimated reduction in risk of superficial venous thrombosis*

Table 12.2 Nurse home visits versus usual care for infant birth weight and emotional/cognitive stimulation

Dependent variables	Nurse-visited group	Mean Comparison group	Mean difference	95% confidence interval
Birth weight, g	3032.2	3050.4	−18.2	−98.7 to 62.4
Emotional/cognitive stimulation (score)	32.3	30.9	1.3	0.4 to 2.2

Table 12.3 Prophylactic use of graduated compression stockings versus no stockings during air travel in general population

Outcomes at <7 days after the flight	Weighted event rates		
	Stockings	No stockings	RRR (95% CI)
Deep venous thrombosis	0.3%	3.69%	92% (77 to 97)
Superficial venous thrombosis	0.55%	0.85%	33% (−87 to 76)

could easily be a chance finding rather than a real effect because the 95% CI around the estimate of the reduction in risk (-97% to 76%) includes increases in risk.

References

1 Murchie P, Campbell NC, Ritchie LD, Thain J. Running nurse-led secondary prevention clinics for coronary heart disease in primary care: qualitative study of health professionals' perspectives. *Br J Gen Pract* 2005;**55**:522–8.

2 Kösters JP, Gøtzsche PC. Regular self-examination or clinical examination for early detection of breast cancer. *Cochrane Database Syst Rev* 2003;(2):CD003373.

3 Davis AR, Westhoff C, O'Connell K, Gallagher N. Oral contraceptives for dysmenorrhea in adolescent girls: a randomized trial. *Obstet Gynecol* 2005;**106**:97–104.

4 Powell H, Gibson PG. Options for self-management education for adults with asthma. *Cochrane Database Syst Rev* 2003;(1):CD004107.

5 Sterne JA. Davey Smith G. Sifting the evidence – what's wrong with significance tests? *BMJ* 2001;**322**:226–31.

6 Goodman SN. Toward evidence-based medicine statistics. 1: The p value fallacy. *Ann Intern Med* 1999;**130**:995–1004.

7 Goodman SN. Toward evidence-based medical statistics. 2: The Bayes factor. *Ann Intern Med* 1999;**130**:1005–13.

8 Tarvainen K. Cadexomer iodine (Iodosorb) compared with dextranomer (Debrisan) in the treatment of chronic leg ulcers. *Acta Chir Scand Suppl* 1988;**544**:57–9.

9 Kitzman H, Olds DL, Henderson CR Jr, Hanks C, Cole R, Tatelbaum R, McConnochie KM, Sidora K, Luckey DW, Shaver D, Engelhardt K, James D, Barnard K. Effect of prenatal and infancy home visitation by nurses on pregnancy outcomes, childhood injuries, and repeated childbearing. A randomized controlled trial. *JAMA* 1997;**278**:644–52.

10 Hsieh HF, Lee FP. Graduated compression stockings as prophylaxis for flight-related venous thrombosis: systematic literature review. *J Adv Nurs* 2005;**51**:83–98.

Chapter 13

DATA ANALYSIS IN QUALITATIVE RESEARCH

Sally Thorne

Unquestionably, data analysis is the most complex and mysterious of all of the phases of a qualitative project and the one that receives the least thoughtful discussion in the literature. For neophyte nurse researchers, many of the data collection strategies involved in a qualitative project may feel familiar and comfortable. After all, nurses have always based their clinical practice on learning as much as possible about the people they work with and detecting commonalities and variations among and between them in order to provide individualized care. However, creating a database is not sufficient to conduct a qualitative study. In order to generate findings that transform raw data into new knowledge, qualitative researchers must engage in active and demanding analytic processes throughout all phases of the research. Understanding these processes is therefore an important aspect not only of doing qualitative research, but also of reading, understanding and interpreting it.

For readers of qualitative studies, the language of analysis can be confusing. It is sometimes difficult to know what the researchers actually did during this phase and to understand how their findings evolved out of the data that were collected or constructed. Furthermore, in describing their processes, some authors use language that accentuates this sense of mystery and magic. For example, they may claim that their conceptual categories 'emerged' from the data[1] – almost as if they left the raw data out overnight and awoke to find that the data analysis fairies had organized the data into a coherent new structure that explained everything! In this chapter, I will try to help readers make sense of some of the assertions that are made about qualitative data analysis so that they can develop a critical eye for discerning when an analytical claim is convincing and when it is not.

Qualitative data

Qualitative data come in various forms. In many qualitative nursing studies, the database consists of interview transcripts from open-ended, focused, but exploratory interviews. However, there is no limit to what might possibly constitute a qualitative database, and, increasingly, we are seeing more and more creative use of such sources as recorded observations (both video and participatory), focus groups, texts and documents, multimedia or public domain sources, policy manuals, photographs, and lay autobiographical accounts.

Qualitative data are not the exclusive domain of qualitative research. Rather, the term can refer to anything that is not quantitative, or rendered into numerical form. Many quantitative studies include open-ended survey questions, semistructured interviews, or other forms of qualitative data. What distinguishes the data in a quantitative study from those generated in a qualitatively designed study is a set of assumptions, principles, and even values about truth and reality. Quantitative researchers accept that the goal of science is to discover the truths that exist in the world and to use the scientific method as a way to build a more complete understanding of reality. Although some qualitative researchers operate from a similar philosophical position, most recognize that the relevant reality, as far as human experience is concerned, is that which takes place in subjective experience, in social context, and in historical time. Thus, qualitative researchers are often more concerned about uncovering knowledge about how people think and feel about the circumstances in which they find themselves than they are in making judgements about whether those thoughts and feelings are valid.

Qualitative analytic reasoning processes

What makes a study qualitative is that it relies relatively heavily upon inductive reasoning processes to interpret and structure the meanings that can be derived from data. Distinguishing inductive from deductive inquiry processes is an important step in identifying what counts as qualitative research. Generally, *inductive reasoning* uses the data to generate ideas (hypothesis generating), whereas *deductive reasoning* begins with the idea and uses the data to confirm or negate the idea (hypothesis testing).[2] In practice, however, many quantitative studies involve much inductive reasoning, whereas good qualitative analysis often requires access to a full range of strategies.[3] A traditional quantitative study in the health sciences typically begins with a theoretical grounding, takes direction from hypotheses or explicit study questions, and uses a predetermined (and auditable) set of steps to confirm or refute the hypothesis. It does this to add evidence to the development of specific, causal, and theoretical explanations of phenomena.[3] In contrast, qualitative research is often guided by the position that an interpretive understanding is only possible by way of uncovering or deconstructing the meanings of a phenomenon (see Chapter 8). As methodological options evolve, we can see increasing enthusiasm for approaches to enquiry that capitalize on the unique angle of vision that derives from both inductive and deductive analytic logic. As a result, there is now an expanding array of blended approaches, such as the 'framework approach' that has evolved within health policy research.[4] Thus, in understanding how to make sense of analytic logic, it can become important to distinguish between an explanation of how something operates (deduction) and why it might operate in the manner that it does (induction), even within the same study.

Because data collection and analysis processes tend to be concurrent, with new analytic steps informing the process of additional data collection and new data informing the analytic processes, it is important to recognize that qualitative data analysis processes are not entirely distinguishable from the data they are purporting to make sense of. The theoretical lens from which a researcher approaches a phenomenon, the strategies she uses to collect or construct data, and the understandings she brings into the research about which of the many possible observations might count as relevant or important data to answer the research question are all analytic processes that influence what becomes data. Analysis also occurs as an explicit step in conceptually interpreting the data set as a whole, using specific analytic strategies to transform the raw data into a new and coherent depiction of the thing being studied. Although many qualitative data analysis computer programs are available on the market today, these are essentially aids to sorting and organizing sets of qualitative data, and none is capable of the intellectual and conceptualizing processes required to transform data into meaningful findings.

Specific analytic strategies

Although a description of the actual procedural details and nuances of every qualitative data analysis strategy is well beyond the scope of this chapter, a general appreciation of the theoretical assumptions underlying some of the more common approaches can be helpful in understanding what a researcher is trying to say about how data were sorted, organized, conceptualized, refined and interpreted.

Constant comparative analysis

Many qualitative analytic strategies rely on a general approach called *constant comparative analysis*. Originally developed for use in the grounded theory methodology of Glaser and Strauss,[5] which itself evolved out of the sociological theory of symbolic interactionism, this strategy involves taking one piece of data (one interview, one statement, one theme) and comparing it with all others that may be similar or different in order to develop conceptualizations of the possible relations between various pieces of data. For example, by comparing the accounts of two different people who had a similar experience, a researcher might pose analytical questions such as *Why is this different from that?* and *How are these two related?* In many qualitative studies, the purpose of which is to generate knowledge about common patterns and themes within human experience, this process continues with the comparison of each new interview or account until all have been compared with each other. A good description of this process is found in the report of a study of the impact of traumatic brain injury on 'sense of self'.[6]

Constant comparison analysis is well suited to grounded theory because this design is specifically used to study those human phenomena for which the researcher assumes that fundamental social processes explain something of human behaviour and experience, such as stages of grieving or processes of recovery. However, many other methodologies draw from this analytical strategy to create knowledge that is more generally descriptive or interpretive, such as coping with cancer or living with illness. Naturalistic inquiry,[7] thematic analysis,[8] and interpretive description[9] are methods that depend on constant comparative analysis processes to develop ways of understanding human phenomena within the context in which they are experienced.

Phenomenological approaches

Constant comparative analysis is not the only approach in qualitative research. Some qualitative methods are not oriented towards finding patterns and commonalities within human experience, but instead seek to discover some of the underlying structure or essence of that experience through the intensive study of individual cases. For example, rather than explain the stages and transitions within grieving that are common to people in various circumstances, a phenomenological study might attempt to uncover and describe the essential nature of grieving and represent it in such a manner that a person who had not grieved might begin to appreciate the phenomenon. The analytic methods that would be used in these studies explicitly avoid cross comparisons and instead orient the researcher towards the depth and detail that can be appreciated only through an exhaustive, systematic and reflective study of experiences as they are lived.

Although constant comparative methods might well permit an analyst to use some pre-existing or emergent theory against which to test all new pieces of data that are collected, these more phenomenological approaches typically challenge researchers to set aside or 'bracket' all such preconceptions so that they can work inductively with the data to generate entirely new descriptions and conceptualizations. There are numerous forms of phenomenological research; however, many of the most popular approaches used by nurses derive from the philosophical work of Husserl on modes of awareness (epistemology) and the hermeneutic tradition of Heidegger, which emphasizes modes of being (ontology).[10] These approaches differ in the degree to which interpretation is acceptable, but both represent strategies for immersing oneself in data, engaging with data reflectively, and generating a rich description that will enlighten readers as to the deeper essential structures underlying a particular human experience. Examples of the types of human experiences that are amenable to this type of inquiry include the suffering experienced by individuals who have a drinking problem[11] and the emotional experiences of parents of terminally ill adolescents.[12] Sometimes authors explain their approaches not by the phenomenological position they have adopted, but by naming the theorist whose specific techniques they are borrowing. Colaizzi[12] and Giorgi[13] are phenomenologists who have rendered the phenomenological attitude into a set of manageable steps and processes for working with such data and have therefore become popular reference sources among phenomenological nurse researchers.

Ethnographic methods

Ethnographic research methods derive from anthropology's tradition of interpreting the processes and products of cultural behaviour. Ethnographers document such aspects of human experience as beliefs, kinship patterns and ways of living. In the health care field, nurses and others have used ethnographic methods to uncover and record variations in how different social and cultural groups understand and enact health and illness. An example of this type of study is an investigation of how older adults adjust to living in a nursing home environment.[14] When a researcher claims to have used ethnographic methods, we can assume that he or she has come to know a culture or group through immersion and engagement in fieldwork or participant observation and has also undertaken to portray that culture through text.[15] Ethnographic analysis uses an iterative process in which cultural ideas that arise during active involvement 'in the field' are transformed, translated, or represented in a written document. It involves sifting and sorting through pieces of data to detect and interpret thematic categorizations, search for inconsistencies and contradictions, and generate conclusions about what is happening and why.

Narrative analysis and discourse analysis

Many qualitative nurse researchers have discovered the extent to which human experience is shaped, transformed and understood through linguistic representation. The vague and subjective sensations that characterize cognitively unstructured life experiences take on meaning and order when we try to articulate them in communication. Putting experience into words, whether verbally, in writing, or in thought, transforms the actual experience into a communicable representation of it. Thus, speech forms are not the experiences themselves, but a socially and culturally constructed device for creating shared understandings about them. *Narrative analysis* is a strategy that recognizes the extent to which the stories we tell provide insights about our lived experiences.[16] For example, it was used as a strategy to learn more about the experiences of women who discover that they have a breast lump.[17] Through analytic processes that help us detect the main narrative themes within the accounts people give about their lives, we discover how they understand and make sense of their lives.

By contrast, *discourse analysis* recognizes speech not as a direct representation of human experience, but as an explicit linguistic tool constructed and shaped by many social or ideological influences. Discourse analysis strategies draw heavily on theories developed in such fields as sociolinguistics and cognitive psychology to try to understand what is represented by the various ways in which people communicate ideas. They capitalize on critical inquiry into the language that is used and the way that it is used to uncover the societal influences underlying our behaviours and thoughts.[18] Thus, although discourse analysis and narrative analysis both rely heavily on speech as the most relevant data form, their reasons for analysing speech differ.

Table 13.1 illustrates the distinctions between the analytic strategies described above using breast cancer research as an example.

Cognitive processes inherent in qualitative analysis

The term 'qualitative research' encompasses a wide range of philosophical positions, methodological strategies, and analytical procedures. Morse[1] has summarized the cognitive processes involved in qualitative research in a way that can help us to better understand how a researcher's cognitive processes interact with qualitative data to bring about findings and generate new knowledge. Morse believes that all qualitative analysis, regardless of the specific approach, involves

- *comprehending* the phenomenon under study
- *synthesizing* a portrait of the phenomenon that accounts for relations and linkages within its aspects
- *theorizing* about how and why these relations appear as they do
- *recontextualizing*, or putting the new knowledge about phenomena and relations back into the context of how others have articulated the evolving knowledge

Table 13.1 General distinctions between selected qualitative research approaches: an illustration using breast cancer research

Method	Research question	Analytic strategy	Research product
Grounded theory	How do women with breast cancer cope with changes to body image?	Constant comparative analysis	Theory regarding basic social processes involved in coping with breast cancer and factors that might account for variations
Phenomenology	What is the lived experience of having breast cancer?	Phenomenological reduction; hermeneutic analysis	Description of the essential structure of the breast cancer experience
Ethnography	How is breast cancer understood and managed in different social contexts?	Representation, inscription, translation, and textualization of culture into writing	Typology of interpretations, relationships, and variations within the breast cancer experience
Narrative analysis	How do women with breast cancer come to know their experience?	Generating, interpreting, and representing women's stories in narrative form	Narrative accounts of women's explanations for their breast cancer experiences

Although the form that each of these steps will take may vary according to such factors as the research question, the researcher's orientation to the inquiry, or the setting and context of the study, this set of steps helps to depict a series of intellectual processes by which data in their raw form are considered, examined, and reformulated to become a research product.

Quality measures in qualitative analysis

In earlier times, it was common for qualitative nurse researchers to claim that such issues as reliability and validity were irrelevant to the qualitative enterprise. Instead, they might say that the proof of the quality of the work rested entirely on the reader's acceptance or rejection of the claims that were made. If the findings 'rang true' to the intended audience, then the qualitative study was considered successful. More recently, nurse researchers have taken a lead among their colleagues in other disciplines in trying to work out more formally how the quality of a piece of qualitative research might be judged. Many of these researchers have concluded that systematic, rigorous and auditable analytical processes are among the most significant factors distinguishing good from poor quality research.[19] Researchers are therefore encouraged to articulate their findings in such a manner that the logical processes by which they were developed are accessible to critical readers, the relation between the actual data and the conclusions about the data is explicit, and the claims made in relation to the data set are rendered credible and believable. Through this short description of analytical approaches, readers will be in a better position to critically evaluate individual qualitative studies and decide whether and when to apply the findings of such studies to their nursing practice.

Summary

Qualitative research is different from quantitative research in many ways, and is more concerned with generating knowledge about how people think, perceive and experience phenomena than the validity of these feelings and experiences. Analysis of qualitative data tends to use inductive rather than deductive reasoning although new approaches, such as the framework approach, increasingly use a blend of induction and deduction. A key feature of qualitative data analysis is the way in which analysis occurs simultaneously with data collection, with the potential for data collection to be influenced by the ongoing analysis. The analysis phase of qualitative research is frequently implicit rather than explicit in research reports and it can be challenging for readers to understand how the analysis took place. There are several commonly used analytical strategies including constant comparative analysis, phenomenological and ethnographic approaches, narrative and discourse analysis. Now that you have an understanding of different approaches to the analysis of qualitative data, Chapter 25 provides a framework for the critical appraisal of qualitative research.

LEARNING EXERCISES

1. Identify an aspect of your field of interest in which new knowledge about subjective experience could be useful to practice.
2. Using the examples in Table 13.1, think about the implications for your qualitative study if you used each of these general approaches to gathering data about your topic.
3. From what you know about the topic, imagine the types of data you might uncover if you began to interview participants or do field research on this topic.
4. Finally, see if you can look ahead to imagine ways in which your current knowledge of this topic might potentially influence or shape your data analysis.
5. Taking the same topic within your own field of interest, try to generate a research question that is deductive. Can you reverse the question and come up with an idea of how a question would be different if you were using an inductive research approach?
6. If you encountered a 'content analysis' study in which the categories used to represent the findings were predetermined from existing knowledge, how would you determine whether the study was most appropriately evaluated using qualitative or quantitative quality criteria? Could you imagine a situation in which such a study might represent high-quality qualitative research? Quantitative research? What would make it of high quality? (This will help you think through your understanding of what constitutes rigorous inductive and deductive logic!)

References

1 Morse JM. 'Emerging from the data': the cognitive processes of analysis in qualitative inquiry. In: Morse JM, editor. *Critical Issues in Qualitative Research Methods*. Thousand Oaks: Sage, 1994:23–43.
2 Holloway I. *Basic Concepts for Qualitative Research*. Oxford: Blackwell Science, 1997.
3 Schwandt TA. *Qualitative Inquiry: A Dictionary of Terms*. Thousand Oaks: Sage, 1997.
4 Pope C, Ziebland S, Mays N. Qualitative research in health care: analysing qualitative data. *BMJ* 2000;**320**:114–16.

5 Glaser BG, Strauss AL. *The Discovery of Grounded Theory: Strategies for Qualitative Research*. Hawthorne: Aldine Transaction, 1967.
6 Nochi M. Struggling with the labeled self: people with traumatic brain injuries in social settings. *Qual Health Res* 1998;8:665–81.
7 Lincoln YS, Guba EG. *Naturalistic Inquiry*. Beverly Hills: Sage, 1985.
8 Taylor SJ, Bogdan R. *Introduction to Qualitative Research Methods: The Search for Meanings*. New York: John Wiley & Sons, 1984.
9 Thorne S, Reimer Kirkham S, MacDonald-Emes J. Interpretive description: a noncategorical qualitative alternative for developing nursing knowledge. *Res Nurs Health* 1997;20:169–77.
10 Ray MA. The richness of phenomenology: philosophic, theoretic, and methodologic concerns. In: Morse JM, editor. *Critical Issues in Qualitative Research Methods*. Thousand Oaks: Sage, 1994:117–33.
11 Smith BA. The problem drinker's lived experience of suffering: an exploration using hermeneutic phenomenology. *J Adv Nurs* 1998;27:213–22.
12 Colaizzi J. The proper object of nursing science. *Int J Nurs Stud* 1975;12:197–200.
13 Giorgi A, editor. *Phenomenology and Psychological Research*. Pittsburgh: Duquesne University Press, 1985.
14 Kahn DL. Making the best of it: adapting to the ambivalence of a nursing home environment. *Qual Health Res* 1999;9:119–32.
15 Boyle JS. Styles of ethnography. In: Morse JM, editor. *Critical Issues in Qualitative Research Methods*. Thousand Oaks: Sage, 1994:159–85.
16 Sandelowski M. We are the stories we tell: narrative knowing in nursing practice. *J Holist Nurs* 1994;12:23–33.
17 Facione NC, Giancarlo CA. Narratives of breast symptom discovery and cancer diagnosis: psychologic risk for advanced cancer at diagnosis. *Cancer Nurs* 1998;21:430–40.
18 Boutain DM. Critical language and discourse study: their transformative relevance for critical nursing inquiry. *ANS Adv Nurs Sci* 1999;21:1–8.
19 Thorne S. The art (and science) of critiquing qualitative research. In: Morse JM, editor. *Completing a Qualitative Project: Details and Dialogue*. Thousand Oaks: Sage, 1997:117–32.

Additional resources

International Institute for Qualitative Methodology: http://www.uofaweb.ualberta.ca/iiqm/. The Institute's website provides a wealth of information related to qualitative journals, conferences, events, and resources, including numerous links to other websites in the field.

Patton MQ. *Qualitative Research and Evaluation Methods*. Third edition. Thousand Oaks: Sage, 2002.

Qualitative Pages: http://sophia.smith.edu/~jdrisko/qualres.htm. This website also provides some very useful links to a wide range of internet resources, including multidisciplinary, international discussion sites that focus on qualitative research issues, and sites describing software for qualitative data analysis.

Sandelowski M. Combining qualitative and quantitative sampling, data collection, and analysis techniques in mixed-method studies. *Res Nurs Health* 2000;23:246–55. This article will be of interest to readers who are trying to discern the difference between qualitative and quantitative analytic logic within the same study.

Sandelowski M, Barroso J. Finding the findings in qualitative studies. *J Nurs Scholarsh* 2002;34:213–19. This article is helpful for readers trying to understand the difference between 'data' and 'findings' in the qualitative context.

Wolcott HF. *Transforming Qualitative Data: Description, Analysis, and Interpretation*. Thousand Oaks: Sage, 1994.

Chapter 14

USERS' GUIDES TO THE NURSING LITERATURE: AN INTRODUCTION

Nicky Cullum

Introduction to critical appraisal

The volume of health care literature has been described in graphic terms. Did you know, for example, that MEDLINE has indexed over 12 million citations in more than 4800 journals since 1966?[1] Clearly, no individual practitioner can read this volume of research: the trick is to quickly filter the research likely to yield valid results from that likely to mislead. Unfortunately, the journal in which a study or review is published is not a reliable guide to the quality of the research. For example, staff of the Evidence-Based Journals office at McMaster University estimated that of approximately 120 journals read for *Evidence-Based Nursing*, *Evidence-Based Medicine* and *ACP Journal Club*, only about 5.4% of approximately 50 000 articles passed evidence-based methodological filters (personal communication, A McKibbon, 20 December 2006).

Anyone who has designed or conducted a research study knows that they are difficult to do well, and disseminating the results is not straightforward either. Researchers like to spread exciting news and may exaggerate the importance and strength of the findings of their research. Clinicians are faced with the challenge of filtering the thousands of articles published each year into manageable information. This challenge is increased because researchers are notoriously bad at communicating in a language that is accessible to anybody other than researchers. It is not surprising that, time and again, nurses tell researchers that they find it extremely difficult, if not impossible, to use research findings in their practice.[2]

But don't despair! Evidence-based practice is possible because (1) there are now several sources of clinical evidence that provide appraised and summarized research for clinicians (see Chapter 4); (2) good search strategies can identify research that has used an appropriate design to answer specific clinical questions (Chapters 5 and 6); and (3) critical appraisal is easy to learn, becomes easier with practice, and critical appraisal checklists, such as those presented in the chapters that follow, are widely available.

When critically appraising a study or review, we aim to answer two broad questions:

1. Are the research design and methods likely to have led to results that will be 'true' (or valid)? This addresses the *internal* validity of the research.

2. If the answer to the first question is 'yes', can I apply the results of this valid research in my own clinical practice? This addresses the *external* validity of the research.

These two broad questions are typically broken down into several much smaller focused questions in critical appraisal checklists.

Clinical scenario

Imagine that you have recently been promoted to a new role in your hospital and now have responsibility for practice development on the medical wards. For the first time in your career, you are able to set aside time for reading and keeping abreast of new research. You think you have about three hours each week and are keen to use those three hours as efficiently as possible. The library is full of medical and nursing journals, but how do you start? One suggestion is that you start by gathering a list of *frequently asked questions* (*FAQs*) that you often ask yourself during your clinical work or are often asked by your colleagues. For example,

- Is it safe for patients with diabetes to inject insulin directly through their clothing without skin cleansing?
- Is it useful to give dietary supplements to critically ill patients on your ward?
- Should you provide education and counselling to patients who have had a myocardial infarction before they are discharged from hospital?

If you apply what you have learned about asking answerable questions (see Chapter 3) to the first question in your list, it becomes: *Is it effective and safe for patients with diabetes to inject insulin through clothing compared with the standard technique of skin cleansing and injection?* The most important lesson to learn about filtering your reading is to read only studies or reviews that have used an appropriate design to answer your particular question. The question about insulin injection is a question of whether a particular treatment (i.e. injection of insulin through clothing) is effective and whether it is safe. In Chapter 7, we learned that randomized controlled trials (RCTs) are the strongest research design for answering this type of question. Systematic reviews of RCTs are better still because they summarize all RCTs done on a particular topic. Searching MEDLINE using PubMed (http://www.ncbi.nlm.nih.gov/entrez/query.fcgi/) with the terms insulin AND inject* AND cloth* AND clinical trial identifies five papers, one of which is a report of a study that appears to directly address our question.[3] The next step is to look at the study or review and decide whether it is valid and clinically applicable. In the early 1990s, the Evidence-Based Medicine Working Group developed an excellent series of critical appraisal checklists, the *Users' Guides to the Medical Literature*.[4] These guides are used as the basis for the 'users' guides' chapters in this book. As you might expect, separate guides exist for different types of clinical questions, as each type of question is best answered using a specific study design. Regardless of the type of study, clinicians should always ask whether the results of the study are valid: that is, *Is the way the study was done likely to give a true result?* The criteria considered under this broad heading of validity vary, depending on whether the question is about treatment, prognosis or harm, or about understanding complex phenomena such as feelings or perceptions. The validity checks can be applied quickly, and with a little practice you will be able to make efficient decisions about whether to read a paper at all (on the principle that if the methods are not valid, there is no point in reading the paper).

For example, the filtering question for a clinical question about whether a treatment works or not is *Was the assignment of patients to treatments randomized?* If a study fails the basic filtering question, you will need to consider carefully whether or not to read on as it is not likely to direct your practice safely.

This approach to filtering your reading helps to limit the amount you do have to read to a manageable amount. If a study passes the validity filtering question and warrants a more detailed review, then there are further questions to help you determine the study validity with greater confidence, and others to help you tease out what the results of the study really mean and whether they apply to your patients.

Returning to your question of injecting insulin through clothing, the PubMed search identified a paper by Fleming *et al.*[3] that compared insulin injection through clothing with conventional techniques. Better still, a search of *Evidence-Based Nursing* (www.evidencebasednursing.com) would have identified that the study by Fleming *et al.* had been summarized in a synopsis, accompanied by a commentary that addressed the question of clinical applicability.[5] The answer seems to be that injecting insulin through clothing appears to be as safe as conventional techniques and more convenient.

Summary

To make the most efficient use of the limited time available to keep abreast of clinical evidence, we should filter our reading so as to read only studies or reviews that are likely to provide valid results for our focused clinical questions. We should always look for high-quality systematic reviews on a topic for which the author has already identified, appraised, and summarized the relevant studies. In Chapter 4, Brian Haynes outlined the 4S approach to searching and showed us how other sources of pre-appraised research, such as the evidence-based journals and *Clinical Evidence*, can also save us work. Where pre-appraised research is not available or not up to date, simple critical appraisal questions can help us to rapidly filter the useful studies from those that contain useless, or even harmful, information and help us make decisions about clinical applicability. Critical appraisal checklists for use in appraising different study designs will form the basis of the chapters that follow.

References

1 PubMed overview. http://www.ncbi.nlm.nih.gov/entrez/query/static/overview.html (accessed 28 February 2006).

2 McCaughan D, Thompson C, Cullum N, Sheldon TA, Thompson DR. Acute care nurses' perceptions of barriers to using research information in clinical decision-making. *J Adv Nurs* 2002;**39**:46–60.

3 Fleming DR, Jacober SJ, Vandenberg MA, Fitzgerald JT, Grunberger G. The safety of injecting insulin through clothing. *Diabetes Care* 1997;**20**:244–7.

4 Oxman AD, Sackett DL, Guyatt GH. Users' guides to the medical literature. 1. How to get started. The Evidence-Based Medicine Working Group. *JAMA* 1993;**270**:2093–5.

5 Injecting insulin through clothing was safe and convenient. *Evidence-Based Nursing* 1998;**1**:12. Abstract of: Fleming DR, Jacober SJ, Vandenberg MA, Fitzgerald JT, Grunberger G. The safety of injecting insulin through clothing. *Diabetes Care* 1997;**20**:244–7.

Chapter 15

EVALUATION OF STUDIES OF TREATMENT OR PREVENTION INTERVENTIONS

Nicky Cullum and Emily Petherick

In Chapter 14, we discussed how critical appraisal is an important step in evidence-based health care because much published health care research is too poor in quality to be safely applied to clinical practice. Critical appraisal is made easier by the availability of quality checklists, which can be used to appraise research studies systematically and efficiently. With practice, readers may no longer even need a checklist and should be able to decide whether an article is worth reading in a matter of moments.

Whether the question you are asking concerns diagnosis, causation, prognosis, or choosing an intervention, there are three fundamental questions that should be considered when deciding whether study or review findings can be applied in practice.[1]

Are the results of the study valid?

This question considers whether the results reported in the study are likely to reflect the true size and direction of treatment effect. Was the research conducted in such a way as to minimize bias and lead to accurate findings, or was it designed, conducted or analysed in such a way as to increase the chances of an incorrect conclusion?

What are the results?

Once you have determined that the results are valid, it is important to gain an understanding of what the results really mean. If a new intervention is shown to be effective, how large is the effect? Is the effect *clinically important*? How precise is the estimate of effect? The *precision* of a result is related to whether the study involved large numbers of people (which increases precision) or small numbers (which reduces precision).

Can I apply the results in practice?

There are two concepts underlying this question. First, you have to decide if the study participants are sufficiently similar to your patients, or whether there is a good reason

Box 15.1 Critical appraisal questions for studies of treatment or prevention interventions

Are the results of the study valid?
- Was the assignment of patients to treatments randomized?
- Was the randomization concealed?
- Was follow-up sufficiently long and complete?
- Were patients analysed in the groups to which they were initially randomized?
- Were patients, clinicians, outcome assessors and data analysts unaware of (blinded to or masked from) patient allocation?
- Were participants in each group treated equally, except for the intervention being evaluated?
- Were the groups similar at the start of the trial?

What are the results?
- How large was the treatment effect?
- How precise is the estimate of treatment effect?

Can I apply the results in practice?
- Are my patients so different from those in the study that the results don't apply?
- Is the treatment feasible in my setting?
- Were all clinically important outcomes (harms as well as benefits) considered?

why it would be inappropriate to apply the results to your patients. Secondly, is the treatment associated with risks or harms that might outweigh the benefits?

In this and subsequent chapters, we will use this basic appraisal framework to critique studies that address different types of clinical questions. Here we will critique a study that evaluates an intervention.

Beginning with a clinical scenario, we will outline a search to identify high-quality, relevant studies and will critique one of the studies using a series of intermediate questions (Box 15.1) that address the three fundamental questions above. These criteria are based on the original *Users' Guides to Medical Literature.*[1]

Clinical scenario

You are a wound care specialist nurse who runs a foot care clinic with podiatrist colleagues. A patient presents at the clinic with a foot wound after having a partial diabetic foot amputation. These wounds are notoriously difficult to heal. However, you have recently read about negative pressure wound therapy on the Internet and believe that this might help your patient's wound to heal much more quickly than conventional wound dressings. You are not sure and arrange to see her in a week, during which time you plan to search for research evidence on this intervention.

The search

You will recall that questions of the effectiveness of preventive and therapeutic interventions are best answered by randomized controlled trials (RCTs), and best of all by systematic reviews of RCTs. A search of the *Cochrane Library* does identify one systematic review of negative pressure for chronic wounds.[2] This review identified one study that assessed the use of negative pressure wound therapy for patients with diabetic foot ulcers; unfortunately, the study included only 10 participants and did not perform any statistical analysis of the results.[3] You conduct a search of MEDLINE (OVID) using the following search strategy:

1. explode 'diabetic foot'/ all subheadings
2. vacuum/
3. 1 AND 2
4. 3 AND (Publication Type = 'randomized-controlled-trial')

The search identifies two RCTs that compare negative pressure wound therapy with standard moist wound care for partial diabetic foot amputation wounds.[3, 4] The first trial, which was the one included in the Cochrane review, included only 10 people, but the second, a much larger trial published more recently, catches your attention.[4] You obtain the article from the library and sit down with your checklist.

Are the results of the study valid?

Was the assignment of patients to treatments randomized?

The purpose of randomization is to create groups that are similar in all respects except exposure to the intervention. Through random assignment of patients to study groups, known and unknown factors that could influence the outcome of the study (e.g. age, sex, and disease severity) are evenly distributed among groups. Methods of randomization vary (e.g. use of computer-generated numbers, tables of random numbers, and coin flipping); the important thing is that the method used ensures that all study participants have the same chance of being assigned to any of the study groups. How can readers judge whether a study was randomized? The best way is to review the methods section of the paper for a description of how the randomization was done and then determine whether the method ensured that each participant had the same chance as every other participant of being allocated to a particular intervention group.

What should you do if there are no relevant randomized trials of the intervention? The next best study is an observational study, in which randomization is *not* used to assemble the study groups. This design can be prone to *selection bias* because the investigators (who are likely to want the intervention to be effective) have control over who goes into each group and might choose the intervention group participants on the basis of their likelihood of experiencing a positive outcome. Comparison of the results of randomized studies with observational studies has shown that observational studies often show larger treatment effects.[5] The authors of the trial of negative pressure wound therapy[4] state that patients were randomly assigned to treatment and that the study sponsors prepared the randomization scheme. We cannot easily judge how the randomization sequence was generated but feel reassured that it was more likely to be true randomization than some *quasi-random method* such as allocation by date of birth or patient record number.

Was the randomization concealed?

The clinician (e.g. nurse, doctor or other health professional) recruiting patients to a study should be unaware of the treatment group to which the next patient will be allocated. This is called *allocation concealment*, and is the focus of Chapter 16. Analysis of previous studies has shown that if recruiters know the allocation schedule in advance, this may (consciously or unconsciously) influence their recruitment behaviour. For example, they might not recruit a patient who would be allocated to the control group or they might alter the sequence of recruitment so that patients who are more severely ill receive the new treatment. Such actions are often taken in the belief (despite the absence of research evidence) that the new treatment is better than either the alternative (old) treatment or no treatment at all. Strategies that conceal allocation include calling a central, coordinating office for each patient assignment; using sequentially numbered, opaque, sealed envelopes; and numbered or coded bottles or containers.[6] In the trial of negative pressure wound therapy, although the authors stated that the study was an RCT, they do not say how allocation was achieved beyond that assignments were placed in sealed envelopes 'to be opened sequentially'.[4] This statement is missing two vital pieces of information. First, the authors do not state whether the envelopes were opaque (and there are tales of clinicians holding envelopes up to the light to determine the allocation).[6] Secondly, the authors do not clearly state that the envelopes were sequentially numbered (and if they are not, researchers have been known to serially open envelopes until they find the allocation they want for a particular participant).[6] In correspondence published subsequent to the original article, the authors clarified that they had, indeed, used sequentially numbered, sealed, opaque envelopes.[7]

Was follow-up sufficiently long and complete?

This appraisal question has two parts: the first refers to how long patients were followed up in order to see what happens to them as a result of their treatment. A certain amount of judgement is required when deciding whether duration of follow-up is sufficient, but clinical practitioners are usually the best people to judge. For example, if a trial is assessing the effect of an intervention for a chronic health problem or prevention of a health problem, the follow-up phase must be long enough that sufficient numbers of participants actually experience the outcome of interest. Short-term follow-up is not helpful in this case because the study may fail to capture sufficient numbers of patients who achieve meaningful outcomes. The trial of negative pressure wound therapy for patients with diabetic foot wounds had a 16-week follow-up period – sufficiently long to see 39% of people in the control group achieve complete healing.[4] Your clinical experience tells you that diabetic amputation sites can take weeks to heal, and although you would have preferred a longer follow-up period in which more patients achieved healing, the 16-week data are informative.

The second part of the question refers to patients dropping out of a study before they reach the endpoint. It may seem obvious that every patient who is recruited to a trial should be accounted for at the end, but this seldom happens. If large numbers of patients are described as 'lost to follow-up', it raises doubt about the validity of the results. Patients drop out of studies for many different reasons, but dropouts do not occur randomly. In this situation, we do not know what happened to the 'lost' participants, and they may have experienced different outcomes from those who remained in the study. It is also possible that loss to follow-up is caused by the intervention itself. For example, patients may disappear from a smoking cessation study because they are embarrassed that they have failed to stop smoking despite the intervention. If more continuing smokers remain in the control arm than in the intervention arm, the treatment looks more effective than it really is. We should be suspicious if dropout rates differ between intervention and control groups. It is reassuring, however, if, in the presence of dropouts or loss to follow-up, the authors have done a *sensitivity analysis* and recalculated the results using different assumptions about what might have happened to the lost patients. For example, researchers might calculate the effect on the overall result of assuming that all the patients lost from the intervention group had a negative outcome and all those lost from the control group had a positive outcome – would the result remain the same? The impact of a range of assumptions about the outcomes of missing patients can be tested in this way. In the presence of some loss to follow-up, we can have much more confidence in the overall result if a sensitivity analysis that tests different assumptions does not overturn the main conclusion. The report of the negative pressure wound therapy trial presents a flow chart indicating what happened to patients in the study: all 162 patients who were randomized seem to appear in the analysis, indicating complete follow-up, which is impressive.[4]

Were patients analysed in the groups to which they were initially randomized?

It may seem counterintuitive, but patients should be analysed in the groups to which they were originally randomized regardless of whether they received or completed the allocated treatment, or even if they received the wrong treatment.[8] This is called *intention-to-treat analysis*. Patients may discontinue their assigned medication because of side effects or because the medication made them feel worse. If patients who discontinued their medication were omitted from the analysis, we would be left with only the patients who were more likely to be compliant and who had better outcomes. The end result would be that the medication would look better than it really is. Readers should look for a statement that intention-to-treat analysis was done, and check that the numbers presented in the analysis are close to the numbers initially randomized. The authors of the negative pressure wound therapy study state that they analysed by intention to treat.[4]

Were patients, clinicians, outcome assessors, and data analysts unaware of (blinded to or masked from) patient allocation?

There are always two, and sometimes four, groups of people involved in a clinical trial (participants, clinicians, outcome assessors, and data analysts), all of whom may be biased if they know which patients were allocated to which treatment. Studies are often labelled as single, double, or triple blind, depending on how many of these groups were unaware of the treatment allocation. However, this rather vague terminology is unhelpful, and researchers should clearly state who was blinded and what steps were taken to minimize bias (see Chapter 18).

If patients are aware of the group to which they have been allocated, they may have a heightened sensitivity to the good (or bad) effects of the treatment. In drug trials, patient awareness is usually avoided through use of a placebo that seems identical to the active treatment. Unfortunately, it is often difficult, or even impossible, to blind patients to nursing interventions, particularly if the intervention has a psychosocial component. If clinicians caring for patients know the allocation, they may unwittingly alter the way they provide other forms of care and may also have a heightened sensitivity to good outcomes or adverse events in a way that biases the evaluation.

Most importantly, the people who measure the outcomes should not be the people who provide usual clinical care. If outcome assessors are aware of group allocation, their measurement of key variables may be influenced. Distortion of outcome measurement is less likely if the measure is objective, such as cotinine concentration as a marker of smoking status.

Although it is not always possible for patients, clinicians and outcome assessors to be blinded to treatment group, it should always be possible for the data analysis to be done using coded data, with no identification of treatment groups.

Readers of randomized trials should look for evidence that patients, clinicians, data analysts and, most importantly, outcome assessors were blinded to patient allocation. If blinding was not possible, researchers should outline the steps they took to minimize bias. In the trial of negative pressure wound therapy, the authors explain that neither participants nor clinicians were blinded to assignment group. Unblinded photographers took standardized digital photographs of the wound, and other investigators (who were unaware of group allocation) measured the wound area from the photographs using digital planimetry.[4] This level of blinded outcome assessment is often the best that can be achieved in wound care trials, and although it is not immune to measurement bias it is more secure than completely open assessment.

Were participants in each group treated equally except for the intervention being evaluated?

Because randomization should ensure that the only systematic difference between study groups is the treatment in question, it is important that this principle is not undermined by extra care given to one group and not the other: this is known as *co-intervention*. Clearly, if patients get an intervention plus some extras, such as closer follow-up or more time with a specialist nurse, it will be impossible to attribute any effects to the intervention itself. If clinicians are unaware of the allocation, then they will not deliver co-interventions to one group and not another. Readers of randomized trials should look carefully at the descriptions of the interventions received by all groups, particularly if clinicians were not blinded to allocation. In the negative pressure wound therapy study,[4] we cannot be confident that trial participants in the different treatment groups received identical co-interventions since none of the caregivers was masked to allocation group. Furthermore, there is evidence that co-interventions were differentially received by participants in the treatment and control groups. For example, the authors reported that fewer patients in the treatment group than in the control group received sharp debridement (21% vs 26%), whereas more patients in the treatment group received surgical closure (16% vs 9%).[4] Both of these interventions are likely to influence the main outcome of time to healing, and decisions were made by clinicians who knew the allocation and may have, even subconsciously, been influenced by this knowledge.

Were the groups similar at the start of the trial?

The process of randomization should ensure that the groups are sufficiently similar at the beginning of a trial. Researchers, however, should reassure themselves and their readers of this by presenting the baseline (or entry) characteristics of participants in each group. The characteristics described should be those that are known to, or believed to, have an influence on the outcome of interest. If the trial has a small sample size, randomization may fail to ensure that some factors are evenly distributed. The researchers may have done statistical tests to see if any significant differences existed in the baseline characteristics of the groups. However, if randomization was done properly, it is already clear that any baseline differences occurred by chance. More important than the significance of any difference is its size and whether the imbalance is likely to have affected the validity of the result. Imbalances in baseline characteristics that exist after randomization can be adjusted for using statistical techniques, and readers should look for evidence of this. Readers can be most confident when results are consistent for analyses done with and without adjustment. In the negative pressure therapy study,[4] the baseline characteristics were presented by allocation group in table format. Broadly speaking, the groups appear fairly evenly balanced, although wounds were slightly larger at baseline in the negative pressure group and of slightly longer duration in the control group. Importantly, even baseline differences that are not statistically significant may influence the results, and it is surprising that the authors of this study did not conduct an adjusted analysis.

The appraisal questions outlined above can be applied to any study that aims to evaluate the effects of a preventive or therapeutic intervention and will help readers to decide whether the results are likely to be valid (i.e. give a true estimate of the effect of the intervention). If you conclude that a study is valid, you should then consider the size of the effect: is the effect of sufficient clinical significance for you to want to use the intervention? In which patients?

What are the results?

The aim of this part of the appraisal is to help readers to judge whether the results of an individual study are important. This decision takes into account the size of the treatment effect and whether the estimate of the treatment effect is precise.

How large was the treatment effect?

The effects of individual treatments are measured using one or more outcome measures. Previous chapters have described how outcome measures can be dichotomous (e.g. yes or no, dead or alive, healed or not healed) or continuous (e.g. length of stay or daily intake of fruits and vegetables) and how these measures are presented and analysed. The key findings of the trial comparing negative pressure wound therapy with standard moist wound care are summarized in Box 15.2. We see that 56% of patients in the negative pressure wound therapy group had healed wounds (*experimental event rate* or *EER*) compared with 39% in the control group (*control event rate* or *CER*) at 16 weeks follow-up.[4] Although the accompanying p-value of 0.040 tells us that the difference between groups was statistically significant, this information has limited usefulness. However, these same data can be expressed in other ways.

Box 15.2 Turning trial results into clinically meaningful information

Proportion of patients in the negative pressure group whose wounds healed 43/77 = 0.56 = 56% (this is the Experimental Event Rate or EER)

Proportion of patients in the control group whose wounds healed 33/85 = 0.39 = 39% (this is the Control Event Rate or CER)

Relative risk of healing in the experimental group relative to the control group = RR = EER/CER = 0.56/0.39 = 1.44

Relative benefit of the experimental treatment over the control treatment = RBI = EER − CER/CER = 0.56 − 0.39/0.39 = 0.17/0.39 = 0.44 (or 44%). In other words, negative pressure wound therapy was associated with a 44% proportional increase in healing compared with the control treatment.

Absolute risk difference, ARD = EER − CER = 0.56 − 0.30 = 0.17. In other words, the experimental treatment (negative pressure wound therapy) resulted in an absolute increase in the percentage of wounds healed of 17%.

Number needed to treat = NNT = 1/ARD = 5.88, which, rounded up to the nearest whole number, is 6. This means that for every six patients with diabetes and an amputation-related foot wound treated with negative pressure, one additional wound will heal by 16 weeks. The smaller the NNT, the more effective the treatment.

The *risk* (or probability) of healing by 16 weeks was 56% or 0.56 in the negative pressure group and 39% or 0.39 in the control group. From this, we can calculate the *relative risk (RR)* of healing in the negative pressure group relative to the control group, which is 0.56/0.39, or 1.44 (note, the term 'risk' is used when referring to the probability of either bad or good outcomes). The RR of healing is greater than 1: this is what we would have expected since the negative pressure group had *more* healing than the control group. We can also calculate the proportional increase in the rates of good outcomes between experimental and control participants in a trial, or the *relative benefit increase*, as (EER − CER)/CER = (0.56 − 0.39)/0.39 = 0.17/0.39 = 0.44; this means a 44% increase in the RR of healing with negative pressure wound therapy. The RR does not take into account the number of patients who would have healed anyway: this is captured by the *absolute risk difference (ARD)*, which is calculated as EER − CER = 0.56 − 0.39 = 0.17 or 17%. This *absolute* difference in risk tells us how much of the effect is a result of the intervention itself. A third approach to presenting the same data is to report the *number needed to treat (NNT)*. The NNT gives the reader an impression of the effectiveness of the intervention by describing the number of people who must be treated with the given intervention in order to prevent one additional bad outcome or to promote one additional good outcome. The NNT is simply calculated as the inverse of the ARD, rounded up to the nearest whole number; in the case of the negative pressure therapy trial,[4] the NNT = 1/17 = 5.88 (95% confidence interval 3.2 to 63.1). If we round up 5.88 to the nearest whole number, the NNT is 6. Put into words, this means that one additional wound would be healed within 16 weeks of therapy for every six patients who are treated with negative pressure wound therapy, and we are 95% sure that the true NNT value lies between 4 and 64. When properly presented, reports of NNTs should incorporate a statement of the duration of follow-up and include the 95%

confidence interval around the NNT estimate. Chapters 12 and 17 provide a more detailed discussion of using NNTs in clinical practice.

When reading reports of statistically significant differences in treatment effects, it is always important to ask oneself whether the difference is *clinically important*. It is quite possible for a statistically significant difference to be unimportant, either because the outcome measure is unimportant or because the difference is too small to be noticed by patients or to warrant a change in practice. For example, a systematic review of antibiotics for sore throat concluded that antibiotics shortened symptom duration by approximately 16 hours,[9] which is probably clinically insignificant when compared with the problems of overuse of antibiotics and the side effects that they may cause.

Many published RCTs do not find statistically significant differences between two treatments. These trials are just as informative as those with significant differences, *if the studies were large enough to detect a significant difference if one existed*. A review of 2000 trials of treatments for schizophrenia reported that the average number of participants in a schizophrenia trial was 65.[10] The authors estimated that only 3% of these studies were large enough to detect a 20% improvement in mental state between groups (which would have required 150 patients in each arm of a trial).[10]

How precise is the estimate of treatment effect?

The true effect of a treatment can never really be known. Instead, we use the results of trials, which are *estimates* of effect. Each estimate is a neighbour of the true treatment effect. The crux is the size of the neighbourhood! *Confidence intervals (CIs)* (often called *confidence limits*) are a statistical device used to communicate the amount of uncertainty surrounding an estimate; in other words, they represent the size of the neighbourhood. The 95% CI represents the range within which we are 95% certain the true value lies. If this range is wide, our estimate lacks precision, and we are unsure of the true treatment effect. Alternatively, if the range is narrow, precision is high, and we can be much more confident. The sample size of a trial is an important determinant of the precision of the result: precision increases with larger sample sizes and thereby reduces the width of the 95% CI. Small studies are likely to produce results with wide CIs (see Chapter 12).

Remember that if the 95% CI of an odds ratio or RR includes 1, there is no statistically significant difference between treatments. Similarly, if the CI of a risk or mean difference includes zero, the difference is not statistically significant. Readers of RCTs can look at the lower limit of the CI around an odds ratio or RR and, using that as the smallest possible effect size, ask themselves *If the effect of the intervention was as small as this, would it be worth having?* If the outcome measures used in a study are continuous, readers can use the same approach, looking carefully at the CI for the estimate of the difference (often a difference in means) and judging whether the smallest difference (the lower end of the CI) would be clinically important. In the negative pressure study,[4] quite a lot of uncertainty remains around the estimate of the NNT. Whereas an NNT of 4 would be very attractive, an NNT of 64 would not (i.e. we might not want to use this treatment in routine care if we had to treat 64 people with negative pressure for 16 weeks in order to heal one additional patient). The cost of the intervention would clearly need to be taken into account.

Can I apply the results in practice?

Are my patients so different from those in the study that the results don't apply?

In considering whether you can use a study's findings in your own patients, look at the characteristics of the patients in the study and how similar they are (or are not) to your own patients. It makes most sense to look for compelling reasons that the results should *not* be applied, rather than looking for evidence that study patients are almost exactly the same as yours.

Is the treatment feasible in my setting?

This is a judgement that depends on factors such as the cost of the intervention (and whether your health care system is prepared to pay for it), the skills and training required to deliver the intervention, and the cost and availability of special equipment.

Were all clinically important outcomes (harms as well as benefits) considered?

It is common for researchers to use various outcome measures to capture different elements of patients' responses to treatment. Typically these might include measures of quality of life and costs as well as direct measures of the ill health treated or prevented. The most important issue for readers of RCTs is that the outcomes reported are likely to be important to the patients or communities targeted by the intervention. It is also important that indirect measures of outcomes are *validated alternatives* that have been shown to be directly related to the outcome of interest. *Indirect, proxy or surrogate outcome* measures are sometimes used by researchers for good reasons. For example, accurate self-reports of smoking behaviour are notoriously difficult to obtain; however, salivary cotinine concentration has been shown to be a valid and reliable alternative because it *relates directly to* smoking behaviour.[11] In the negative pressure study,[4] the outcome measured was the number of wounds completely healed after 16 weeks of treatment. This outcome is highly objective, requires no complex measurement procedure, and is likely to be an outcome that matters to patients. Table 15.1 gives further examples of surrogate outcome measures.

Adverse events or side effects experienced by trial participants should be clearly detailed in reports of RCTs. However, because such events are relatively rare, and trials are usually quite small, larger observational studies are better suited to collecting this type of data.

Increasingly, health systems are placing greater importance on the measurement of the cost-effectiveness of interventions. Readers might therefore look for information relating to costs, and particularly cost-effectiveness, either in a trial report or a separate publication. Chapter 21 addresses the critical appraisal of reports of economic evaluations. The authors of the negative pressure RCT[4] did not report other important outcomes such as quality of life (the treatments may have a differential effect on this), costs, or wound recurrence, and you would likely require more information on these aspects before implementing negative pressure therapy.

Table 15.1 Examples of surrogate or proxy outcome measures

Focus of study	Hypothetical trial	Surrogate or proxy outcome measure	Patient-oriented outcome
Pressure ulcer prevention	Comparison of two alternative pressure-relieving surfaces	Interface pressure between patient and support surface	Incidence of new pressure ulcers on either surface
Preoperative fasting	Comparison of 12-hour fast with 2-hour fast	Volume of gastric contents at induction of anaesthesia	Risk of aspiration pneumonia
Surgical gloves to prevent postoperative infection	Comparison of double-gloving with a single pair of gloves to be worn by surgical team	Risk of puncture to the innermost glove	Incidence of surgical site infections

Resolution of the clinical scenario

Although this is a fairly good quality study, you feel that the wide CIs around the NNT estimate and the absence of data on cost-effectiveness leave you unable to justify negative pressure wound therapy as a first-line treatment for your patient, although it could be considered for patients with amputation wounds that require encouragement to heal.

LEARNING EXERCISES

1. Bandage A and Bandage B are alternative compression bandages for treating venous leg ulcers. In an RCT comparing the two bandages, 60% of patients had healed ulcers after 12 weeks of treatment with Bandage A compared with 75% of patients treated with Bandage B. Calculate the relative benefit increase associated with Bandage B compared with Bandage A. Then, calculate the ARD and the NNT.
2. Collect examples of trials in your area of interest. Practise using a critical appraisal checklist to assess some of these trials, and practise the calculations outlined above.

Solutions to learning exercises
1. *Proportion of participants healed with Bandage A = 0.6 or 60%*
   Proportion of participants healed with Bandage B = 0.75 or 75%
   RR of healing with Bandage B vs Bandage A = 0.75/0.60 = 1.25; i.e. Bandage B was associated with a 25% proportional increase in healing over Bandage A.
   ARD = risk of healing with Bandage B minus risk of healing with Bandage A = 0.75 − 0.60 = 0.15. The NNT is 1/0.15 = 6.7, which, rounded up to the next whole number, is 7. In other words, for every seven people treated with Bandage B instead of Bandage A for 12 weeks, an additional person will have their venous ulcer healed.

References

1 Oxman AD, Sackett DL, Guyatt GH. Users' guides to the medical literature. 1. How to get started. The Evidence-Based Medicine Working Group. *JAMA* 1993;**270**:2093–5.
2 Evans D, Land L. Topical negative pressure for treating chronic wounds. *Cochrane Database Syst Rev* 2001;(1):CD001898.
3 McCallon SK, Knight CA, Valiulus JP, Cunningham MW, McCulloch JM, Farinas LP. Vacuum-assisted closure versus saline-moistened gauze in the healing of postoperative diabetic foot wounds. *Ostomy Wound Manage* 2000;**46**:28–32, 34.
4 Armstrong DG, Lavery LA, for the Diabetic Foot Study Consortium. Negative pressure wound therapy after partial diabetic foot amputation: a multicentre, randomised controlled trial. *Lancet* 2005;**366**:1704–10.
5 Kunz R, Oxman AD. The unpredictability paradox: review of empirical comparisons of randomised and non-randomised clinical trials. *BMJ* 1998;**317**:1185–90.
6 Schulz KF, Grimes DA. Allocation concealment in randomised trials: defending against deciphering. *Lancet* 2002;**359**:614–18.
7 Armstrong DG, Lavery LA. Negative pressure therapy in diabetic foot wounds – authors' reply. *Lancet* 2006;**367**:726–7.
8 Hollis S, Campbell F. What is meant by intention to treat analysis? Survey of published randomised controlled trials. *BMJ* 1999;**319**:670–4.
9 Del Mar CB, Glasziou PP, Spinks AB. Antibiotics for sore throat. *Cochrane Database Syst Rev* 2006;(4):CD000023.
10 Thornley B, Adams C. Content and quality of 2000 controlled trials in schizophrenia over 50 years. *BMJ* 1998;**317**:1181–4.
11 Abrams DB, Follick MJ, Biener L, Carey KB, Hitti J. Saliva cotinine as a measure of smoking status in field settings. *Am J Public Health* 1987;**77**:846–8.

Chapter 16

ASSESSING ALLOCATION CONCEALMENT AND BLINDING IN RANDOMIZED CONTROLLED TRIALS: WHY BOTHER?

Kenneth F. Schulz

Chapter 15 outlined the primary and secondary questions for evaluating studies of health care interventions. One of the primary questions for assessing the validity of a study's findings is whether the assignment of patients to treatments was randomized and whether randomization was concealed. One of the secondary questions is whether patients, clinicians, outcome assessors and data analysts were unaware of (blinded to or masked from) patient allocation. This chapter discusses why allocation concealment and blinding are such critical criteria to consider when assessing the validity of studies that evaluate interventions.

Allocation concealment

Random allocation to intervention groups remains the only method of ensuring that the groups being compared are on an equivalent footing at the beginning of a study, thus eliminating selection and confounding biases. This has allowed randomized controlled trials (RCTs) to play a key part in advancing health care practice.

The success of randomization depends on two interrelated processes.[1, 2] The first entails generating a sequence by which the participants in a trial are allocated to intervention groups. To ensure unpredictability of that allocation sequence, investigators should generate it by a random process (e.g. computer-generated numbers, random number tables, or coin flipping). The second process, *allocation concealment*, shields those involved in a trial from knowing upcoming assignments in advance.[3, 4] Without this protection, investigators have been known to change who gets the next assignment, making the comparison groups less equivalent.[5, 6]

Suppose, for example, that an investigator creates an adequate allocation sequence using a random number table. However, the investigator then affixes the list of that sequence to a bulletin board, with no allocation concealment. Those responsible for admitting participants could ascertain the upcoming treatment allocations and then route participants with better prognoses to the experimental group and those with poorer prognoses to the control group, or vice versa. Bias would result. Inadequate allocation concealment also exists, for example, when assignment to groups depends on whether a participant's hospital number is odd or even, or depends on translucent envelopes that allow discernment of assignments when held up to a light bulb.

Strategies to conceal allocation include calling a central, coordinating office for each patient assignment at the time that the participant presents for study inclusion; using sequentially numbered, opaque, sealed envelopes; and using numbered bottles or containers. A study by Richter et al.[7] evaluated the effectiveness of on-demand β_2-agonist inhalation in reducing the number of asthma episodes in patients with moderate to severe asthma. The investigators ensured unpredictability of the allocation sequence by using a computerized random number generation process. To shield those responsible for entering patients into the trial from knowing upcoming assignments, they used sequentially numbered, opaque, sealed envelopes. Unfortunately, their article neglected to state the 'sequentially numbered aspect'. On average, such articles yield exaggerated results, as discussed below.[5] Thus, their original report creates a false impression of poor allocation concealment. However, the authors confirmed, when contacted, that they used numbered envelopes. Each envelope contained the group assignment for one patient.

Recent studies have shown that poorly designed RCTs and poorly reported RCTs yield biased results. For example, in a study of 250 controlled trials from 33 meta-analyses in pregnancy and childbirth, investigators found that alleged RCTs with inadequate and unclear allocation concealment yielded larger estimates of treatment effects (on average 41% and 33%, respectively) than trials in which authors reported adequate concealment.[5] Investigators found similar results for trials in digestive diseases, circulatory diseases, mental health, and stroke.[8] Trials that used inadequate or unclear allocation concealment yielded, on average, 37% larger estimates of effect than trials that used adequate concealment. These exaggerated estimates of treatment effects reveal meaningful levels of bias. If a study were designed to detect an improvement in quality of life of 25% or 50% from a particular treatment, biases of 30% to 40% would overwhelm estimates of the treatment effect. The elimination of bias is crucial in trials designed to detect moderate effects.

Allocation concealment should not be confused with blinding. Allocation concealment focuses on preventing selection and confounding biases, safeguards the assignment sequence *before and until* allocation, and can *always* be successfully implemented.[1] By comparison, blinding concentrates on preventing study participants and personnel from determining the group to which participants have been assigned (which leads to *ascertainment bias*), safeguards the sequence *after* allocation, and cannot always be implemented.[1, 9]

Blinding

Blinding or *masking* involves keeping patients, clinicians, outcome assessors, and/or data analysts unaware of patient allocation to avoid bias. For example, if unblinded, patients may have a heightened sensitivity to the good (or bad) effects of a treatment, clinicians may unwittingly alter the way they provide care or look for good or adverse outcomes; outcome assessors may distort outcome measurement; and data analysts may alter their approach to analysing the data. Ideally, although not usually possible in studies evaluating nursing interventions, all four groups are blinded. In the study by Richter et al. described above, two of the groups were blinded: outcome assessors and data analysts. The authors explained that blinding of patients was not possible because patients could easily identify the (side) effects of β_2-agonists. There was no mention of clinician blinding.[7]

Double-blinding (variably but usually defined as blinding patients, clinicians and outcome assessors – see Chapter 18) also appears to reduce bias. The study of 250 controlled trials from 33 meta-analyses in pregnancy and childbirth found that trials that were not double-blinded yielded larger estimates of treatment effect than trials in which authors reported double-blinding (odds ratios exaggerated, on average, by 17%).[5] Another recent analysis similarly indicated the importance of double-blinding.[10] However, although double-blinding seems to prevent bias, its effect appears weaker than that of allocation concealment. Indeed, Moher *et al.* found that double-blinding had little influence on estimates of effect.[8]

Reporting of methods

Investigators must not only minimize bias but must also communicate those efforts to readers. Readers should not have to assume or guess which methods were used. Yet, assessments of the reporting quality of published trials have consistently found major flaws.[3, 11–17] Only 9% of trials in specialist journals and 15% in general journals reported both an adequate method of generating random sequences and an adequate method of allocation concealment.[3, 11, 18] Of trials reported as double-blind, only 45% described similarity of the treatment and control regimens, and only 26% provided information on protection of the allocation schedule.[19] Most reports simply provide no information on methods.

With so little relevant information, many readers resort to inappropriate markers of trial quality. Two noteworthy examples highlight this concern. First, many designate a trial as high quality if it is double-blind, as if double-blinding is the essential requirement of an RCT. Although double-blinding can reflect good methods, it is not the sole criterion of quality. Adequate allocation concealment actually appears to be the more important indicator. Moreover, many trials cannot be double-blinded. Such trials must be judged on other merits and not on an inapplicable standard based on double-blinding. To further complicate matters, a study recently found that the term 'double-blind' was interpreted differently by both readers and experts.[20] Surveys of physicians and review of recent textbooks including definitions of blinding revealed numerous unique interpretations of the term; for example, some thought it meant that patients and clinicians were blinded, whereas others thought that patients and outcome assessors were blinded.[20] This has led to the recommendation that the terms single-blinded, double-blinded, and triple-blinded be abandoned and replaced with descriptions specifically stating *which* of the groups were unaware of allocation (see Chapter 18).[20]

Secondly, some assume that good quality trials contain arms of equal sizes, whereas poor quality trials contain arms of unequal sizes. This standard has marginal value only if investigators used a restricted randomization generation scheme that aimed for equality. Otherwise, exactly equal numbers in treatment groups in a simple randomized trial may mean that some process *other* than randomization was used (e.g. allocation of every second patient to the intervention group).

Although RCT reporting remains weak, it is improving. Methodologists, editors, and clinicians addressed the prevailing flaws in reporting by publishing the Consolidated Standards of Reporting Trials (CONSORT) statement.[21] Currently, 200 journals have adopted the standards,[22] including such high profile health care journals as *JAMA, BMJ, Lancet, Pediatrics*, and *Archives of Internal Medicine*. These journals were five of the highest contributors of articles that were abstracted in *Evidence-Based Nursing* in 2005 (personal communication, Susan Marks, 20 December 2006). *Nursing Research* is noteworthy as the single nursing journal that has explicitly adopted the CONSORT standards.[22] Even with these improvements, readers of RCTs should be wary of the information provided in many current trial reports.

Summary

As users of RCT results, we must understand the potential for humans to interject bias. Judging the quality of trials on the basis of allocation concealment and blinding reflects current empirical research.

LEARNING EXERCISES

Using any database (e.g. PubMed, CINAHL), find four randomized trials relevant to an aspect of your nursing practice.
1. For each trial, grade the allocation as **A** (concealed), **B** (not concealed) or **C** (unclear). Ensure that you are clear about which aspect of the text you used in deciding on your answers.
2. For those (if any) studies to which you allocated a **B** grade, think about what impact the lack of allocation concealment may have had on the outcomes of the trial. How does this affect your views of the validity of the results?
3. For each trial, assess the blinding and identify which groups, if any, were blinded and which were not.
4. If any of the studies were graded **B** for allocation concealment and also did not have any blinding, think about the impact this may have had on the outcomes of the trial. How do these threats to validity affect your interpretation of the study results?

Note

This chapter was adapted from an editorial that originally appeared in *ACP Journal Club* 2000;**132**:A11–12.

References

1 Schulz KF. Subverting randomization in controlled trials. *JAMA* 1995;**274**:1456–8.
2 Schulz KF. Randomized trials, human nature, and reporting guidelines. *Lancet* 1996;**348**:596–8.
3 Schulz KF, Chalmers I, Grimes DA, Altman DG. Assessing the quality of randomization from reports of controlled trials published in obstetrics and gynecology journals. *JAMA* 1994;**272**:125–8.
4 Chalmers TC, Levin H, Sacks HS, Reitman D Berrier J, Nagalingam R. Meta-analysis of clinical trials as a scientific discipline. I: Control of bias and comparison with large co-operative trials. *Stat Med* 1987;**6**:315–28.
5 Schulz KF, Chalmers I, Hayes RJ, Altman DG. Empirical evidence of bias. Dimensions of methodological quality associated with estimates of treatment effects in controlled trials. *JAMA* 1995;**273**:408–12.
6 Pocock SJ. Statistical aspects of clinical trial design. *Statistician* 1982;**31**:1–18.
7 Richter B, Bender R, Berger M. Effects of on-demand β_2-agonist inhalation in moderate-to-severe asthma. A randomized controlled trial. *J Intern Med* 2000;**247**:657–66.

8 Moher D, Pham B, Jones A, Cook DJ, Jadad AR, Moher M, Tugwell P, Klassen TP. Does quality of reports of randomised trials affect estimates of intervention efficacy reported in meta-analyses? *Lancet* 1998;**352**:609–13.

9 Schulz KF. Unbiased research and the human spirit: the challenges of randomized controlled trials. *CMAJ* 1995;**153**:783–6.

10 Khan KS, Daya S, Collins JA, Walter SD. Empirical evidence of bias in infertility research: overestimation of treatment effect in crossover trials using pregnancy as the outcome measure. *Fertil Steril* 1996;**65**:939–45.

11 Altman DG, Doré CJ. Randomization and baseline comparisons in clinical trials. *Lancet* 1990;**335**:149–53.

12 Moher D, Fortin P, Jadad AR, Juni P, Klassen T, Le Lorier J, Liberati A, Linde K, Penna A. Completeness of reporting of trials published in languages other than English: implications for conduct and reporting of systematic reviews. *Lancet* 1996;**347**:363–6.

13 Williams DH, Davis CE. Reporting of assignment methods in clinical trials. *Control Clin Trials* 1994;**15**:294–8.

14 Sonis J, Joines J. The quality of clinical trials published in *The Journal of Family Practice*, 1974–1991. *J Fam Pract* 1994;**39**:225–35.

15 Mosteller F, Gilbert JP, McPeek B. Reporting standards and research strategies for controlled trials: agenda for the editor. *Control Clin Trials* 1980;**1**:37–58.

16 DerSimonian R, Charette LJ, McPeek B, Mosteller F. Reporting on methods in clinical trials. *N Engl J Med* 1982;**306**:1332–7.

17 Tyson JE, Furzan JA, Reisch JS, Mize SG. An evaluation of the quality of therapeutic studies in perinatal medicine. *J Pediatr* 1983;**102**:10–13.

18 Schulz KF, Chalmers I, Altman DG, Grimes DA, Doré CJ. The methodologic quality of randomization as assessed from reports of trials in specialist and general medical journals. *Online J Curr Clin Trials* 1995;Doc No 197:[81 paragraphs].

19 Schulz KF, Grimes DA, Altman DG, Hayes RJ. Blinding and exclusions after allocation in randomised controlled trials: survey of published parallel group trials in obstetrics and gynaecology. *BMJ* 1996;**312**:742–4.

20 Devereaux PJ, Manns BJ, Ghali WA, Quan H, Lacchetti C, Montori VM, Bhandari M, Guyatt GH. Physician interpretations and textbook definitions of blinding terminology in randomized controlled trials. *JAMA* 2001;**285**:2000–3.

21 Begg C, Cho M, Eastwood S, Horton R, Moher D, Olkin I, Pitkin R, Rennie D, Schulz KF, Simel D, Stroup DF. Improving the quality of reporting of randomized controlled trials. The CONSORT statement. *JAMA* 1996;**276**:637–9.

22 CONSORT journals. http://www.consort-statement.org/Endorsements/Journals/journals. html (accessed 22 November 2006).

Chapter 17

NUMBER NEEDED TO TREAT: A CLINICALLY USEFUL MEASURE OF THE EFFECTS OF NURSING INTERVENTIONS

Alba DiCenso

After establishing that the results of a study of the effectiveness of a nursing intervention are valid (see Chapter 15), the next step is to determine the size of the effect and whether the effect is clinically important. When determining the clinical significance of effective nursing interventions, findings can be expressed in three ways: as a change in relative risk, a change in absolute risk, and as the *number needed to treat (NNT)*. The final step, the application of the findings to an individual patient, requires knowledge about both the study and the patient. This involves consideration of the extent to which the patient resembles those who were enrolled in the study and the patient's risk for the event for which the intervention was designed.[1] This chapter will outline the differences between relative risk reduction, absolute risk reduction and NNT, and will highlight the advantages of NNTs in clinical decision-making with individual patients.

A randomized controlled trial of a telephone intervention to reduce mortality and hospital admission in people with chronic heart failure illustrates the usefulness of the NNT.[2] In this trial, the investigators randomized 1518 patients with stable heart failure to one of two groups: 760 patients were allocated to receive an education booklet, frequent standardized telephone follow-up by nurses, and usual care (intervention group), and 758 patients were allocated to usual care only (control group). Addressing the validity of the trial, the design involved *randomization* of patients to the intervention or control groups; allocation to groups was *concealed*, ensuring that the cardiologists identifying eligible patients were unaware of whether patients would be entered into the intervention or control group; data analysis was based on the *intention-to-treat principle*, in which patient outcomes were attributed to the group to which the patient was originally assigned, even if the patient dropped out of the study or, for other reasons, did not actually receive the planned intervention; and finally, *loss to follow-up* at 16 months was only 0.5%.

Turning to the results, 16.8% of patients who received the telephone intervention were admitted to hospital for worsening heart failure (we will call this the *experimental event rate* or *EER*), whereas 22.3% of those in the usual care control group were admitted (we will call this the *control event rate* or *CER*). This difference was statistically significant.

A traditional measure of the effect of an intervention is the *relative risk reduction (RRR)*, defined as the proportional reduction in rates of harmful outcomes between experimental and control participants in a trial, calculated as (CER − EER)/CER.* The unadjusted RRR is (22.3% − 16.8%)/22.3% or 24.7%; that is, the telephone intervention reduced the risk of being admitted for worsening heart failure by 24.7%.

The RRR has limitations because it fails to discriminate huge absolute effects of the intervention from those that are trivial.[3] For example, if the hospital admission rates for worsening heart failure were 10 times less than those observed in this trial, and only 2.23% of control group patients and 1.68% of intervention group patients were admitted to hospital, the RRR would still be 24.7% (see Table 17.1). This is because the RRR ignores how rarely or commonly the outcome in question occurs in the patients entering the trial (known as the *baseline risk*). Restricting reporting of efficacy to only RRRs can lead to unnecessarily treating people with low susceptibilities. For example, an estimated RRR of 50% might be statistically significant and clinically important for people at moderate-to-high risk of a particular adverse event. However, for patients with a low probability of the event, the risk reduction might not be sufficient to warrant the side effects and costs of the intervention.[4, 5]

In contrast to the non-discriminating RRR, the absolute difference in the rates of hospital admission due to worsening heart failure between control group and experimental group patients (i.e. CER − EER) clearly *does* discriminate between these extremes; this measure is called the *absolute risk reduction (ARR)* and is defined as the absolute arithmetic difference in rates of harmful outcomes between experimental and control patients (this measure is also sometimes known as the *absolute risk difference* or *ARD*).† In the telephone intervention trial, the ARR = CER − EER = 22.3% − 16.8% = 5.5%. In the hypothetical example provided above, in which 1.68% of experimental group patients and 2.23% of control group patients were admitted due to worsening heart failure, the ARR = CER − EER = 2.23% − 1.68% = 0.55% (see Table 17.1). The absolute difference takes into account the baseline risk of patients (e.g. 22.3% in the telephone intervention trial and 2.23% in the hypothetical example) and provides more detailed information than the RRR. However, because the

Table 17.1 Measures of clinical significance

	Scenario 1	Scenario 2
Control group event rate (CER)	22.3%	2.23%
Experimental group event rate (EER)	16.8%	1.68%
Relative risk reduction (RRR) = (CER − EER)/CER	24.7%	24.7%
Absolute risk reduction (ARR) = CER − EER	5.5%	0.55%
Number needed to treat (NNT) = 100%/ARR	19	182

* In this chapter, we use RRR to illustrate intervention effects. Two other terms which are used to illustrate intervention effects are *relative benefit increase (RBI)*, defined as the proportional increase in rates of good outcomes between experimental and control participants, and *relative risk increase (RRI)*, defined as the proportional increase in rates of harmful outcomes between experimental and control participants. Both of these are calculated identically to RRR (i.e. [CER − EER]/CER).[7]
† Although we use ARR to illustrate intervention effects in this chapter, two other terms that reflect absolute differences are *absolute benefit increase (ABI)*, defined as the absolute arithmetic difference in rates of good outcomes between experimental and control participants, and *absolute risk increase (ARI)*, defined as the absolute arithmetic difference in rates of harmful outcomes between experimental and control participants. Both of these are calculated identically to ARR (i.e. CER − EER).[7]

ARR is a dimensionless, abstract number that may be difficult to incorporate into clinical practice, we divide the ARR into 1 (or 100%) to generate the NNT.[6]

The *NNT* is the number of people who need to receive the experimental intervention in order for one additional person to achieve a favourable outcome (e.g. healing of a leg ulcer) over a predefined period of time.[7] In the telephone intervention trial, we generate the number of patients with heart failure for whom we would provide the telephone intervention in order to prevent one additional admission for worsening heart failure within 16 months of the intervention. The NNT is 1/ARR or 100%/5.5% or 1/0.055 = 18.2; we usually round this number upwards (because we can't have part of a person!), and we can now say that, for every 19 people with heart failure who receive the telephone intervention, one admission for worsening heart failure will be averted. Using the hypothetical example provided above in which the ARR was 0.55% rather than 5.5%, the NNT is 100%/0.55% or 1/0.0055 = 181.8 or 182 people with heart failure who would need to receive the telephone intervention in order to prevent one additional person from experiencing admission for worsening heart failure (see Table 17.1). If the ARR is large, only a small number of people need to receive the intervention to observe a benefit in at least some of them, and if the ARR is small, many people need to receive the intervention to observe a benefit in only a few.[8]

How can NNTs help me in clinical decision-making?

The NNT is a useful measure for making decisions about the effort expended with a particular intervention to achieve a single positive outcome (e.g. pain reduction).[9] It is a meaningful way of expressing the magnitude of the effect of an intervention over usual care. Knowing the NNT helps clinicians determine whether the likely benefits of the intervention are worth the potential harm and costs.[10] For example, we would be comfortable providing 10 people with a safe, low-cost intervention to prevent one person from experiencing a pressure ulcer (an NNT of 10), but more reluctant to treat 10 000 people with a risky, high-cost intervention to prevent one person from experiencing a pressure ulcer (an NNT of 10 000).[11] Decisions regarding different interventions for the same condition and outcome can be facilitated by comparing NNTs for the various options.[12]

The remainder of this chapter will focus on important points to keep in mind when calculating or interpreting NNTs.

NNTs are only useful for interventions that produce dichotomous outcomes

Because we are calculating the number of people who need to be treated, the only outcomes that lend themselves to this are dichotomous outcomes, which are counts of the number of people who experience and do not experience an event (e.g. alive or dead, recovered or not recovered). NNTs cannot be calculated when the outcome is presented as a mean value such as mean blood pressure or mean length of stay. In the telephone intervention trial described above, one outcome was the number of people who were admitted to hospital for worsening heart failure, an outcome that lends itself nicely to the calculation of NNT. In trials reporting continuous outcomes, the investigators will sometimes dichotomize these outcomes by reporting the percentage of study participants who attain a threshold value (e.g. the percentage of people who attain ≥50% improvement in a depression score on a scale such as the Hopkins Symptom Checklist Depression Scale[13]). While outcomes in the telephone intervention trial included quality of life as measured by the Minnesota Living with Heart Failure questionnaire, only mean scores were reported, precluding the calculation of NNTs for this outcome.

NNTs should always be interpreted in the context of their precision

The reported NNT is a point estimate that represents the most likely value of the NNT in a population prognostically similar to study participants.[9] To express the precision of the point estimate, NNTs should be accompanied by 95% *confidence intervals (CIs)* that represent upper and lower limits within which the true NNT would be expected to lie 95% of the time. In the telephone intervention trial, the investigators did not present NNTs or their accompanying CIs; we have calculated the CI around the NNT of 19 to be 11 to 69. To interpret this information, we would consider the best estimate of the number of people who would need to receive the telephone intervention to avert one hospital admission for worsening heart failure to be 19. However, it is possible that we might see a benefit of the intervention after treating as few as 11 people, or perhaps not until 69 people have received the intervention. The intent of this chapter is to inform readers about the interpretation of NNTs and corresponding CIs; details about the calculation of CIs around NNTs can be found elsewhere.[14, 15]

Interpretation of NNTs must always consider the follow-up time associated with them

Because the number of reported events in a study has occurred by following the study participants for a specified period of time, this must be reflected in the interpretation of the NNT. For example, in the telephone intervention study, participants were followed up for an average of 16 months. The NNT for admission for worsening heart failure at 16 months was 19 (95% CI 11 to 69). Put into words, 19 people with heart failure would need to receive the telephone intervention to prevent one additional admission for worsening of heart failure after 16 months and the true NNT could be as low as 11 and as high as 69.

Clinical decision-making must consider adverse outcomes as well as positive effects

Interventions that lead to beneficial effects may often be associated with adverse effects as well. To determine the effect of the adverse events, we calculate the *number needed to harm* or *NNH*, which is defined as the number of people who, if receiving the experimental intervention, would lead to one additional person being harmed compared with people who receive the control intervention.[7] Like the NNT, NNH is calculated as 1/absolute difference (or 100%/absolute difference expressed as a percentage) and is accompanied by a CI.

A large trial of low-dose aspirin for the primary prevention of cardiovascular disease in women[16] illustrates the need to consider both the benefits and adverse effects of a treatment. After 10 years, 19 934 women randomized to 100 mg of aspirin every other day experienced fewer strokes than the 19 942 women randomized to placebo. The event rate for stroke was 1.1% in the intervention group (EER) and 1.3% in the control group (CER). This difference was statistically significant. The unadjusted RRR is (CER − EER)/CER = (1.3% − 1.1%)/1.3% = 15.4%, meaning that aspirin reduced the relative risk of stroke by 15%. The ARR is 1.3% − 1.1% = 0.2%. The NNT is 100%/0.2% or 1/0.002 = 500, which means we would need to treat 500 women with aspirin for 10 years to prevent one additional woman from experiencing a stroke.

Although this appears to be an important beneficial effect, it must be considered in conjunction with the adverse effects. Women in the aspirin group had a higher incidence of gastrointestinal bleeding over the 10-year period (4.6% in the aspirin group vs 3.8% in the placebo group). This absolute risk increase of 4.6% − 3.8% = 0.8% generates an NNH over 10 years of 125, meaning that for every 125 women who take aspirin over 10 years, one will experience gastrointestinal bleeding. Clinicians and patients must decide when the effects of an intervention are large enough to more than offset its adverse effects.

NNTs will vary with baseline risk

NNTs vary with baseline risk: the lower the baseline risk, the higher the NNT will be. Let's consider two hypothetical examples to illustrate how the baseline risk of people for whom we provide care may influence our decision to implement an effective intervention. The first focuses on prevention of adolescent pregnancy. Let's say that a study completed in the United Kingdom shows the effectiveness of an adolescent pregnancy prevention programme. Two nurses, one in the United States (US) and one in the Netherlands, are considering whether to implement this programme in their countries. The NNTs will vary dramatically in these two countries because the baseline risk of adolescent pregnancy in the US is the highest of all developed countries, whereas the baseline risk of adolescent pregnancy in the Netherlands is one of the lowest in the world. As a result, the NNT to prevent one additional pregnancy in the US will be dramatically lower than the NNT to prevent one additional pregnancy in the Netherlands. Consequently, the nurse in the US might justifiably decide to go ahead with the intervention, whereas the nurse in the Netherlands might be equally justified in choosing not to implement the programme.

In the second example, consider a study that has shown the effectiveness of a falls prevention programme for older people. The NNT will be much lower for those at high risk of falling, such as those who have had previous falls and are cognitively impaired. By considering baseline risk and calculating NNTs for older people at high and low risk of falls, we can make decisions about who should be offered the falls prevention programme. This becomes especially important when the intervention is costly or has associated risks.

For people at very high risk of the target event, the NNT will tend to be low, and treatment is likely to be justified. For people at very low risk of the target event, the

NNT is likely to be high enough to raise doubts about whether treatment is warranted, even when the outcome being prevented is serious.[11] For example, people at high risk of dying from coronary heart disease who are treated with drugs to lower cholesterol concentrations will experience a greater reduction in the risk of dying than those at lower risk – that is, 30 people at high risk might have to be treated for 5 years to save one life, but 300 people at low risk would have to be treated to save one life.[17] Thus, a treatment that might be worth implementing in a person at high risk may not be worth implementing in a person at lower risk.[17]

How do we determine the baseline risk of a specific patient to whom we are considering offering the intervention? First, we can assign our patient the same event rate as that experienced by the control group in the trial. Although this is simple, it is only sensible if our patient is very similar to the average participant in the control group. Secondly, if the study presents the data for subgroups of study participants, and one subgroup shares similar characteristics with our patient, we can assign our patient the control group rate for that subgroup. Thirdly, we can look for a prospective study that examined the prognosis of untreated people similar to our patient and use its results to determine a baseline risk rate.[3]

Once we have estimated the baseline risk of our patient, the NNT can be calculated in two ways. The first makes use of a nomogram (Figure 17.1) designed by Chatellier et al.[18] To use this nomogram, a straight line is drawn from the point on the left-hand column of the nomogram corresponding to the baseline risk for our patient (absolute risk in the absence of treatment) to the point on the centre column corresponding to the RRR calculated from the trial. The point of intercept of this line with the right-hand column gives the NNT (see Box 17.1). By taking the upper and lower limits of the CI around the RRR, we can obtain the upper and lower limits of the NNT. This allows us to assess the precision of the NNT and the magnitude of effectiveness on the most optimistic and most pessimistic limits of the CI.

Because we may not always have the nomogram with us, an alternate method to calculate NNT might be preferable. We can determine the relation between our patient's baseline risk and that of the average control group study participant. The relation is expressed numerically as a decimal fraction that we will call 'f'. For example, if our patient has twice the baseline risk of the average control group participant, then $f = 2$; if our patient has half the baseline risk, then $f = 0.5$; if our patient has the same baseline risk, then $f = 1$. The NNT for our patient is simply the reported NNT divided by f.[5, 19] For instance, in the telephone intervention trial, if a clinician felt that patient A was at one-half ($f = 0.5$) the risk of hospital admission for worsening heart failure compared with the average control group participant, the patient-specific NNT would be calculated by dividing the study NNT of 19 by 0.5 resulting in an NNT

Box 17.1 Using the nomogram to determine numbers needed to treat (NNTs)

Using the data in Table 17.1, practise using the nomogram in Figure 17.1. Begin with Scenario 1 and locate the control group event rate (22.3%) on the left-hand column. Using a straight edge, connect the point corresponding with the control event rate (CER) to the point on the centre column that corresponds to the relative risk reduction (RRR) (24.7%). The point of intercept of this line with the right-hand column gives the NNT (19). Repeat this exercise using the data from Scenario 2.

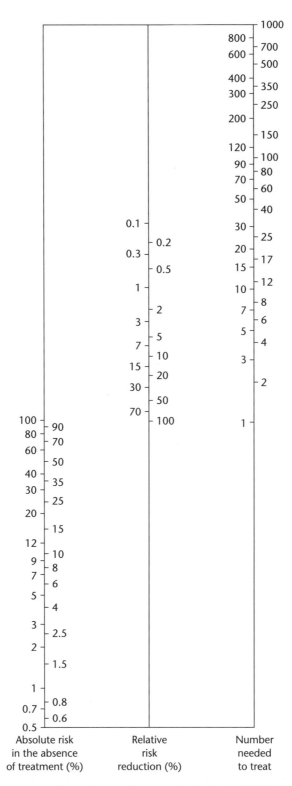

Figure 17.1 Nomogram to determine numbers needed to treat (NNTs). Reproduced with permission of BMJ Publishing Group from Chatellier *et al.* 1996.[18]

of 38 for patient A. In other words, the telephone intervention would need to be given to 38 people with baseline risks of patient A to prevent one additional hospital admission for worsening heart failure.

Summary

The NNT and its 95% CI are useful in interpreting the clinical significance of valid study results and making intervention decisions. The NNT provides information about the benefit of an intervention by taking into account the underlying risk without the intervention and the risk reduction resulting from the intervention. An NNT should be accompanied by information about the length of the observation period. The NNH should be considered along with the NNT to assess both the benefit and harm of an intervention. Once a patient has been informed about the benefits and risks of a specific intervention, the patient's preferences and values should guide the decision to receive or not receive the intervention.

LEARNING EXERCISES

1. Identify a randomized controlled trial (RCT) that evaluates an intervention of interest to your clinical practice and that reports at least one dichotomous outcome. Calculate the impact of the intervention by determining the change in relative risk, the change in absolute risk, the number needed to treat (NNT), and, if relevant data are available, the number needed to harm (NNH).
2. Review the calculations with a colleague explaining what the numbers mean in your own words.
3. Explain to your colleague the limitation of the relative risk reduction (RRR) as a measure of the effect of an intervention.
4. Assume that the baseline risk for the outcome of interest in the patients for whom you provide care is half the baseline risk of the control group in the RCT. Assuming the same RRR, estimate how this will change the NNT. Use the nomogram to check the accuracy of your estimate.

References

1 Guyatt GH, Cook DJ, Jaeschke R. How should clinicians use the results of randomized trials? *ACP J Club* 1995;**122**:A12–13.
2 GESICA Investigators. Randomised trial of telephone intervention in chronic heart failure: DIAL trial. *BMJ* 2005;**331**:425.
3 Sackett DL. On some clinically useful measures of the effects of treatment. *Evidence-Based Medicine* 1996;**1**:37–8.
4 Sackett DL, Cook RJ. Understanding clinical trials. *BMJ* 1994;**309**:755–6.
5 Cook RJ, Sackett DL. The number needed to treat: a clinically useful measure of treatment effect. *BMJ* 1995;**310**:452–4.
6 Tramer MR, Walder B. Number needed to treat (or harm). *World J Surg* 2005;**29**:576–81.
7 DiCenso A, Guyatt G, Ciliska D, editors. *Evidence-based Nursing: A Guide to Clinical Practice*. St. Louis: Elsevier Mosby, 2005.
8 Barratt A, Wyer PC, Hatala R, McGinn T, Dans AL, Keitz S, Moyer V, For GG. Tips for learners of evidence-based medicine: 1. Relative risk reduction, absolute risk reduction and number needed to treat. *CMAJ* 2004;**171**:353–8.
9 Weeks DL, Noteboom JT. Using the number needed to treat in clinical practice. *Arch Phys Med Rehabil* 2004;**85**:1729–31.

10 Dalton GW, Keating JL. Number needed to treat: a statistic relevant for physical therapists. *Phys Ther* 2000;**80**:1214–19.

11 Sinclair JC, Cook RJ, Guyatt GH, Pauker SG, Cook DJ. When should an effective treatment be used? Derivation of the threshold number needed to treat and the minimum event rate for treatment. *J Clin Epidemiol* 2001;**54**:253–62.

12 Osiri M, Suarez-Almazor ME, Wells GA, Robinson V, Tugwell P. Number needed to treat (NNT): implication in rheumatology clinical practice. *Ann Rheum Dis* 2003;**62**:316–21.

13 Simon GE, Ludman EJ, Tutty S, Operskalski B, Von Korff M. Telephone psychotherapy and telephone care management for primary care patients starting antidepressant treatment: a randomized controlled trial. *JAMA* 2004;**292**:935–42.

14 Altman DG. Confidence intervals for the number needed to treat. *BMJ* 1998;**317**:1309–12.

15 Bender R. Calculating confidence intervals for the number needed to treat. *Control Clin Trials* 2001;**22**:102–10.

16 Ridker PM, Cook NR, Lee IM, Gordon D, Gaziano JM, Manson JE, Hennekens CH, Buring JE. A randomized trial of low-dose aspirin in the primary prevention of cardiovascular disease in women. *N Engl J Med* 2005;**352**:1293–1304.

17 Davey Smith G, Song F, Sheldon TA. Cholesterol lowering and mortality: the importance of considering initial level of risk. *BMJ* 1993;**306**:1367–73.

18 Chatellier G, Zapletal E, Lemaitre D, Menard J, Degoulet P. The number needed to treat: a clinically useful nomogram in its proper context. *BMJ* 1996;**312**:426–9.

19 McAlister FA, Straus SE, Guyatt GH, Haynes RB. Users' guides to the medical literature: XX. Integrating research evidence with the care of the individual patient. *JAMA* 2000;**283**:2829–36.

Chapter 18

THE TERM 'DOUBLE-BLIND' LEAVES READERS IN THE DARK

P.J. Devereaux

'Double-blind' is the term researchers frequently use, and readers frequently accept, as a key marker of validity in randomized controlled trials (RCTs). Clinical trial experts and clinicians, when asked, all claim to 'know' what 'double-blind' means. Unfortunately, it means diverse things to those questioned.[1] The term lacks consistency in its use and interpretation, a critical flaw for any technical term if it is to be understood. As a result of this limitation, we have advocated abandoning the current blinding lexicon (i.e. single blinded, double blinded, and triple-blinded) and recommended transparent reporting of the blinding status of each group involved in the execution, monitoring, and reporting of clinical trials.

Blinding (or *masking*) in RCTs is the process of withholding information about treatment allocation from those who could potentially be influenced by this information. The scientific community has long considered blinding an important safeguard against bias. Benjamin Franklin, in 1784, was probably the first to use blinding in scientific experimentation.[2] Louis XVI commissioned Franklin to evaluate mesmerism, the most popular unconventional 'healing fluid' of the 18th century. Franklin applied a blindfold to participants to remove their knowledge of when mesmerism was and was not applied. Blinding eliminated the intervention's effects and established mesmerism as a sham.[2] From this work, the scientific community recognized the power of blinding to enhance objectivity, and it quickly became, and remains, a commonly used strategy in scientific research.

The groups that can potentially introduce bias into an RCT through knowledge of the treatment allocation are shown in Table 18.1. Individuals in the seven groups listed in the table are likely to have, or develop, opinions about the efficacy of the intervention under investigation. Because of these opinions, unblinded individuals can systematically bias trial findings through conscious or subconscious mechanisms. When unblinded, participants may introduce bias through use of other effective interventions, differential reporting of symptoms,[3] psychological or biological effects of receiving a placebo (although studies demonstrate conflicting evidence),[4, 5] or dropping out. Unblinded health care providers can distort trial results if they differentially prescribe effective co-interventions, influence compliance with follow-up, or influence patient reports.[3] Unblinded data collectors can introduce bias through differential encouragement during performance testing, differential timing or frequency of outcome measurements, and variable recording of outcomes.[6, 7] Unblinded outcome

Table 18.1 Groups that can potentially be blinded in randomized controlled trials

Group	Description
Participants	Individuals who are randomly assigned to the interventions under evaluation
Health care providers	Physicians, nurses, physiotherapists, or other personnel who care for the participants during the study period or administer the interventions
Data collectors	Individuals who collect data for the study outcomes. Data collection could include administering a questionnaire, taking a physical measurement, or eliciting symptoms
Outcome adjudicators	The individuals who ultimately decide whether a participant has experienced the outcome(s) of interest
Data analysts	The individuals who conduct the data analysis
Data safety and monitoring committee	The committee that reviews the data to advise on the continuing safety of the trial and persistent uncertainty of the efficacy of the intervention under evaluation
Manuscript writers	The individuals who write versions of the manuscript before the breaking of the randomization code: in a fully blinded study, one version is written with the assumption that group A received the experimental intervention, and the other is written with the assumption that group B received the experimental intervention.

adjudicators may introduce bias in their assessments of outcomes, this being most likely during assessment of subjective outcomes.[3] Unblinded data analysts have the potential to introduce systematic bias through decisions on patient withdrawals, post-hoc selection of outcomes or analytic approaches, selection of time points that demonstrate the maximum or minimum effects, and many other decisions.[8] Unblinded members of the data safety and monitoring committee may introduce bias at the time of interim analyses through their recommendations to stop or continue a study.[8] Blinding of authors, while seldom done,[8, 9] may reduce biases in the presentation and interpretation of results.

Case reports document individual examples of the biases described above.[7, 8, 10, 11] However, no high-quality methodological study has evaluated whether blinding of individual groups systematically affects the estimate of effect in RCTs. Investigators have published four high-quality methodological studies (i.e. studies that assessed RCTs from meta-analyses, thereby controlling for the confounders of disease state and intervention), but they assessed the influence of investigators' statements that trials were double blinded on the estimates of effect.[12–15] Although two studies[12, 14] showed lower estimates of effect in RCTs reported as double blinded, the other studies[13, 15] did not find an association between reporting of double blinding and estimates of effect. The groups that were actually blinded in these studies probably varied and are certainly open to question. Heterogeneity in the groups that were blinded in studies reported as double blinded may explain these discrepant findings.

Although the true magnitude of bias introduced through unblinding remains (and is likely to remain) uncertain, health care providers should consider the blinding status of each group when assessing study validity. Unfortunately, suboptimal reporting of blinding status in full-text publications and secondary journals has hindered readers.[16, 17] Authors have commonly relied on conventional blinding terminology (i.e. single blinded, double blinded, and triple blinded) to convey blinding status.[1] We have demonstrated great variability in physician interpretations and textbook definitions of these terms.[1] Furthermore, a recent study surveyed researchers to determine which groups were actually blinded in their trials that were reported as double blind.[18] Survey respondents provided 18 different combinations of groups actually blinded in trials that were reported as double blind. As well, approximately 1 in 5 trials reported as double blind had not blinded patients, health care providers, or data collectors. As a result of these limitations of the term double blind, authors have recommended, and the editors of several journals have abandoned, the current blinding terminology and adopted transparent reporting of the blinding status of the groups listed in Table 18.1. As a result of this policy, readers can make more informed decisions about the validity of the studies upon which they base their practice.

Although this chapter focuses on blinding in RCTs, the issue is also relevant for other study designs where knowledge of group membership may affect the results. For example, in cohort or case-control studies where researchers abstract chart data to identify outcomes or predisposing factors, readers should determine whether the abstractors were blinded to group membership. Unblinded data abstractors may lead to variable recording of outcomes or predisposing factors. As in RCTs, blinding is not always possible. Nevertheless, when assessing the validity of a study, readers should consider the blinding status of all groups that could introduce bias through their knowledge of group membership.

Summary

Blinding, or masking, those involved in an RCT to treatment allocation is considered an important strategy in minimizing bias. Within trials there are potentially seven groups who could be blinded, from participants and health care providers through to data monitoring committees and manuscript writers. The potential consequences of unblinding vary depending on the role of that individual in the trial and no high quality study has yet evaluated whether the blinding of different groups systematically affects the results of RCTs. One of the challenges readers face when interpreting the results of published RCTs is determining the level of blinding for each group since this is often poorly reported using vague terminology such as 'single blind' and 'double blind'. We make a plea for authors to be more precise in their reports of blinding and for readers to be thorough in their consideration of who was and was not blinded and the potential biases that may have been introduced as a consequence.

LEARNING EXERCISES

1. Do a search and find five trials published in the last year. How many of the five trials identify which groups were blinded? How many simply refer to 'single blinding' or 'double blinding'?

2. What difference would it make to your ability to use the results of a trial, if 'double blind' actually referred to the data analysts and the manuscript writers, as opposed to the patients and outcome assessors?
3. Find one trial that clearly tells you who was blinded in the study. With a colleague, discuss the following questions, each with regard to patients, health care providers, data collectors and outcome assessors:
   (a) Was the group in question blinded?
   (b) If not, would it have been possible to blind them in such a study?
   (c) If the group in question was not blinded, what is the potential impact on outcomes?

Note

This chapter is reproduced with permission of the American College of Physicians from an editorial by Devereaux PJ, Bhandari M, Montori VM, Manns BJ, Ghali WA, Guyatt GH. Double blind, you are the weakest link – good-bye! *ACP J Club* 2002;**136**:A11–12; *Evidence-Based Medicine* 2002;**7**:4–5; and Double blind, you have been voted off the island! *Evidence-Based Mental Health* 2002;**5**:36–7.

References

1 Devereaux PJ, Manns BJ, Ghali WA, Quan H, Lacchetti C, Montori VM, Bhandari M, Guyatt GH. Physician interpretations and textbook definitions of blinding terminology in randomized controlled trials. *JAMA* 2001;**285**:2000–3.
2 Kaptchuk TJ. Intentional ignorance: a history of blind assessment and placebo controls in medicine. *Bull Hist Med* 1998;**72**:389–433.
3 Altman DG, Schulz KF, Moher D, Egger M, Davidoff F, Elbourne D, Gotzsche PC, Lang T. The revised CONSORT statement for reporting randomized trials: explanation and elaboration. *Ann Intern Med* 2001;**134**:663–94.
4 de la Fuente-Fernandez R, Ruth TJ, Sossi V, Schulzer M, Calne DB, Stoessl AJ. Expectation and dopamine release: mechanism of the placebo effect in Parkinson's disease. *Science* 2001;**293**:1164–6.
5 Hrobjartsson A, Gotzsche PC. Is the placebo powerless? An analysis of clinical trials comparing placebo with no treatment. *N Engl J Med* 2001;**344**:1594–602.
6 Jadad AR. *Randomised Controlled Trials: A User's Guide.* London: BMJ Books, 1998:20–36.
7 Guyatt GH, Pugsley SO, Sullivan MJ, Thompson PJ, Berman L, Jones NL, Fallen EL, Taylor DW. Effect of encouragement on walking test performance. *Thorax* 1984;**39**:818–22.
8 Gotzsche PC. Blinding during data analysis and writing of manuscripts. *Control Clin Trials* 1996;**17**:285–90.
9 Dong BJ, Hauck WW, Gambertoglio JG, Gee L, White JR, Bubp JL, Greenspan FS. Bioequivalence of generic and brand-name levothyroxine products in the treatment of hypothyroidism. *JAMA* 1997;**277**:1205–13.
10 Karlowski TR, Chalmers TC, Frenkel LD, Kapikian AZ, Lewis TL, Lynch JM. Ascorbic acid for the common cold. A prophylactic and therapeutic trial. *JAMA* 1975;**231**:1038–42.
11 Noseworthy JH, Ebers GC, Vandervoort MK, Farquhar RE, Yetisir E, Roberts R. The impact of blinding on the results of a randomized, placebo-controlled multiple sclerosis clinical trial. *Neurology* 1994;**44**:16–20.
12 Schulz KF, Chalmers I, Hayes RJ, Altman DG. Empirical evidence of bias. Dimensions of methodological quality associated with estimates of treatment effects in controlled trials. *JAMA* 1995;**273**:408–12.
13 Moher D, Pham B, Jones A, Cook DJ, Jadad AR, Moher M, Tugwell P, Klassen TP. Does quality of reports of randomised trials affect estimates of intervention efficacy reported in meta-analyses? *Lancet* 1998;**352**:609–13.

14 Kjaergard LL, Villumsen J, Gluud C. Reported methodologic quality and discrepancies between large and small randomized trials in meta-analyses. *Ann Intern Med* 2001;**135**:982–9.

15 Juni P, Altman DG, Egger M. Systematic reviews in health care: assessing the quality of controlled clinical trials. *BMJ* 2001;**323**:42–6.

16 Devereaux PJ, Manns BJ, Ghali WA, Quan H, Guyatt GH. The reporting of methodological factors in randomized controlled trials and the association with a journal policy to promote adherence to the Consolidated Standards of Reporting Trials (CONSORT) checklist. *Control Clin Trials* 2002;**23**:380–8.

17 Devereaux PJ, Manns BJ, Ghali WA, Quan H, Guyatt GH. Reviewing the reviewers: the quality of reporting in three secondary journals. *CMAJ* 2001;**164**:1573–6.

18 Haahr MT, Hrobjartsson A. Who is blinded in randomized clinical trials? A study of 200 trials and a survey of authors. *ClinTrials* 2006;**3**:360–5.

Chapter 19

EVALUATION OF SYSTEMATIC REVIEWS OF TREATMENT OR PREVENTION INTERVENTIONS

Donna Ciliska, Nicky Cullum and Susan Marks

Chapter 15 focused on critical appraisal of primary studies of treatment or prevention. This chapter will deal with critical appraisal of systematic reviews of treatment or prevention interventions.

What is a systematic review?

Basing clinical decisions on a single research study can be a mistake for several reasons. Individual studies may have inadequate sample sizes to detect clinically important differences between treatments (leading to false negative results), the results of apparently similar studies may vary because of chance, and subtle differences in the study designs and participants may lead to different or even discrepant findings. A *systematic review* (sometimes called an overview) is a rigorous summary of all research evidence that relates to a specific question; the question may be one of causation, diagnosis or prognosis but often addresses the effectiveness of an intervention. Systematic reviews differ from unsystematic reviews in that they attempt to overcome possible biases at all stages by following a rigorous methodology for searching, research retrieval, appraisal of retrieved research for relevance and validity (quality), data extraction, data synthesis, and interpretation. One way that bias is reduced is by the use of explicit, pre-set criteria to select studies for inclusion on the basis of relevance and validity. A second way is by having two or more people independently make study selection decisions, compare their decisions, and discuss discrepancies before moving on to independently extract data from the studies. Explicit details of the methods used at every stage are recorded. Many, but not all, systematic reviews incorporate *meta-analysis* (the quantitative combination of the results of similar studies). Meta-analysis produces an overall summary statistic that represents the effect of the intervention across different studies. Because meta-analysis in effect combines the samples of each contributing study to create one larger study, the overall summary statistic is much more precise than the effect size in any one contributing study.

Systematic reviews have the potential to overcome several barriers to utilization of research by clinicians. Nurses have difficulties using research because of lack of access and time to retrieve numerous research reports and lack of skills to appraise and synthesize the articles once retrieved. Systematic reviews offer nurses a solution in the form of a summary of research-based knowledge on a topic, which takes into account the validity of the primary research studies. Nevertheless, not every systematic review is of high quality, and the critical appraisal step remains essential.

Clinical scenario

> You work in an outpatient paediatric clinic and often see children whose parents are frustrated and concerned about their child's night-time bed wetting (nocturnal enuresis). They ask if you would recommend the use of night-time alarm systems that they have seen advertised. Should you recommend the use of these alarms for their children with non-organic nocturnal enuresis?

The search

As described in Chapter 4, an efficient literature search strategy begins with a search for relevant research that has already met quality criteria and has been summarized in a *synopsis* or included in a *synthesis* (or systematic review) of primary studies. The evidence-based journals publish exactly this type of synopsis. You search the *Evidence-Based Nursing* website (www.evidencebasednursing.com) using the term 'enuresis'. You find an abstract and commentary for a systematic review by Glazener and Evans published in 2001.[1] The abstract, entitled 'Review: alarm interventions reduce nocturnal enuresis in children', reports that alarms reduce enuresis compared with no intervention or other interventions. This looks promising. You retrieve the full Cochrane review from the *Cochrane Library* by simply entering the term 'enuresis' in the search box for 'Title, abstract, or keywords'; alternatively, you could have searched by author. You happily find that the review was updated in 2005.[2] You now need to assess the quality of the review: can you confidently use this review to inform practice? The questions relevant to the critical appraisal of systematic reviews[3, 4] are summarized in Box 19.1 and will be applied to the updated review by Glazener *et al.*[2]

Are the results of the systematic review valid?

Is this a systematic review of randomized trials?

Good systematic reviews determine at the outset to include those studies that used the most appropriate design to answer the clinical question. Questions about the effectiveness of treatment or prevention are best answered by randomized controlled trials (RCTs), whereas questions about harm or prognosis are best answered by cohort studies (see Chapter 7). The review by Glazener *et al.* included 53 randomized or quasi-randomized trials (3152 children): 17 comparisons of alarms with no intervention and 59 comparisons of different alarms or of alarms with drugs, behavioural interventions, or various combinations thereof.[2]

Box 19.1 Critical appraisal questions for systematic reviews of treatment or prevention interventions

Are the results of the systematic review valid?

- Is this a systematic review of randomized trials?
- Does the systematic review include a detailed and exhaustive description of the strategies used to find all relevant trials?
- Does the systematic review include a description of how the validity of individual studies was assessed?
- Were individual patient data or aggregate data used in the analysis?

What are the results?

- Are the results consistent from study to study?
- How large is the treatment effect?
- How precise is the estimate of treatment effect?

Can I apply the results in practice?

- Are my patients so different from those in the studies included in the review that the results don't apply?
- Is the treatment feasible in my setting?
- Were all clinically important outcomes (harms as well as benefits) considered?
- What are my patient's values and preferences for both the outcome we are trying to prevent and the side effects that may arise?

Does the systematic review include a detailed and exhaustive description of the strategies used to find all relevant trials?

It is usually necessary to search several electronic bibliographic databases and to use other strategies, such as hand searching of journals and consultation with experts, to ensure that every relevant primary study is identified. A search confined only to MEDLINE and CINAHL will be biased towards studies that were published in English and those that found significant differences between interventions (i.e. if a reviewer only finds the two studies that found a difference and not the 10 that did not, she is likely to draw misleading conclusions).[5] Therefore, a search strategy is considered thorough if it includes several databases, if the reference lists of relevant papers were searched, if key journals were searched by hand, and if key informants were contacted. Hand searching contributes to the completeness of retrieval, as occasionally the people who index articles for databases such as MEDLINE may use inappropriate keywords or may miss articles or even entire journal issues. Glazener et al.[2] searched the Cochrane Incontinence Review Group's specialized register, which includes searches of 20 databases and hand searches of three relevant journals and relevant conference proceedings. The most recent search date was November 2004. References were also checked for additional studies.[2] The review by Glazener et al.[2] could be considered to have an extensive search strategy; the only source that they did not report accessing was key informants.

Every systematic review should grow from a focused question, which itself leads to the development of inclusion criteria and a sensitive and specific search strategy.

After the articles are retrieved, it is necessary to be pedantic about the *application* of inclusion and exclusion criteria. The review by Glazener et al.[2] identified an overall objective of determining the effects of alarms for treatment of enuresis in children. Inclusion criteria were randomized or quasi-randomized trials that compared use of alarms with a control condition (no intervention, behavioural interventions, drugs, or combinations thereof) in children <16 years of age with non-organic nocturnal enuresis. Trials of children with organic causes for bed wetting were excluded, as were trials of daytime wetting.[2]

Does the systematic review include a description of how the validity of individual studies was assessed?

An unsystematic narrative review often reports on study findings without considering the methodological strength of the studies. Differences in study quality might explain differences in results because studies of poorer quality tend to overestimate the effectiveness of interventions.[6] Authors of systematic reviews sometimes use quality rating scales to compare outcomes by study strength. If a large number of studies met the initial inclusion criteria, the authors may decide to apply a quality rating threshold for inclusion of studies in the review, or to give greater weight to stronger studies.

A pre-specified quality checklist helps to ensure that reviewers appraise each study consistently and thoroughly – another means of minimizing bias. Having two or more raters, as well as a specified mechanism for dealing with differences of opinion, helps to reduce both mistakes and bias and increases readers' confidence in the systematic review. Quality rating tools applied to individual studies usually include criteria such as those presented in Chapter 15.

The review by Glazener et al.[2] applied explicit, pre-specified validity criteria including level of concealment of allocation at randomization, comparability of groups at baseline, blinding of outcome assessment, use of intention-to-treat analysis, and extent of follow-up. The authors were explicit about the quality criteria used in this review.

Were individual patient data or aggregate data used in the analysis?

Less commonly, authors may request individual patient data from the investigators of individual studies. In this case, rather than using the summary statistics (e.g. relative risks or odds ratios) from each study, individual patient data may be combined across studies to allow comparisons of outcomes for subgroups, defined, for example, by age or severity of illness. Glazener et al.[2] did not use individual patient data.

What are the results?

Are the results consistent from study to study?

Although we would not expect to find the same magnitude of effect in all studies, we would be more confident in using the results of a review if the results of individual studies were qualitatively similar – that is, all showing a positive effect or all showing no effect. But what if treatment effect differs across studies? Many systematic reviews identify studies with important differences in terms of the types of patients; the timing, duration and intensity of the intervention; or the outcome measures. The reviewers make decisions about whether meta-analysis is appropriate by using a combination of judgement and a statistical test for *heterogeneity* – a test of the extent to which differences between the results of individual studies are greater than you would expect if all studies were measuring the same underlying effect and the observed differences were only because of chance. The more significant the test of heterogeneity, the less likely that the observed differences are because of chance alone; this would indicate that some other factor (e.g. study design, patients, intervention, or outcomes) is responsible for observed differences in treatment effects across studies.[3]

Although the value of judgement in deciding whether statistical synthesis is appropriate cannot be overemphasized, the statistical test for heterogeneity has low power and may fail to identify important differences in study results. Readers of reviews must also make judgements, using their clinical expertise, about whether meta-analysis of specific results makes clinical and methodological sense. Glazener et al.[2] chose to statistically combine five RCTs that compared alarms with no intervention for the outcome of 'numbers not achieving 14 consecutive dry nights or relapsing' (subsequently referred to as 'treatment failure or relapse'). All five trials had similar populations, interventions and outcome measures, and the results were similar in direction and size of differences between the treatment and control groups. The test for heterogeneity was not significant (p = 0.62).[2]

Different statistical approaches can be used in meta-analysis. *Fixed effects models* are most commonly used when no significant heterogeneity exists between studies; this model assumes that the true effect of the treatment is the same in each study, with differences in results arising because of chance. A *random effects model* assumes that the study results vary around some overall average treatment effect, and the calculation of the summary statistic incorporates an estimate of between-study variation.[7] Glazener et al.[2] used a fixed effects model in their analyses, which is appropriate since the test for heterogeneity was not significant (p = 0.62).

How large is the treatment effect?

Comparing a simple count of the number of studies that found a positive effect of an intervention with the number that found no effect or a harmful effect would be misleading. This would assume that all studies had equal validity, power, duration, dosage, etc., to potentially have the same effect. Meta-analysis, when appropriate, can assign different weights to individual study estimates so that those with greater precision, or higher quality, will make a greater contribution to the summary estimate. Glazener et al.[2] used meta-analysis to determine the relative risk (RR) of treatment failure or relapse in the intervention versus the control group and used the graphical display common to Cochrane reviews to summarize their findings (Figure 19.1). It is useful to learn how to interpret these figures as they provide much information at a quick glance.

First, focus on the far left column. Looking down you will see a row for each of the five studies included in this comparison, referenced by the name of the first author and year the study was done. The list begins with the study by Bollard (1981a) and ends with the study by Wagner (1985). Looking along each study (row), we see a shaded box with a horizontal line through it. We can determine whether an intervention is more or less effective than its comparator without reading the actual numbers. In each row, the box indicates the summary statistic of the particular study: in this case, the box represents the RR, and the horizontal line indicates the 95%

Review: Alarm interventions for nocturnal enuresis in children
Comparison: 01 ALARM vs CONTROL
Outcome: 04 Numbers not achieving 14 dry nights or relapsing

Study	Treatment n/N	Control n/N	Relative Risk (Fixed) 95 % CI	Weight (%)	Relative Risk (Fixed) 95% CI
01 alarm vs control					
Bollard 1981a[1]	7/15	15/15		18.8	0.47 [0.27, 0.80]
Bollard 1981b[2]	10/20	20/20		25.0	0.50 [0.32, 0.78]
Sloop 1973[3]	14/21	20/21		25.0	0.70 [0.51, 0.96]
Wagner 1982[4]	7/12	12/12		15.0	0.58 [0.36, 0.94]
Wagner 1985[5]	7/13	13/13		16.3	0.54 [0.33, 0.89]
Subtotal (95% CI)	81	81		100.0	0.56 [0.46, 0.68]

Total events: 45 (Treatment), 80 (Control)
Test for heterogeneity chi-square = 2.61, df = 4, p = 0.62, I^2 = 0.0%
Test for overall effect z = 5.73, p < 0.00001

0.2   0.5   1   2   5
favours alarm   favours control

Figure 19.1 Graphical display of results of meta-analysis. Reproduced with permission of John Wiley & Sons and Catherine Glazener from Glazener CM, Evans JH, Peto RE. Alarm interventions for nocturnal enuresis in children. *Cochrane Database Syst Rev* 2005;(2):CD002911.

[1] Bollard J, Nettelbeck T. A comparison of dry-bed training and standard urine-alarm conditioning treatment of childhood bedwetting. *Behaviour Research & Therapy* 1981;**19**(3):215–26.

[2] Bollard J. A 2-year follow-up of bedwetters treated by dry-bed training and standard conditioning. *Behaviour Research & Therapy* 1982;**20**(6):571–80.

[3] Sloop EW, Kennedy WA. Institutionalized retarded nocturnal enuretics treated by a conditioning technique. *American Journal of Mental Deficiency* 1973;**77**(6): 717–21.

[4] Wagner W, Johnson SB, Walker D, Carter R, Wittner J. A controlled comparison of two treatments for nocturnal enuresis. *Journal of Pediatrics* 1982;**101**(2): 302–307.

[5] Wagner WG, Matthews R. The treatment of nocturnal enuresis: a controlled comparison of two models of urine alarm. *Journal of Developmental & Behavioral Pediatrics* 1985;**6**(1):22–6.

confidence interval (CI) around that RR. Recall that an RR of 1 means that there is no difference in the event rates of the treatment and control groups for treatment failure or relapse; the risks are the same. An RR on the right side of the vertical line representing 1 (i.e. an RR >1) would favour the control condition (i.e. fewer children in the control group with treatment failures or relapses), and an RR on the left side of the vertical line would favour the treatment (i.e. fewer children in the treatment group with treatment failures or relapses).

Readers can get an idea of the heterogeneity of the study results simply by looking at the extent to which the lines are scattered. In this case, the results of each of the five studies are on the left side of 1 – that is, all estimates of RR were <1, and the CIs overlapped considerably. If the boxes for different studies were on both sides of 1 and had non-overlapping CIs, you would have less confidence in using the results of this review in a clinical decision. Applying this information, the study in the first row by Bollard (1981a) has an associated RR on the left side of 1, indicating that fewer children in the alarm group had treatment failures or relapses than children in the control group. Because the CI does not cross the vertical line (i.e. does not include 1), this difference is statistically significant. Looking down the list, all five studies reported a statistically significant reduction in treatment failures when alarms were used.

The result of combining all five studies is found at the bottom of Figure 19.1. The overall summary statistic, in this case the combined RR, is depicted as a diamond, which also encompasses the 95% CI. The edges of the diamond do not cross or touch 1, indicating a statistically significant difference in favour of alarms. When outcomes are *dichotomous* (e.g. alive or dead, dry or wet), meta-analyses generally use RRs or odds ratios as the summary statistic; alternatively, when outcomes are *continuous* (e.g. blood pressure, blood glucose concentrations, or weight), the summary statistic is the *mean effect size* or *mean difference*.[8] Each of these statistics may be weighted or unweighted. When the mean effect size or mean difference is reported, the vertical line of no difference is at 0 rather than 1.

Although the summary statistic is the most important bottom line, more can be learned from Figure 19.1. The second column from the left (Treatment *n*/N) gives the number in the treatment group who experienced the outcome of interest (treatment failure or relapse) (*n*) out of the total number in the treatment (alarm) group (N). The third column (Control *n*/N) gives the same information for the control group in each study. The fifth column of numbers (Weight %) tells us how much a particular study contributed to the overall summary statistic, with more weight given to studies of greater precision. The column on the far right – Relative Risk (fixed) 95% CI – provides the RRs and accompanying 95% CIs for each individual study corresponding to the box and horizontal line for that study.

You can also calculate other summary statistics, such as the relative risk reduction (RRR) and number needed to treat (NNT), using the estimates provided in Figure 19.1. The structured abstracts included in some of the evidence-based synopsis journals (e.g. *Evidence-Based Nursing*) usually include these statistics. Chapters 11, 12 and 17 explain these measures of effect in detail.

In Figure 19.1, we see that the summary RR is 0.56, 95% CI 0.46 to 0.68. We can calculate the RRR by subtracting the RR from 1 (i.e. 1 − 0.56 = 0.44 or 44%). In a similar way, we can calculate the 95% CI around the RRR: 1 − 0.46 = 0.54 or 54% and 1 − 0.68 = 0.32 or 32%. That is, the 95% CI around the RRR of 42% is 32% to 54%, indicating that the true RRR may be as low as 32% or as large as

54%). The NNT to prevent one additional treatment failure or relapse for alarms versus usual care was 3 (95% CI 2 to 4). In other words, to prevent one additional treatment failure or relapse (i.e. not achieving 14 consecutive dry nights or relapsing after treatment completion), you would need to treat three children with alarms, and we are 95% certain that the true NNT may be as low as two children and as high as four children. One of the limitations of using NNTs derived from meta-analyses is that the patients in individual trials may vary considerably – particularly in terms of how susceptible they were to the outcome of interest.[7] In many reviews, the length of follow-up varies across the primary studies, making the NNT difficult to interpret. In the analysis shown in Figure 19.1, length of follow-up was not reported in one study and varied from 44 days to 12 months in the other four studies. Furthermore, decisions about whether or not to use enuresis alarms would also involve consideration of risks, costs, and patient preference and acceptability.

How precise is the estimate of treatment effect?

As described in Chapter 11, CIs around the RR and the RRR indicate the *precision* of the estimate of the true treatment effect, which can never be really known. Wide CIs indicate less precision in the estimate. The convention is to use the 95% CI, which represents the range within which we are 95% certain that the true value lies. Precision increases with larger sample sizes, although this is difficult to see in our example of the review by Glazener et al.[2] because the five studies had similar sample sizes (range 24 to 42 children).

The CI for the summary RR is fairly narrow (0.46 to 0.68).[2] The CI is useful for decision-making because we can look at the limit closest to 1 (no effect) and ask ourselves: *If the effect was as small as this, would it be worthwhile?* In the review by Glazener et al.[2] the risk, or probability, of treatment failure or relapse in the alarm group is 56% of the risk of treatment failure or relapse in the control group. The 95% CI indicates that the true risk of treatment failure or relapse in the alarm group may be only 46% of the risk in the control group, or the risk may be as high as 68%. To determine your confidence in adopting the intervention, you should consider the boundary of the CI closest to 1. If the risk of treatment failure or relapse in the alarm group really is almost 70% of the risk in the control group, would you still want to implement the intervention, given its cost, inconvenience, and side effects?

Can I apply the results in practice?

Are my patients so different from those in the studies included in the review that the results don't apply?

As when evaluating a treatment assessed in an individual trial (Chapter 15), you need to consider the characteristics of the patients in the individual studies included in a review, and the extent to which they are similar to your own patients. Why might the results not be applicable to your patients? In the five trials included in Figure 19.1, participants were somewhat more likely to be boys and ranged in age from 6 to 16 years[2] and so are similar to some of the patients you see in your clinic. The review should also provide sufficient details about the intervention to enable implementation in your own setting.

Is the treatment feasible in my setting?

Use of nocturnal alarms seems a clinically feasible intervention in terms of the ability of care providers to recommend alarm systems. Feasibility for this scenario, however, would relate to the ability of parents to either buy the alarm system or have it provided to them.

Were all clinically important outcomes (harms as well as benefits) considered?

Researchers try to look at both positive and negative outcomes that are important to patients and the health care system. Such outcomes might include mortality, morbidity, quality of life, patient satisfaction, and cost-effectiveness. Data on harm may not be systematically collected and fully reported in primary studies, and few systematic reviews of treatments undertake thorough searches for the relevant harm data that are likely to be reported in cohort studies. Glazener *et al.*[2] simply described different outcomes that were reported in 13 primary studies, such as alarm malfunction, false alarms, fright, failure to awaken the child, and awakening others. Costs were not reported. This review did not incorporate a formal economic evaluation, although they did provide a cost estimate based on the British National Formulary of £33.60 for an alarm (including batteries and sensors); sensors would need replacing after each wetting (£12/sensor).

What are my patient's values and preferences for both the outcome we are trying to prevent and the side effects that may arise?

Each family will have to decide if the potential benefits of dry nights (e.g. a child's positive feelings about himself and reduced bed changes and laundry) are worth the cost of the alarm and the potential effects of loss of sleep for the child and the rest of the family. Clinicians can recommend the use of alarms based on potential benefits, but informal cost–benefit considerations will also figure into the decision-making of families.

Resolution of the clinical scenario

Before answering the question in the scenario, we must now ask ourselves *Is this a good review?* Our assessment based on the criteria summarized in Box 19.1 suggests that the answer is 'yes'. Glazener *et al.*[2] addressed clear, focused questions; did a fairly extensive search for studies; included randomized and quasi-randomized trials; applied pre-defined inclusion, exclusion and validity criteria; and did a meta-analysis to calculate RRs and odds ratios for most of the main outcomes. The review found that alarms reduce non-organic nocturnal enuresis more than no treatment in children. As a clinician, you feel quite confident in letting families know that alarms have the potential to help reduce enuresis, while also informing them of the potential negative outcomes (i.e. costs, failed alarms, sleep interruptions) with less certainty.

LEARNING EXERCISES

1. With two or three colleagues, search for a systematic review on a topic of interest in PubMed, using 'Clinical Queries' and 'Find Systematic Reviews'. Each of you should try to find a review

that includes a 'blobogram' (i.e. a graphical presentation of results similar to that shown in Figure 19.1). Practise interpreting the findings from the 'blobograms' before you read the conclusions of the review. Does your interpretation match that of the authors?
2. See if you can find more than one review on a given topic. Use the critical appraisal criteria in Box 19.1 to decide which is the strongest review. Explain why you would have more confidence in that review.

References

1 Review: alarm interventions reduce nocturnal enuresis in children. *Evidence-Based Nursing* 2001;4:110. Abstract of Glazener CMA, Evans JHC. Alarm interventions for nocturnal enuresis in children. *Cochrane Database Syst Rev* 2001;(1):CD002911.
2 Glazener CM, Evans JH, Peto RE. Alarm interventions for nocturnal enuresis in children. *Cochrane Database Syst Rev* 2005;(2):CD002911.
3 Sackett DL, Strauss SE, Richardson WS, Rosenberg W, Haynes RB. *Evidence-Based Medicine. How to Practice and Teach EBM.* Second edition. London: Churchill Livingstone, 2000.
4 DiCenso A, Guyatt G, Ciliska D, editors. *Evidence-Based Nursing: A Guide to Clinical Practice.* St. Louis: Elsevier Mosby, 2005.
5 Egger M, Smith GD. Bias in location and selection of studies. *BMJ* 1998;316:61–6.
6 Kunz R, Oxman AD. The unpredictability paradox: review of empirical comparisons of randomised and non-randomised clinical trials. *BMJ* 1998;317:1185–90.
7 Smeeth L, Haines A, Ebrahim S. Numbers needed to treat derived from meta-analyses – sometimes informative, usually misleading. *BMJ* 1999;318:1548–51.
8 Sheldon T. Estimating treatment effects: real or the result of chance? *Evidence-Based Nursing* 2000;3:36–9.

Additional resources

Books

DiCenso A, Guyatt G, Ciliska D, editors. *Evidence-Based Nursing: A Guide to Clinical Practice.* St. Louis: Elsevier Mosby, 2005.
McKibbon A, Eady A, Marks S. *PDQ Evidence-Based Principles and Practice.* Hamilton: BC Decker Inc, 1999.

Articles

Greenhalgh T. Papers that summarise other papers (systematic reviews and meta-analyses). *BMJ* 1997;315:672–5.
Oxman AD, Cook DJ, Guyatt GH, for the Evidence-Based Medicine Working Group. Users' guides to the medical literature. VI How to use an overview. *JAMA* 1994;272:1367–71.

Online resources

BMJ series: www.bmj.com/cgi/content/full/315/7109/672
Centre for Health Evidence. Users' guides to evidence-based practice. www.cche.net/principles/content_all.asp
National Health Service. Critical Appraisal Skills Program and Evidence-Based Practice. 10 questions to help you make sense of reviews. http://www.phru.nhs.uk/casp/critical_appraisal_tools.htm#s/reviews

Chapter 20

EVALUATION OF STUDIES OF SCREENING TOOLS AND DIAGNOSTIC TESTS

Andrew Jull

Nursing gives constant attention to difference. Assessment and screening are integral to this activity. Studies evaluating screening tools and diagnostic tests are increasing in number, but the quality of many studies remains poor.[1] Thus, nurses should be able to critically appraise evidence from such studies to ensure that the highest quality tools are used. In this chapter, we outline a framework[2] to critique a study evaluating a screening tool for depression. The aim of any screening instrument is to quickly identify cases that would benefit from further investigation. This differs from the aim of a diagnostic test, which is to 'rule in' or 'rule out' a differential diagnosis, or if 'ruling in' the diagnosis, to shift a person's probability over a threshold so that practitioners can recommend a treatment or treatment options. However, the framework outlined here can also be applied to studies of diagnostic tests.

Clinical scenario

> You have recently read an article that suggests home health nurses have considerable difficulty in identifying patients with depression.[3] This ability varied by level of experience, but overall performance was low. These findings confirm your own observations, and you begin to give some thought to whether your district nursing service should screen new patients for depression. You decide that a first step would be to identify whether there are any screening instruments that could be used in your setting.

The search

Constructing a clinical question for screening tools and diagnostic tests using the PICO format is not too dissimilar to building a question for intervention studies (Chapter 15). The proposed test is the Intervention (or exposure), if it is known (see Box 20.1); otherwise a broad search term can be used. It is not strictly necessary to identify the comparison test for the search; this is especially the case for areas such as mental health where there may be more than one reference test or *gold standard* for

Box 20.1 Clinical question

> Population: community-dwelling patients
> Intervention: screening tools
> Comparison: gold standard or other reference test
> Outcome: improved identification of depression

Box 20.2 Screening questions for depression

> - During the past month have you often been bothered by feeling down, depressed, or hopeless? (yes/no)
> - During the past month have you often been bothered by little interest or pleasure in doing things? (yes/no)
> - Is this something with which you would like help? (yes/yes, but not today/no)

Box 20.3 Critical appraisal questions for studies of screening tools and diagnostic tests

> **Are the results of the study valid?**
> - Was there an independent blind comparison with a reference (gold) standard of diagnosis?
> - Was the diagnostic test evaluated in an appropriate spectrum of patients (similar to those we would meet in clinical practice)?
> - Was the reference standard applied regardless of the test results?
> - Was the test validated in a second, independent group of patients?
>
> **What are the results?**
> **Can I apply this test in practice?**
> - Is the test available, affordable, accurate, and precise in my setting?
> - Can we generate clinically sensible estimates of patients' pretest probabilities?
> - Will the resulting post-test probabilities affect patient management?

comparison. Questions about the effectiveness of screening tools are best answered by cross-sectional studies. Such studies can be quite difficult to locate, but the key-word phrase 'sensitivity and specificity' is useful, as is the subheading /di (for diagnosis). You do the following search on MEDLINE (OVID):

1. Depression/di
2. Depressive disorder/di
3. Primary health care
4. Family practice
5. Community health services
6. 1 OR 2
7. (3 or 4 or 5) AND 6

The search identifies 567 articles. Limiting the search to full-text English language papers published in the past five years produces a more manageable 60 citations. One of the citations identified is a study of the performance of a previously validated, two-question instrument[4] when an additional 'help' question is added.[5] The authors, Arroll *et al.*, concluded that the tool was useful and that the addition of a 'help' question (see Box 20.2) decreased the number of false positives. However, you need to reassure yourself that the study is valid, and begin to review the questions for critically appraising studies of screening tools and diagnostic tests that are summarized in Box 20.3.

Are the results of the study valid?

Was there an independent blind comparison with a reference (gold) standard of diagnosis?

There are two aspects to this question. First, the accuracy of any tool is best determined by comparing its results with those obtained from a widely accepted reference test. This is also referred to as a *gold standard* test. Thus, palpating a child's forehead for fever could be compared with a reading from a mercury thermometer to obtain a true estimation as to whether a child has a major fever. There are times when a gold standard may not exist, or the gold standard may be so invasive that comparisons using such a test are unlikely. On such occasions, the reference standard should be a widely accepted test that has well-defined attributes and is likely to be superior to the instrument being evaluated. It is not enough that the test simply be widely accepted. For instance, comparing palpation with a widely used measure that is less accurate than a mercury thermometer (e.g. tympanic thermometry) would provide an inaccurate estimation of how many patients actually had a fever.[6] Even if the study used a mercury thermometer or a device with similar accuracy, readers must still be reassured that an acceptable technique of thermometry was applied. For example, using mercury thermometry via an axillary route is likely to provide an unreliable estimate of temperature. If >1 assessor was used, the study should also provide an estimate of the level of agreement between assessors. In Arroll *et al.*, the reference test used to diagnose depression was the Composite International Diagnostic Interview (CIDI). CIDI is a standardized tool developed by the World Health Organization for use in research to diagnose mental disorders according to ICD-10 and DSM-IIIR criteria. Only one assessor was used to complete the CIDI, and therefore an assessment of inter-rater agreement was not necessary.

The second aspect of the question guards against *expectation bias*. It is important, when evaluating an instrument, that clinicians form their own views of a participant's condition, without knowledge of the results of previous tests or the views of colleagues. Prior knowledge can influence an assessment. Unblinded assessments can overestimate correct diagnoses by as much as 30% compared with blinded assessments.[7] Therefore, it is imperative that clinicians making an assessment using the gold standard or reference test are kept separate from those using the other instrument, and that the two groups of clinicians are not aware of each other's assessments. In the study by Arroll *et al.*, there was only one assessor. However, participant questionnaires were self-administered, so the assessor was kept blind to participant responses until the questionnaires had been completed. Evaluation of participant responses was completed by the investigators. This method is common in screening tests for mental health problems.[8–10]

Was the diagnostic test evaluated in an appropriate spectrum of patients (similar to those we would meet in clinical practice)?

The main challenge when evaluating a screening instrument is to apply it to the indicated population.[11] Tests are often developed using an accessible population of patients known to have the target disorder and a group of healthy controls. For example, the normal values of an Ankle Brachial Pressure Index were established by testing 110 patients with known occlusive peripheral arterial disease and comparing their test values with those of 25 healthy controls.[12] If an instrument does not discriminate between those with and without the disorder at this stage, then it is unlikely to be clinically useful. But, the value of an instrument lies in its ability to distinguish those that have the disorder in the full spectrum of patients in a clinical setting. In terms of assessment, it is easier to identify patients with florid presentation from those without the condition than from those with a mild presentation. A screening instrument can only be useful if it can differentiate between those likely to have the disorder and those who do not have the disorder in a real clinical population. In order to evaluate this ability, studies should enrol consecutive participants to minimize the potential for selection bias and enhance generalizability. Arroll *et al.* approached 1094 consecutive patients attending six general practice clinics (19 general practitioners). The inclusion criteria were very inclusive: participants were only excluded if they currently had a prescription for a psychoactive drug or withheld consent. Consent was obtained in the waiting room, and 1025 patients consented to participate; 89 patients were excluded based on the criterion for psychoactive drug prescription. The participation rate was high at 86% (936/1094).

Was the reference standard applied regardless of the test results?

To avoid *verification* or *workup bias*, participants need to receive both tests regardless of the outcome of the first test. If the first test is negative, and the participant does not receive the gold standard test to verify this result, then the study results will be distorted.[7] In some instances, participants who have a negative test may decide not to have the gold standard test, especially if the gold standard test is an invasive procedure.[13] Test results may also be uninterpretable.[14] Rather than exclude such participants, investigators can follow them up over an appropriate time period and monitor for symptoms of the target disorder. In the study by Arroll *et al.*, all consenting participants completed both tests, including people who were already receiving psychoactive drugs; this latter group was then excluded from the analysis.

Was the test validated in a second, independent group of patients?

For readers to be reassured that study findings are not the result of idiosyncrasies in the initial cohort of participants or the individual skills of assessors, the tool should be evaluated in a second, independent group of patients.[2] If the findings are replicated, health care providers can have more confidence in the accuracy of the test results.

For example, initial investigation of the CRAFFT test to screen for substance abuse in 99 adolescents was promising but required validation in a larger sample.[15] The tool was later validated in a study of 538 patients in a young adult medical practice.[10] The study by Arroll et al.[5] is the validation of a two-question screening instrument that had only previously been tested in an outpatient clinic population.[4] The investigators included an extra question to reduce false positives, and this question had not been previously validated, nor was it validated in a second sample by Arroll et al. We would therefore be more reassured if we found a study replicating the instrument including Arroll's extra question.

What are the results?

All of us, at any given point in time, have a probability of having particular disorders. This probability is the baseline prevalence of each disorder in the community. But we are all different. Think about two patients, both presenting with a small leg ulcer involving the medial malleolus, with ankle flare, presence of haemosiderin pigmentation, and a history of varicose veins. One patient is a 71-year-old woman, who is otherwise healthy, and the second is a 55-year-old man with type 2 diabetes. Although venous aetiology accounts for up to 70% of all leg ulcers,[16] an experienced nurse knows that the *baseline or pretest probability* of the ulcer having a purely venous aetiology in these two patients is different. For the 71-year-old woman with an uncomplicated presentation, the pretest probability of having a venous ulcer is likely to be between 50% and 70%. Following simple assessments (e.g. measurement of the ratio of ankle:brachial pressure index) of her blood supply to rule out other causes, an experienced nurse is likely to recommend that the patient start compression treatment. Alternatively, the pretest probability for venous ulceration is likely to be considerably lower in the 55-year-old man with type 2 diabetes. Venous disease is present in only 6–9% of leg ulcers in patients with diabetes.[17] Simple assessments to rule out other causes of the ulcer may not convince the clinician that the ulcer is venous. Treatment for venous ulceration involves applying high compression bandaging to the affected limb, but the bandaging can create an ischaemic leg or foot if the patient has arterial insufficiency (more common in diabetes). The clinical hazard of misdiagnosis and ischaemia has increased the threshold for beginning treatment, and the low pretest probability means that the nurse may prefer to refer this patient for further testing before being reassured that compression is safe.

The above example shows that, no matter what the outcome of an assessment or test is, it cannot tell a nurse whether a patient does or does not have the disorder. It can only reveal the probability of having or not having the disorder.[18] The ability of a test to discriminate between people more likely to have a disorder and those less likely to have a disorder is determined by its *likelihood ratio (LR)*. The reference test in the study by Arroll et al. indicated that 47 patients had depression. Answering 'yes' to the 'help' question and one other question correctly identified 45 of these 47 patients (45/47 or 0.96) as being likely to be depressed. However, the instrument also incorrectly classified 94 patients as being likely to be depressed from the 889 patients whom the reference test ruled out as not depressed (94/889 or 0.11) (Table 20.1). The ratio between these two likelihoods is the LR. When considering LRs, it is the percentages or proportions of patients that the instrument correctly and incorrectly identifies as having the disorder that is considered, not the actual

Table 20.1 Results of a two-question tool as a case-finding instrument for depression. Table created using data from Arroll *et al.* 2005[5]

Test results	Depression		Likelihood ratio
	Present	Absent	
Present	0.96	0.11	8.7
Absent	0.04	0.89	0.04
Total	1.00	1.00	—

Table 20.2 Size of likelihood ratios (LRs) and associated utility of changes in probability. Table created using data from Jaeschke *et al.* 2002[18]

Size of LRs	Utility
+LR > 10 or –LR < 0.1	Generates large changes from pretest to post-test probability
+LR 5 to 10 or –LR 0.1 to 0.2	Generates moderate shifts in pretest to post-test probability
+LR 2 to 5 or –LR 0.2 to 0.5	Generates small changes in pretest to post-test probability
+LR 1 to 2 or –LR 0.5 to 1	Generates little or no shift in pretest to post-test probability

numbers of patients. Thus, the ratio of true positive results (i.e. those that the instrument correctly identifies as being depressed) to false positive results (i.e. those that the instrument incorrectly identifies as being depressed) is 0.96/0.11, or 8.7. This is the *likelihood ratio for a positive test result (+LR)* being correct. From the +LR of 8.7, we can infer that a positive result from the 'help' question and one other question is about nine times more likely to be a true-positive than a false-positive result.

Just as the +LR can be calculated, the likelihood of the instrument being wrong when it returns a negative result can also be calculated. The screening questions missed two of the 47 depressed patients (2/45 or 0.04) but correctly identified 795 patients as being unlikely to be depressed out of the 889 patients (795/889 or 0.89) in which depression was absent. The ratio of false-negative results (i.e. those that the instrument incorrectly identifies as not being depressed) to true-negative results (i.e. those that the instrument correctly identifies as not being depressed) is 0.04/0.89, or 0.04. This is the *likelihood ratio for a negative test result (–LR)* being wrong. From the –LR of 0.04, we can infer that very few patients are likely to be depressed when the screening instrument returns a negative result.

The usefulness of LRs is revealed when we look at their ability to shift a patient from a pretest probability to a *post-test probability*. In doing so, the results help reduce the clinical uncertainty associated with screening or diagnosis. A rough guide to the magnitude of LRs and their effects on post-test probability is shown in Table 20.2.

The challenge of working out the changes in probability of a patient having a disorder after a test is eased by the use of a simple nomogram (Figure 20.1).[19] By running a straight line through the pretest probability (left-hand column) and the LR (centre column), the post-test probability can be determined from the point at which the line intersects the right-hand column. A pretest probability could simply be the prevalence of depression in the community, which has been estimated to be 5% of the adult population.[20] If the patient in our scenario answers 'yes' both to the

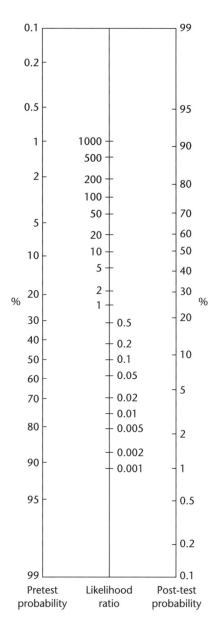

Figure 20.1 Nomogram for determining post-test probabilities.[19] Copyright © 1975 Massachusetts Medical Society. All rights reserved.

'help' question and to one of the other questions, we can extend a line from a pretest probability of 5% through approximately 9 (+LR 8.7) on the central line to obtain a post-test probability of about 30% that the patient actually has depression. However, if our patient answers 'no' to both questions, we can extend a line from 5% through 0.05 (−LR 0.04) to obtain a post-test probability of approximately 0.03% of being wrong if we accept that our patient is not depressed. Thus, we can be confident that if a patient does not answer 'yes' to the help question and one of the other questions, he or she is very unlikely to be depressed. On the other hand, a post-test probability of approximately 30% is high enough to consider referral for further testing.

Arroll *et al.* provided the LRs for the questions in their study. Older studies often do not report LRs, but instead report the sensitivity and specificity of the tests. The *sensitivity* of a test is the proportion of patients with the target disorder who have a positive test result, whereas the *specificity* is the proportion of patients without the target disorder who have a negative test result. LRs are easily obtained if the sensitivity and specificity of a test are known. The sensitivity and specificity of the screening instrument are 0.96 and 0.89, respectively. A +LR is obtained by the following formula:

sensitivity/(1 − specificity) or 0.96/(1 − 0.89) = 0.96/0.11 = 8.7

Similarly, the −LR can be obtained using a slightly different formula:

(1 − sensitivity)/specificity or (1 − 0.96)/0.89 = 0.04/0.89 = 0.04

Sometimes sensitivity and specificity are presented as percentages (i.e. 96% and 89%). The same formulas can be used, substituting 100 for 1 when subtracting. For further explanation of how sensitivity and specificity are calculated, consult any clinical epidemiology text.

Can I apply the test in practice?

We have determined that the study by Arroll *et al.* is valid and decided that the results indicate that the instrument (1) may be useful for identifying patients who may benefit from referral for further testing when the patient responds positively to the questions, and (2) is useful for ruling out depression when the patient responds negatively to the questions. The next step is to determine whether it can be used with your own group of patients.

Is the test available, affordable, accurate, and precise in my setting?

LRs can be stable, but they are derived from selections of patients and thus may not be as accurate for patients who are selected in different ways. Therefore, we need to be assured that a test will maintain its accuracy in the clinical setting in which we work. In an earlier question about validity, we needed to be assured that the instrument was tested in patients with mild, moderate and severe conditions as well as those without the disorder. Now we need to be assured of the similarity of the study population to patients in our own setting. It is uncommon to find a report that describes a population of patients exactly like our own, so we need to examine the demographics of the study participants to decide whether they are so dissimilar to our own that we should rule out using the study. For instance, an earlier iteration of the screening instrument used in the study by Arroll *et al.* was validated in a population that had a high prevalence of depression (18%) and consisted mainly of US male veterans, two-thirds of whom were unemployed.[3] Arroll *et al.* did not report the demographics of their study population, so we can only presume a broad similarity between the patients that district nurses encounter and those seen in general practice. Given the high participation rate and the number of practices included in the study, this presumption seems quite safe. In order to test this presumption, the corresponding author can be (and was) contacted. The author's reply was that the average age of patients was 46 years (range 16–92 years), 73% were women, and ethnicity was predominantly New Zealand European (85%). The ethnic mix of the remaining participants was Maori, Pacific Island, Asian, or other (personal communication, Bruce Arroll). Again, there is no reason why this information should preclude application of the screening instrument to the populations encountered by district nurses.

When considering the accuracy of diagnostic tests as opposed to screening tools, another concern is that many instruments report only one +LR and one –LR, although a test can behave differently depending on the severity of the disorder. Higher LRs can be found with florid conditions and lower ones with earlier presentations of the disorder. For instance, a serum ferritin concentration ≤18 μ/l has a much higher LR (41.5) than serum ferritin concentrations >18–45 μ/l (3.12) for diagnosis of iron deficiency anaemia in elderly people.[14]

Can we generate clinically sensible estimates of patients' pretest probabilities?

Pretest probability is the probability that a presenting patient has a particular disorder. Sackett *et al.*[2] identify five different sources for estimating pretest probability: clinical experience, prevalence statistics, practice databases, studies specifically focused on determining pretest probabilities, and the original study itself. Clinical experience will generate what is essentially a 'guesstimate', and false heuristics may influence such an estimate. In the absence of other sources, this method can be employed. However, better sources are prevalence statistics drawn from regional or national morbidity data or from studies investigating the prevalence of a disorder. These estimates are only as good as the sources of the data or the settings of the prevalence studies. If a prevalence study is set in a referral centre, the results can be misleading if applied to primary care settings. Practice databases, whether local, regional, or national, are also only as good as their data sources. Reliance on voluntary reporting can deliver inaccurate data. Studies investigating pretest probabilities are few in number and difficult to retrieve. An alternative is to use the prevalence of the disorder reported in the study being critically appraised.

The prevalence of depression in Arroll *et al.* was 5% (47/936), which is similar to estimated rates in adult populations.[20] Therefore, it seems sensible to use 5% as a pretest probability, unless the patient has comorbidities that might increase the pretest probability. For example, a systematic review of prevalence studies of depression in people with diabetes found that the mean rate of current depression was 14% – almost three times that of the general population.[21]

Will the resulting post-test probabilities affect patient management?

The major concern here is whether the results will move a patient across a threshold that would stop further testing for the suspected disorder. This would occur when a disorder has been ruled out, when a referral for further testing or treatment is made, or when treatment is initiated. For example, if the pretest probability for depression is 5%, and a patient's response to the screening instrument is negative, the post-test probability of depression would be so low that that no further testing would be warranted. If a patient's response was positive (and remembering that the post-test probability was slightly >30%), it would still be too low to move the patient over a treatment threshold. However, referral for further investigation needs to be considered. On the other hand, if the pretest probability of depression was higher, as it would be in patients with diabetes, then referral for further investigation should be mandatory as the post-test probability would be about 60%.

Resolution of the clinical scenario

The study by Arroll *et al.* has reasonably strong validity, the setting seems broadly similar, and you have no reason to believe that the rate of depression in the population served by district nursing would be so dissimilar as to rule out using the results of the study. You suspect that the mean age of participants (46 years) is younger than you might expect in a district nursing population. However, the age range (16–92 years) seems applicable, and again, possible age differences do not seem a justifiable reason to rule out the study. You resolve to raise the issue of screening for depression with your Practice Development Committee, with a view to implementing the tool used in the study by Arroll *et al.* You also start to consider plans for implementation and what additional information might be necessary to support such planning. You decide to canvass your colleagues for their views on the common diseases encountered in their practices. This will help you to identify additional diseases for which you may need to identify pretest probabilities.

LEARNING EXERCISES

1. Calculate the positive and negative likelihood ratios for a test with a sensitivity of 96% and specificity of 89%.
2. Using the likelihood ratios from exercise 1 and the nomogram in Figure 20.1, determine the post-test probabilities for a positive test on following range of prevalences: 5%, 12%, 23%.

Solutions to learning exercises
1. +LR 8.7, −LR 0.04
2. 31%, 54%, 72%

References

1 Reid MC, Lachs MS, Feinstein AR. Use of methodological standards in diagnostic test research. Getting better but still not good. *JAMA* 1995;**274**:645–51.
2 Sackett DL, Straus SE, Richardson WS, Rosenberg W, Haynes RB. *Evidence-Based Medicine. How to Practice and Teach EBM.* Second edition. London: Churchill Livingstone, 2000.

3 Brown E, McAvay G, Raue PJ, Moses S, Bruce ML. Recognition of depression among elderly recipients of home care services. *Psychiatr Serv* 2003;**54**:208–13.

4 Whooley MA, Avins AL, Miranda J, Browner WS. Case-finding instruments for depression. Two questions are as good as many. *J Gen Inter Med* 1997;**12**:439–45.

5 Arroll B, Goodyear-Smith F, Kerse N, Fishman T, Gunn J. Effect of addition of a "help" question to two screening questions on specificity for diagnosis of depression in general practice: diagnostic validity study. *BMJ* 2005;**331**:884–6.

6 Jensen BN, Jensen FS, Madsen SN, Lossl K. Accuracy of digital tympanic, oral, axillary, and rectal thermometers compared with standard rectal mercury thermometers. *Eur J Surg* 2000;**166**:848–51.

7 Lijmer JG, Mol BW, Heisterkamp S, Bonsel GJ, Prins MH, van der Meulen JH, Bossuyt PM. Empirical evidence of design-related bias in studies of diagnostic tests. *JAMA* 1999;**282**:1061–6.

8 Cotton MA, Ball C, Robinson P. Four simple questions can help screen for eating disorders. *J Gen Intern Med* 2003;**18**:53–6.

9 Luck AJ, Morgan JF, Reid F, O'Brien A, Brunton J, Price C, Perry L, Lacey JH. The SCOFF questionnaire and clinical interview for eating disorders in general practice: comparative study. *BMJ* 2002;**325**:755–6.

10 Knight JR, Sherritt L, Shrier LA, Harris SK, Chang G. Validity of the CRAFFT substance abuse screening instrument among adolescent clinic patients. *Arch Pediatr Adolesc Med* 2002;**156**:607–14.

11 van der Schouw YT, Verbeek AL, Ruijs SH. Guidelines for the assessment of new diagnostic tests. *Invest Radiol* 1995;**30**:334–40.

12 Yao ST, Hobbs JT, Irvine WT. Ankle systolic pressure measurements in arterial disease affecting the lower extremities. *Br J Surg* 1969;**56**:676–9.

13 The PIOPED Investigators. Value of the ventilation/perfusion scan in acute pulmonary embolism. Results of the Prospective Investigation of Pulmonary Embolism Diagnosis (PIOPED). *JAMA* 1990;**263**:2753–9.

14 Guyatt GH, Patterson C, Ali M, Singer J, Levine M, Turpie I, Meyer R. Diagnosis of iron-deficiency anemia in the elderly. *Am J Med* 1990;**88**:205–9.

15 Knight JR, Shrier LA, Bravender TD, Farrell M, Van der Bilt J, Shaffer HJ. A new brief screen for adolescent substance abuse. *Arch Pediatr Adolesc Med* 1999;**153**:591–6.

16 Nelzen O, Bergqvist D, Lindhagen A. Venous and non-venous leg ulcers: clinical history and appearance in a population study. *Br J Surg* 1994;**81**:182–7.

17 Baker SR, Stacey MC, Jopp-McKay AG, Hoskin SE, Thompson PJ. Epidemiology of chronic venous ulcers. *Br J Surg* 1991;**78**:864–7.

18 Jaeschke R, Guyatt G, Lijmer J. Diagnostic tests. In: Guyatt G, Rennie D, editors. *Users' Guides to the Medical Literature. A Manual for Evidence-Based Clinical Practice.* Chicago: American Medical Association, 2002;121–40.

19 Fagan TJ. Letter: Nomogram for Bayes theorem. *N Engl J Med* 1975;**293**:257.

20 Ohayon MM, Priest RG, Guilleminault C, Caulet M. The prevalence of depressive disorders in the United Kingdom. *Biol Psychiatry* 1999;**45**:300–7.

21 Gavard JA, Lustman PJ, Clouse RE. Prevalence of depression in adults with diabetes. An epidemiological evaluation. *Diabetes Care* 1993;**16**:1167–78.

Chapter 21

EVALUATION OF STUDIES OF HEALTH ECONOMICS

Deborah Braccia, Suzanne Bakken and Patricia W. Stone

As health care technology continues to expand, the cost of using all effective clinical services exceeds available resources. Due to the scarcity of resources, decisions about the implementation of new services are often based on economic evidence. Economic evidence seeks to inform resource allocation decisions, such as those made by health care providers and funders, guideline developers, and individual practitioners. Unfortunately, not all economic evidence is high quality. To determine whether economic evidence provides a sound basis for decision-making, nurses need to apply the critical appraisal questions summarized in Box 21.1.

Box 21.1 Critical appraisal questions for economic evaluations

Are the results valid?
- Is the appropriate economic evaluation method used?
- Are the alternative courses of action appropriate and well-defined?
- Is the perspective of the analysis stated, and are appropriate costs considered?
- If cost-utility analysis methods are used, are the utilities (patient preferences) reasonable?
- Are the events used comprehensive, and are the probabilities of events derived from credible sources?
- Are data on costs and outcomes appropriately discounted?
- Is uncertainty in the data adequately addressed?

What are the results of the economic evaluation?
- How do the resulting costs or costs per unit of health gained compare with other interventions?
- Are the conclusions likely to change with sensible changes in costs and outcomes? (i.e. are the results robust?)

Can I apply the results in practice?
- Do the costs in the report apply in my setting?
- Will the intervention (or new model of care) be effective in my setting?

Clinical scenario

You have recently completed a midwifery programme and joined a community-based birthing centre. The centre has been under increased pressure to cut costs. As a member of an interdisciplinary team charged with examining ways to reduce costs, you review a battery of tests to determine if routine screening tests used during the course of pregnancy are justified in terms of the current standard of care and existing evidence. You note that all pregnant women at your centre are routinely screened for hepatitis C virus. If a woman is found to be HCV positive, elective caesarean section is recommended as the delivery route in order to avert perinatal transmission. The standard of care at the institution in which you trained was to not screen asymptomatic pregnant women at low risk for hepatitis C infection.

At the next interdisciplinary team meeting, you bring up the difference in hepatitis C screening recommendations used by the centre and the institution in which you trained. Before making any changes to the battery of screening tests used by the centre, the team wants to know what evidence exists in the published literature about routine screening of asymptomatic, low-risk, pregnant women for hepatitis C virus. Specifically the questions are (1) Is hepatitis C virus screening justified in asymptomatic, low-risk pregnant women? and (2) Is hepatitis C virus screening of asymptomatic, low-risk pregnant women and elective caesarean section to avert perinatal transmission, cost-effective?

The team searches MEDLINE and CINAHL using the keywords 'costs', 'hepatitis C', 'pregnancy', and 'screening'. This search identifies a cost-effectiveness analysis by Plunkett and Grobman[1] that directly addresses the questions of interest. You retrieve the article and apply the critical appraisal questions summarized in Box 21.1.

Are the results of this economic evaluation valid?

Although the number of published economic evaluations is increasing,[2] many experts question the methodological rigour of these analyses.[3, 4] Therefore, it is important for nurses to be able to assess the validity of these complex analyses.

All rigorous economic evaluations consider *opportunity costs*, that is, the value of the benefit gained from using the resources for the next best alternative use. For example, the opportunity cost to a local health department of funding a community health screening programme for elderly people may be the benefits foregone of not being able to fund a prenatal programme for at-risk pregnant women (because the available resources were used to fund the elderly screening programme instead). As well as opportunity costs, economic evaluations should consider the *incremental* (i.e. extra) benefit that would be gained for the *incremental* (i.e. extra) *cost*. A classic example illustrating incremental cost and effectiveness is the sixth-stool guaiac test used to screen for colorectal cancer in people >40 years of age. The average cost per case of cancer detected using ≤5 tests has been calculated to be US$2541, but the incremental cost of the extra sixth test is estimated to be between US$47 and US$127 million.[5] This is because the probability of detecting an additional case of cancer with the sixth test (the incremental effectiveness) was so low that millions of dollars (the incremental costs) would be spent before identifying one more person with cancer.

Is the appropriate economic evaluation method used?

Five different analytic tools are commonly used to assess the economic impact of new and established health care interventions or technologies (Table 21.1). Briefly, costs

Table 21.1 Five different types of economic evaluations

Economic evaluation	Definition
Cost-effectiveness analysis (CEA)	An analytic tool in which incremental costs and effects are aggregated into a ratio, and effects are measured in a common natural unit
Cost–utility analysis (CUA)	A specific form of CEA in which effects are measured in dollars per quality adjusted life-years (QALY) gained
Cost–benefit analysis (CBA)	An analytic tool for estimating the net social benefit of a strategy and in which both costs and effects are measured in currency
Cost-minimization analysis (CMA)	An analytic tool for estimating the costs of strategies when the effects are equal
Cost–consequence analysis (CCA)	An analytic tool in which incremental costs and consequences are listed without any attempt to aggregate them

should be measured in the same way in all analyses; the methods differ in terms of how effects (outcomes) are measured. Each of the five methods will be discussed in further detail below.

Cost-effectiveness analysis

In *cost-effectiveness analysis*, the health outcomes of each alternative analysed must be reported in the same unit, such as life-years (LYs) gained or cases avoided. Additionally, costs and effects are summarized in a *cost–effectiveness ratio*, which is calculated using the following formula:

$$\text{Cost–effectiveness ratio} = (C_1 - C_2)/(E_1 - E_2)$$

where C_1 is the cost of the new intervention, C_2 is the cost of the comparator, E_1 is the effect of the new intervention, and E_2 is the effect of the comparator.

In cost-effectiveness analysis, analysts often use a *decision analytic approach* (i.e. a complex mathematical modelling technique) that captures the long-term costs and effectiveness.

An increasing number of cost-effectiveness analyses relevant to nursing have been published on topics such as the cost-effectiveness of neonatal nurse practitioners[6] and the cost-effectiveness of a free-standing birth centre.[7] However, like many published cost-effectiveness analyses, the methods used in these analyses have been found wanting due to their lack of adherence to methodological recommendations, such as using a standard outcome measure (e.g. costs per LY gained).[8]

An advantage of using a common unit for analysis is that comparisons can be made across groups or settings. Results of separate analyses from various health care settings can then, at least in theory, be compared across patient populations.[9, 10] However, a disadvantage of using cost per life-year gained is that one year of life in an altered health state is considered equal to any other year of life. Only length of survival is considered and not quality of life issues such as suboptimal health states (e.g. life with perfect health is valued the same as life with aphasia).

Cost–utility analysis

Cost–utility analysis is a special type of cost-effectiveness analysis that includes measures of both the quantity and quality of life. Outcome measures that consider both quality and quantity of life include disability-adjusted life-years (DALYs), healthy year equivalents (HYE), and quality-adjusted life-years (QALY), which are the most common. To compute QALYs, analysts value different health outcomes using *utilities* (also called *preference weights* or *quality adjustments*). The utilities are then multiplied by the amount of time experienced in a given health state. Utilities are generally measured on a scale from 0 to 1. Perfect health is given a value of 1 and death is given a value of 0. It is unrealistic to expect that a person would sustain the same quality of life consistently over time. People move in and out of health states. For example, a person has a stroke and then recovers. Individual QALYs are calculated by multiplying the time spent in each health state by the utility of that health state. These are then summed to arrive at an overall QALY. Some experts recommend using cost–utility analyses because they take into account both the quantity and quality of life and use a standardized measurement and therefore allow decision-makers to directly compare the efficiency of alternative ways of spending health care resources.[11–14]

Cost–benefit analysis

In *cost–benefit analysis*, outcomes are measured according to a monetary unit. A single currency figure, representing costs minus benefits, is calculated. The challenge with this approach is that many health care situations are difficult to quantify financially and require a value judgement. Furthermore, there are ethical concerns surrounding the assignment of a monetary amount to the value of human life.[15, 16] Because of these issues, the use of cost-effectiveness analysis and cost–utility analysis has been more prevalent in the health care literature than cost–benefit analysis.[3] An advantage of using cost–benefit analysis in health care is that the results can be compared with other areas of governmental investment (e.g. school education or transportation safety).

Cost-minimization analysis

The central assumption of a true *cost-minimization analysis* is that the competing interventions or strategies have equivalent health outcomes and therefore only the costs are compared. The decision then focuses on the selection of the least expensive strategy to achieve the same outcome. For example, a randomized trial compared an inpatient education programme and usual care in adults admitted to hospital with acute asthma.[17] The clinical outcomes were considered to be the same irrespective of the intervention, and the resources used (e.g. outpatient appointments, emergency department visits and hospitalizations) were calculated. In this case, the inpatient education programme was the least costly intervention. However, the circumstances under which cost-minimization analysis is an appropriate method of analysis are rare because there are few situations in which we can be confident that clinical outcomes are equivalent (i.e. few studies are adequately powered to detect such equivalence).

Cost–consequence analysis

In a *cost–consequence analysis*, the consequences of two or more alternatives are measured as well as the costs. The consequences of each alternative are listed, and decision-makers can form their own opinions about the relative importance of the findings. For example, researchers compared the outcomes and costs of a modified therapeutic community intervention with usual care in substance abusers who were homeless and mentally ill.[18] The incremental costs of the therapeutic community compared with usual care were calculated, and the outcomes of each model of care were listed. Conclusions about the choice of intervention based on costs and outcomes were left to readers, which is appropriate for this type of analysis.

Returning to the study by Plunkett and Grobman,[1] we see that the authors assessed the cost-effectiveness of routine hepatitis C virus screening in low-risk pregnant women. The report described the study as a cost-effectiveness analysis, but because the effects were measured in QALYs gained, the design can further be described as a cost–utility analysis, which is appropriate for the question.

Are the alternative courses of action appropriate and well defined?

When determining the validity of any economic evaluation, readers must decide if the strategies being analysed are appropriate and well defined. Consider, for example, a study to determine if a transprofessional care management approach produced savings in service delivery dollars compared with the traditional treatment approach for people with AIDS who were terminally ill and receiving home care.[19] The researchers did not identify any benefits in specific clinical outcome measures but did find an 8% reduction in average delivery costs for patients receiving transprofessional care management. Of key importance in this study was that the new intervention (i.e. transprofessional care management) was clearly described and appropriately compared with usual care.

Another mistake is to view an intervention as 'all or nothing'. For example, not all patients with a particular diagnosis need case management; instead, case management may be most cost-effective in patients at high risk for particular outcomes. However, such knowledge may not be gained unless the subpopulations with different risk levels are identified. In their evaluation of routine hepatitis C virus screening for pregnant women, Plunkett and Grobman[1] clearly specified the alternatives (no screening; screening and treatment; or screening, treatment, and elective caesarean section to avert perinatal transmission of hepatitis C virus), and the appropriate costs for each of the alternatives were considered in the analysis.

Is the perspective of the analysis stated, and are appropriate costs considered?

Table 21.2 lists some of the resources that are often measured in economic evaluations. When assessing costs, three components drive the measurement: (1) the

Table 21.2 Resources frequently measured in economic evaluations of health care

Direct health care	Direct non-health care
Intervention	Transportation
Hospitalization	Family/caregiver time
Outpatient visits	Social services
Long-term care	Patient productivity
Other health care	
Patient time receiving care	

perspective of the analysis, (2) the resources considered for that perspective, and (3) how the value (or cost) of the resources was determined.

The perspective of the analysis

The appropriate resources to consider vary depending on the perspective from which the analysis is conducted and the question being asked.[20, 21] For example, an intensive care unit manager may only be interested in costs incurred in the unit (e.g. resources consumed while patients are in the unit and length of stay in the unit). However, a hospital administrator would be interested in the resources used during the entire hospital stay. Often, both resources related to the intervention itself and those associated with net downstream health care utilization are of interest. For example, an insurer or national health care service would be interested in the direct costs associated with an initial hospitalization (e.g. resources related to supplies and staffing) as well as downstream resources used (e.g. readmissions to hospital, outpatient visits, and other treatments). Furthermore, when conducting an analysis from a *societal perspective*, costs and effects are included regardless of who accrues them. Therefore, non-health care resources are included.

Ideally, all economic evaluations should be conducted from a societal perspective. However, because of the difficulty of assessing societal perspectives and the specific concerns of decision-makers, analyses are often conducted using more narrow perspectives. The danger in using a narrow perspective is that costs may simply be shifted. For example, the cost savings related to a decreased length of hospital stay may be shifted to the family, in terms of extra caregiver burden. In the study by Plunkett and Grobman,[1] the authors clearly stated that the evaluation was conducted from the perspective of the health care system.

Valuing the resources or costs

Analysts value resources in different ways.[22, 23] It is important to note that in health care environments, charges generally do not equal true costs. Third-party payers negotiate payment for services rendered based on the cost of the service and an agreed profit margin. This occurs in both for-profit and not-for-profit institutions. In order for health care institutions to generate more revenue, fee-for-service customers are often asked to pay full charges (i.e. a higher rate of pay). This is called *institutional cost shifting*. Therefore, in the United States, many analysts use *cost-to-charge ratios*, which are calculated by dividing the total costs in a given cost centre by the total charges for the same resource. Cost-to-charge ratios are recognized as a gross adjustment to charges. They are better than using charges alone but not as accurate as cost accounting systems.

Additionally, because one dollar in 1980 does not have the same purchasing power as a current dollar, to be valid, the costs from different years must be calculated and placed into a standard year format. Standardization of all costs to the same currency and year is essential. Plunkett and Grobman[1] measured direct costs in 2003 US dollars and included pretest and post-test counselling, hepatitis C virus screening tests, and delivery.[1] Annual costs related to a diagnosis of hepatitis C, including stage of liver disease, treatment, liver transplantation, and hepatocellular carcinoma costs, were also provided.

If cost–utility analysis methods are used, are the utilities (patient preferences) reasonable?

Methods for eliciting utilities vary and are the focus of a unique body of science and research.[24–27] However, a systematic review concluded that the same, or a similar, health state is often valued differently (i.e. mild angina had a low value of 0.7 and a high value of 0.95), and values are often based on the opinion of researchers rather than rigorous assessments of patient or community-based preferences.[28] Therefore, careful attention is warranted when assessing preference weight scores and how they were derived. Increasingly, utilities are being collected for a variety of health states.[29, 30] Stated utility variables used in the study of hepatitis C virus screening included stages of liver disease, hepatocellular carcinoma, liver transplantation, and delivery methods. All utility variables were derived from the published literature, except for delivery methods. Because no utility scores for delivery methods were found in the published literature, scores were derived by a panel of five experts using the 'time trade-off' technique. Although use of community preferences is recommended over experts, the utility scores are reasonable.

Are the events used comprehensive, and are the probabilities of events derived from credible sources?

For each alternative (e.g. intervention) considered, there are probabilities of events occurring (e.g. the desired outcome and/or side effects). Decision-makers need to determine whether the events included in an economic evaluation are comprehensive; this can be accomplished by collaborating with clinical experts or (where relevant) by using their own clinical expertise. The reliability of the evidence should also be considered. Some economic evaluations are conducted alongside randomized controlled trials, whereas others are estimates based on previously published evidence (e.g. randomized controlled trials and meta-analyses). In addition, because an economic evaluation may include modelling of longer term outcomes, analysts often gather probabilities of these events from a variety of sources, including observational data.

In the study by Plunkett and Grobman,[1] the clinical events described were comprehensive, and the probabilities of these events were well documented. Probability values for disease progression, receipt of treatment for hepatitis C, delivery methods, and prenatal transmission were obtained from the published literature. For simplicity, the authors chose to enter all pregnant women into the model at age 30 years, and this was the only probability variable not derived from the published literature.

Are data on costs and outcomes appropriately discounted?

Once all costs and benefits have been calculated for an economic evaluation, future costs and benefits are *discounted to present value*. Discounting reflects the principles of time preference and opportunity costs. *Time preference* suggests that people place greater value on something they have today than on something they will have in the future. Interest rates reflect these same principles: if you forego the opportunity of buying something today and invest the money, you will enjoy a higher rate of return in the future. Therefore, future costs and benefits are discounted to present value using the formula $F/(1 + r)^n$, where F = the future value, r = the discount rate, and n = the number of years.[31] Currently, most experts recommend using a 3% discount rate for both costs and effects.[11] In the study by Plunkett and Grobman,[1] future costs and QALYs were converted into present value by discounting at a 3% annual rate.

Is uncertainty in the data adequately addressed?

Decision-making in health care is inevitably done in a context of uncertainty. Health economists undertake sensitivity analyses and construct cost-effectiveness acceptability curves to explore the impact of uncertainty in economic evaluations. This involves varying the value of important variables over a reasonable set of parameters[11, 32] and allows the investigator to determine what the results might be under different assumptions. For example, in a *univariate sensitivity analysis*, a parameter such as a utility weight is varied to determine the degree of influence that a particular variable (in this case, utility weight) has on the result of the analysis. Although univariate sensitivity analyses can be informative, looking at one variable alone is usually inadequate. *Multivariate sensitivity analysis* and *cost-effectiveness acceptability curves* examine multiple sources of uncertainty at the same time and can generate more accurate estimates of cost-effectiveness under varying conditions and, thus, better inform decision-makers. Assessing uncertainty is an important element of a sound economic evaluation. In the study of hepatitis C virus screening,[1] uncertainty in the model was adequately addressed using the sensitivity analyses and simulation trials on the Markov model.

What are the results of the economic evaluation?

Once it has been determined that the results of the economic analysis are likely to be valid (i.e. the study is an unbiased assessment), the clinical significance of the results should be determined. Nurses should consider whether an intervention will provide a benefit at an acceptable cost. For example, for a cost-minimization analysis, one should consider whether the difference in cost is sufficient to warrant switching from one intervention to another (bearing in mind that the process of implementation itself has associated costs, and these may be substantial). For a cost–utility analysis, one should consider how the costs/QALY compare with those of other interventions. In their economic analysis, Plunkett and Grobman[1] showed that hepatitis C virus screening, treatment and caesarean delivery in low-risk, asymptomatic, pregnant women was not cost-effective compared with no screening. The cost–effectiveness ratio was $1 170 000 per QALY.

How do the resulting costs or costs per unit of health gained compare with other interventions?

Rather than using an arbitrary threshold for costs/QALY above which an intervention would not be funded, one can compare the reported cost with the costs of other interventions currently being offered (or considered) in a given clinical setting by referring to league tables. *League tables* list cost-effectiveness results from several different studies and, in theory, allow readers to compare the cost-effectiveness of different interventions. Many league tables are available in the published literature. However, because of wide variations in the methods used in the original analyses that are summarized, these tables can be misleading if taken at face value.[33] In one league table, all results were standardized to a common currency, and attempts were made to ensure correct calculation of cost–effectiveness ratios to improve comparability of the results across analyses.[34] However, the assumptions made in the individual analyses, such as the choice of comparator, were not assessed.

Are the conclusions likely to change with sensible changes in costs and outcomes (i.e. are the results robust)?

Readers of economic evaluations often wish to judge the robustness of the results given different assumptions or scenarios. For example, in a trial comparing a brief smoking cessation intervention with usual care in hospital inpatients, 4.3% more patients successfully quit smoking with the brief intervention than with usual care, at an incremental cost of US$159 per smoker.[35] However, self-reported smoking status data may not be accurate because respondents are likely to give socially desirable responses. In the smoking cessation trial, only 52% of participants provided blood samples for biochemical confirmation of abstinence. Therefore, the estimated quit rate in this study may be overestimated. However, the authors did a sensitivity analysis and found that even when the quit rate was varied from 8.0% to 0.6%, the intervention was still cost-effective, varying between $US909 and $US53 347/LY gained.

Can I apply the results in practice?

When appraising any research evidence, it is important to consider the applicability or generalizability of the results to your own setting. In an economic evaluation, the applicability of both cost and benefit estimates are assessed.

Do the costs in the report apply in my setting?

Costs may vary due to local prices and different practice patterns. Sensitivity analyses should cover a range of costs that may account for such differences.

Will the intervention (or new model of care) be effective in my setting?

As always, readers should consider how their own patients are similar to, or different from, those in the study. Patient preferences for the outcomes and utilities used in the analysis should also be assessed.

Resolution of the clinical scenario

The key aspects of the economic analysis by Plunkett and Grobman[1] are summarized in Table 21.3. The analysis showed that it is not cost-effective to routinely screen for hepatitis C virus in asymptomatic, low-risk, pregnant woman. Based on this economic evidence, the interdisciplinary team will recommend that routine screening for hepatitis C virus not be done in low-risk pregnant women.[1] However, the practice of screening pregnant woman who have risk factors for hepatitis C will continue until the team can review the evidence supporting this practice.

Table 21.3 Summary of an economic analysis of routine hepatitis C virus screening in pregnancy

Feature	Study by Plunkett and Grobman[1]
Overall study design	Cost-effective analysis; more specifically, a cost–utility analysis using a decision-analytic model (decision tree with Markov analysis)
Perspective of analysis	Health care system
Alternatives compared	Three approaches to manage asymptomatic hepatitis C virus infection in low-risk pregnant women: (1) no screening; (2) screening and treatment; (3) screening, treatment, and elective caesarean section to avert perinatal transmission of hepatitis C virus
Effect measures	cost–effectiveness ratio < US$50 000/ QALY
Source of effectiveness data	Threshold commonly used in the published literature
Source of quality of life (utility) weights	Utility values by mode of delivery were derived using the time trade-off technique from a panel of five experts. All other utilities were derived from the published literature
Estimates of resource use	
Source of cost data	Published literature, only direct cost used
Discounting	Costs and QALYs are discounted at a 3% annual rate in the base case analysis
Addressing uncertainty	The Markov model was validated by running 10 000 simulation trials and comparing results with longitudinal data from five prospective cohort studies and recently published empirically calibrated models of hepatitis C virus screening. One-way sensitivity analyses were performed on all model variables. Multivariate analyses were performed on variables of interest
Year of currency	2003 US dollars
Source of funding	Government
Country of study	United States

LEARNING EXERCISE

Identify some economic evaluations relevant to your area of interest and work through the critical appraisal checklist in Box 21.1.

References

1 Plunkett BA, Grobman WA. Routine hepatitis C virus screening in pregnancy: a cost-effectiveness analysis. *Am J Obstet Gynecol* 2005;**192**:1153–61.
2 Elixhauser A, Halpern M, Schmier J, Luce BR. Health care CBA and CEA from 1991 to 1996: an updated bibliography. *Med Care* 1998;**36**:MS1–9, MS18–147.
3 Gerard K, Smoker I, Seymour J. Raising the quality of cost-utility analyses: lessons learnt and still to learn. *Health Policy* 1999;**46**:217–38.

4 Neumann PJ, Stone PW, Chapman RH, Sandberg EA, Bell CM. The quality of reporting in published cost-utility analyses, 1976–1997. *Ann Intern Med* 2000;**132**:964–72.

5 Neuhauser D, Lweicki AM. What do we gain from the sixth stool guaiac? *N Engl J Med* 1975;**293**:226–8.

6 Bissinger RL, Allred CA, Arford PH, Bellig LL. A cost-effectiveness analysis of neonatal nurse practitioners. *Nurs Econ* 1997;**15**:92–9.

7 Stone PW, Walker PH. Cost-effectiveness analysis: birth center vs. hospital care. *Nurs Econ* 1995;**13**:299–308.

8 Chang WY, Henry BM. Methodologic principles of cost analyses in the nursing, medical, and health services literature, 1990–1996. *Nurs Res* 1999;**48**:94–104.

9 Graham JD, Corso PS, Morris JM, Segui-Gomez M, Weinstein MC. Evaluating the cost-effectiveness of clinical and public health measures. *Annu Rev Public Health* 1998;**19**:125–52.

10 Tengs TO, Wallace A. One thousand health-related quality-of-life estimates. *Med Care* 2000;**38**:583–637.

11 Gold MR, Siegel JE, Russell LB, Weinstein MC, editors. *Cost-Effectiveness in Health and Medicine.* Oxford: Oxford University Press, 1996.

12 Weinstein MC, Siegel JE, Gold MR, Kamlet MS, Russell LB. Recommendations of the Panel on Cost-Effectiveness in Health and Medicine. *JAMA* 1996;**276**:1253–8.

13 Siegel JE, Weinstein MC, Russell LB, Gold MR. Recommendations for reporting cost-effectiveness analyses. Panel on Cost-Effectiveness in Health and Medicine. *JAMA* 1996;**276**:1339–41.

14 Russell LB, Gold MR, Siegel JE, Daniels N, Weinstein MC. The role of cost-effectiveness analysis in health and medicine. Panel on Cost-Effectiveness in Health and Medicine. *JAMA* 1996;**276**:1172–7.

15 Kenkel D. On valuing morbidity, effectiveness analysis, and being rude. *J Health Econ* 1997;**16**:749–57.

16 Pauly MV. Valuing health care benefits in money terms. In Sloan F, editor. *Valuing Health Care: Costs, Benefits, and Effectiveness of Pharmaceuticals and other Medical Technologies.* Cambridge: Cambridge University Press, 1995:99–124.

17 George MR, O'Dowd LC, Martin I, Lindell KO, Whitney F, Jones M, Ramondo T, Walsh L, Grissinger J, Hansen-Flaschen J, Panettieri RA Jr. A comprehensive educational program improves clinical outcome measures in inner-city patients with asthma. *Arch Intern Med* 1999;**159**:1710–16.

18 French MT, Sacks S, De Leon G, Staines G, McKendrick K. Modified therapeutic community for mentally ill chemical abusers: outcomes and costs. *Eval Health Prof* 1999;**22**:60–85.

19 Cherin DA, Huba GJ, Brief DE, Melchior LA. Evaluation of the transprofessional model of home health care for HIV/AIDS. *Home Health Care Serv Q* 1998;**17**:55–72.

20 Stone PW. Dollars and sense: a primer for the novice in economic analyses (Part II). *Appl Nurs Res* 2001;**14**:110–12.

21 Stone PW. Dollars and sense: a primer for the novice in economic analyses (Part I). *Appl Nurs Res* 2001;**14**:54–5.

22 Lave JR, Pashos CL, Anderson GF, Brailer D, Bubolz T, Conrad D, Freund DA, Fox SH, Keeler E, Lipscomb J. Costing medical care: using Medicare administrative data. *Med Care* 1994;**32**:JS77–89.

23 Stone PW, Chapman RH, Sandberg EA, Liljas B, Neumann PJ. Measuring costs in cost-utility analyses. Variations in the literature. *Int J Technol Assess Health Care* 2000;**16**:111–24.

24 Hornberger J, Lenert LA. Variation among quality-of-life surveys. Theory and practice. *Med Care* 1996;**34**:DS23–33.

25 Bosch JL, Hammitt JK, Weinstein MC, Hunink MG. Estimating general-population utilities using one binary-gamble question per respondent. *Med Decis Making* 1998;**18**:381–90.

26 Patrick DL, Starks HE, Cain KC, Uhlmann RF, Pearlman RA. Measuring preferences for health states worse than death. *Med Decis Making* 1994;**14**:9–18.

27 Lohr KN, Aaronson NK, Alonso J, Burnam MA, Patrick DL, Perrin EB, Roberts JS. Evaluating quality-of-life and health status instruments: development of scientific review criteria. *Clin Ther* 1996;**18**:979–92.

28 Bell CM, Chapman RH, Stone PW, Sandberg EA, Neumann PJ. An off-the-shelf help list: a comprehensive catalog of preference scores from published cost-utility analyses. *Med Decis Making* 2001;**21**:288–94.

29 Badia X, Diaz-Prieto A, Rue M, Patrick DL. Measuring health and health state preferences among critically ill patients. *Intensive Care Med* 1996;**22**:1379–84.

30 Fryback DG, Dasbach EJ, Klein R, Klein BE, Dorn N, Peterson K, Martin PA. The Beaver Dam Health Outcomes Study: initial catalog of health-state quality factors. *Med Decis Making* 1993;**13**:89–102.

31 Stone PW. Methods for conducting and reporting cost-effectiveness analysis in nursing. *Image J Nurs Sch* 1998;**30**:229–34.

32 Fenwick E, Claxton K, Sculpher M. Representing uncertainty: the role of cost-effectiveness acceptability curves. *Health Econ* 2001;**10**:779–87.

33 Gerard K, Mooney G. QALY league tables: handle with care. *Health Econ* 1993;**2**:59–64.

34 Chapman RH, Stone PW, Sandberg EA, Bell C, Neumann PJ. A comprehensive league table of cost-utility ratios and a sub-table of 'panel-worthy' studies. *Med Decis Making* 2000;**20**:451–67.

35 Meenan RT, Stevens VJ, Hornbrook MC, La Chance PA, Glasgow RE, Hollis JF, Lichtenstein E, Vogt TM. Cost-effectiveness of a hospital-based smoking cessation intervention. *Med Care* 1998;**36**:670–8.

36 Pearson ML. Guideline for prevention of intravascular device-related infections. Part I. Intravascular device-related infections: an overview. The Hospital Infection Control Practices Advisory Committee. *Am J Infect Control* 1996;**24**:262–77.

Chapter 22

EVALUATION OF STUDIES OF PROGNOSIS

Ellen Fineout-Overholt and Bernadette Mazurek Melnyk

When patients first receive a diagnosis of a disease or condition, their initial questions often focus on *what can be done?* – that is, questions about treatments or interventions. Patients also want to know what will happen to them in the short and long term, in terms of disease progression, survival and quality of life. These are questions of prognosis. For example, the family of a patient who has had a first ischaemic stroke will want to know if the patient will die, if current disabilities such as paralysis or aphasia will continue and for how long, what kind of life the patient can expect to have after discharge from hospital, and the likelihood of a recurrent stroke. The answers to some of these questions will likely influence decision-making about treatment. If a patient is likely to die in the short term, families may be unwilling to initiate invasive treatments or those associated with pain or other adverse effects. Similarly, some conditions, such as the common cold, are self-limiting and will resolve in time without treatment. In such cases, patients will often forgo treatment, especially if it is costly or has unpleasant side effects.

Nurses, in various contexts, may be faced with questions of prognosis. It is therefore important for nurses to understand how to assess and interpret evidence related to disease prognosis. This chapter will focus on the critical appraisal of studies of prognosis. The specific questions that will guide this appraisal, initially outlined by Laupacis *et al.*[1] are summarized in Box 22.1.

Definition of prognosis

Prognosis refers to the expected outcomes of a disease or condition and the probability with which they are likely to occur.[1, 2] Expanding the definition further, prognosis includes the effects of a disease or condition over time and the estimated chance of recovery or ongoing associated morbidity, given a set of variables, which are called prognostic factors or prognostic indicators. *Prognostic factors* are variables that predict which patients are likely to do better or worse over time.[2] For example, in Perth, Western Australia, the Perth Community Stroke Study team examined the factors that predicted death and disability at 5 years in patients with a first-ever stroke who survived the first 30 days.[3] Patients were assessed at baseline for 26 variables. At 5 years, 45% of patients had died, and 36% had new disabilities. Factors that

Box 22.1 Critical appraisal questions for studies of prognosis[1]

Are the results valid?

- Was there a representative and well defined sample of patients at a similar point in the course of the disease?
- Was follow-up sufficiently long and complete?
- Were objective and unbiased outcome criteria used?
- Did the analysis adjust for important prognostic factors?

What are the results?

- How large is the likelihood of the outcome event(s) in a specified period of time?
- How precise are the estimates of likelihood?

Can I apply the results in practice?

- Were the study patients similar to my own?
- Will the results lead directly to selecting or avoiding therapy?
- Are the results useful for reassuring or counselling patients?

predicted death or disability (i.e. prognostic factors) included age, moderate or severe hemiparesis, and disability at baseline. More specifically, patients who had moderate hemiparesis at baseline were almost three times more likely to die or be disabled at 5 years, whereas those with severe hemiparesis were over four times more likely to die or be disabled.[3] Thus, prognostic factors can help us to predict which patients are more or less likely to experience a given outcome.

Study designs for questions of prognosis

Questions of prognosis can be addressed by case-control studies or cohort studies. As well, randomized controlled trials implicitly address questions of prognosis, as each arm of a trial (treatment and control) is a cohort.[2] Let's consider the following question: which patients are most likely to die 30 days after a first acute myocardial infarction (MI)? A case-control study design might involve identifying a group of patients with a first MI who had died (cases) and a group who had survived (controls) and then identifying the characteristics (prognostic factors) that distinguish between the two groups (e.g. age or sex). Limitations of case-control studies include the risk that selection of cases and controls may be biased, such that the groups differ systematically in unknown ways.[1] Furthermore, retrospective collection of data on prognostic factors relies on the accuracy of people's memories or the accuracy of medical charts.[1] Such limitations decrease the strength of the evidence in guiding clinical decision-making.[2]

Prognostic questions are best addressed using cohort study designs, which are not subject to the same problems as case-control studies. In our example, a cohort study would involve identifying a group of patients (cohort) at the time of their first MI, collecting baseline data on various characteristics that might be associated with the outcome (mortality), and then following up the cohort over time to see which patients die and which survive. Cohort studies may also include a control group. In our example, the control group could include people who have not had an MI and are followed up over the same time period.

Clinical scenario

You work in a primary care clinic. Your first patient of the day is an 8-month-old girl, Amy, who was recently discharged from hospital after an episode of meningitis. Her parents are concerned about whether Amy is likely to have any developmental problems or disabilities as a result of the meningitis. You don't know the answer, but offer to find out.

The search

You begin by formulating your clinical question as a basis for the search for evidence: *In young children who have meningitis, is it likely that there will be long-term neurological, cognitive, behavioural, or developmental consequences?* You decide to begin searching for pre-appraised evidence and search *Evidence-Based Nursing* online because the content includes only studies and reviews that meet specific methodological criteria. You begin searching by typing the terms 'meningitis' and 'prognosis' into the 'Word(s) Anywhere in the Article' field and identify an abstract[4] of a study by Bedford *et al.*[5] on infants in England and Wales who had meningitis and were followed up for 5 years. You retrieve the full article, and as you begin to read you use the questions summarized in Box 22.1 to assess the quality of the study and the relevance of the findings to your question.

Are the results of the study valid?

Was there a representative and well-defined sample of patients at a similar point in the course of the disease?

It is important to have a representative sample of patients in order to minimize bias. *Bias* refers to systematic differences from the truth.[2] In a prognosis study, bias can lead to systematic overestimates or underestimates of the likelihood of specific outcomes.[2] For example, if patients were recruited from tertiary care centres, which typically deal with patients who have rare or severe conditions, the sample would not likely be representative of patients presenting in primary care settings.[2] Authors should clearly indicate how a sample was selected and the criteria used to diagnose the condition.[2] It is also important that patients included in a prognosis study all have a similar prognostic risk so that meaningful conclusions can be drawn about the expected outcomes.

Prognosis study samples should comprise an *inception cohort* of patients who are at a similar, clearly described point in the disease process. Inception cohorts often include patients with a first onset of a disease or condition (e.g. a first-ever myocardial infarction) or those who have recently been diagnosed. The stage of a disease will clearly influence outcomes. For example, studies of 5-year mortality rates in women with breast cancer could include women diagnosed with different stages of breast cancer. We might expect higher 5-year mortality rates for women diagnosed with advanced-stage cancer than those diagnosed at an earlier stage. When it is not possible to achieve a homogeneous sample (e.g. patients are at disparate points in their illness trajectories), the authors should report the data by disease stage or some other indicator of severity (e.g. APACHE II scores).

Let's return to our clinical example and consider the study by Bedford *et al.*[5] on 5-year follow-up of infants with meningitis. The sample comprised 1717 children (index children) who had survived an episode of acute meningitis during their first year and 1485 age- and sex-matched controls identified from the general practices of each index child. An earlier report of this study described the identification and selection of the sample.[6] Monthly cards were sent to 566 consultant paediatricians which asked if they had managed any cases of acute infantile meningitis during the previous month. Clinical and laboratory information was collected on standard forms sent to the paediatrician and consultant microbiologist involved in the management of the case. Death certificates for all infants recorded as having died of meningitis were obtained from the Office of Population Census and Surveys. Initial inclusion criterion for the study was 'intention to treat' by the paediatrician. Infants who had viable bacteraemia, viruses, or detectable bacterial antigen in the cerebrospinal fluid (CSF) or a white cell count in the CSF greater than $20 \times 10^6/l$ were included. Infants who had clinical conditions that were highly suggestive of meningitis, but were too ill to have a lumbar puncture, were also included. Infants with spina bifida and ventricular shunt infections were excluded.

Thus, the original sample included children with confirmed meningitis (defined by objective criteria) except for those too ill for lumbar puncture. The children were initially identified by treating paediatricians and followed up through their general practitioners. The control group of age- and sex-matched children was selected from the general practices attended by index children. This suggests that the sample is representative of children in general practice settings. Although it was not explicitly stated that only infants with a first case of meningitis were included (inception cohort), this was probably the case given that all infants had contracted the disease before the age of one year.

Was follow-up sufficiently long and complete?

The follow-up period should be long enough to detect the outcomes of interest.[1] That is, the appropriate length of follow-up will depend on the outcome of interest. For example, to determine the risk of severe disability in patients with a chronic disease such as rheumatoid arthritis, a 10-year follow-up period would yield more meaningful results than a 6-month follow up. In contrast, severity of West Nile infection after a bite from an infected mosquito will be evident within a few days. In addition to the length of follow-up, readers of prognosis studies need to consider the completeness of follow-up.[1] If a large percentage of patients from the original sample are not available for follow-up, the likelihood of bias may increase. That is, participants who are not available for follow-up may have systematically higher or lower risks of particular outcomes than those who are available for follow-up.[2] Study participants may become unavailable during follow-up because they move to different geographic locations or lose interest in participating in the study, or because they die. Study authors need to account for all patients included in the original sample and to provide information about the characteristics of patients who are lost to follow-up. Patients who die need to be identified through death certificates or health databases. Excluding patients who die, or are lost to follow-up for other reasons, would underestimate the positive or negative outcomes of disease.

Applying these criteria to the study by Bedford et al.[5] we see that infants who had meningitis in their first year were followed up to 5 years of age. The outcomes of interest, cognitive or behavioural disabilities, are likely to be identifiable by this time, particularly with the onset of formal schooling. Indeed, Bedford et al.[5] included information on type of schooling to determine degree of disability. The initial sample included 1880 children with meningitis, of whom 163 died, and 1485 children in the control group. Data were available at 5-year follow-up for 1584 of the 1717 surviving children (92%) who had meningitis and 1391 of 1485 children in the control group (94%). The authors accounted for all children included in the original sample, specifying the reasons for missing data in both the index children and the control group. Reasons included emigration, loss to follow-up, and lack of response by both parents and general practitioners to questionnaires. The high follow-up rates of 92% and 94% help to minimize the possibility of bias resulting from large numbers of participants not being included in the analysis.

Were objective and unbiased outcome criteria used?

Outcomes should be defined at the beginning of a prognosis study, and objective measures should be used when possible.[2] Objectivity of outcomes can be described along a continuum of judgement.[1] Some outcomes, such as death, are objective: they are easily measured and require no judgement (a person is either dead or alive). Other outcomes, such as disability or quality of life, are more difficult to quantify, and their measurement may be subject to liberal judgement by outcome assessors.[1] The assessment of these more subjective outcomes could be influenced by knowledge of which prognostic factors were present at baseline. For example, a person assessing disability in patients with rheumatoid arthritis may be influenced by knowledge of the patient's previous activity level, believing that those who were less active are more likely to have severe disability. To minimize the possibility of bias, it is especially important that those people assessing more subjective outcomes be blinded to the prognostic indicators of participants or that self-administered questionnaires be used.[1] Blinding of outcome assessors may not be needed when outcomes are objective or unequivocal (e.g. death).[1]

Returning to the study by Bedford et al.[5] we note that the main outcome of interest was disability. Data were collected using questionnaires completed by general practitioners and families of participants. General practitioners were asked about the child's neuromotor development, learning, vision, hearing, speech and language, behaviour, and seizure disorders. Parents reported on the child's health, development and schooling. The questionnaires were specifically developed for this study, and no information was given about testing of the reliability or validity of the questionnaires. Obviously, general practitioners and parents were aware of whether the child had had an episode of meningitis and of the presence of specific prognostic factors, and this knowledge could have influenced their responses to questions about certain outcomes. The authors used data from both general practitioner and parent questionnaires to assign each child to one of four categories of disability based on an existing model: no disability (no developmental problems); mild disability (middle ear disease, strabismus, febrile convulsions, and behavioural problems); moderate disability (mild neuromotor disabilities, intellectual impairment, moderate sensorineural hearing loss, mild to moderate visual impairment, treatment-controlled epilepsy, and uncomplicated hydrocephalus); and severe disability (severe neuromotor and intellectual impairment, severe seizure disorders, and severe visual or auditory impairment).

The authors did not report whether the person(s) responsible for assigning levels of severity were blinded to knowledge about whether a given child had had meningitis or the presence of specific prognostic factors. Again, such knowledge could have influenced decisions about assigning a severity level, especially in areas where considerable judgement was needed to interpret responses on the questionnaires. Thus, a possibility exists that bias may have influenced reporting by general practitioners and parents and the determination of levels of disability by study personnel.

Did the analysis adjust for important prognostic factors?

As previously stated, studies of prognosis usually collect data on several prognostic factors that are thought to influence the outcome of interest. Decisions about which prognostic factors are most relevant are usually based on clinical experience and an understanding of the biology of the disease.[2] When analysing the results of a prognosis study, authors usually identify different groups of patients based on these prognostic factors and adjust for these different factors in the analysis.[1] Such adjustment is important to identify which factors best predict outcomes. For example, Camfield *et al.* followed up an inception cohort of 692 children with epilepsy for up to 22 years to identify factors associated with all-cause mortality.[7] The mortality rate was 6% at 20 years after onset compared with a rate of 0.88% in the general population. Initial analyses seemed to indicate that children who had onset at birth and those with secondary generalized epilepsy were more likely to die after 20 years. However, these differences disappeared when the analyses adjusted for the presence of severe neurological disorder. That is, children with epilepsy who had severe neurological deficits had a substantially increased risk of death after 20 years (an increase of 210%) compared with the general population; children with epilepsy who did not have neurological deficits had a similar risk of death to that of the general population. Onset at birth and type of epilepsy were not, in fact, associated with differential mortality rates. Without the inclusion of 'neurological disorder' as a prognostic factor in the analysis, one could have mistakenly assumed that children who developed epilepsy at birth and those with secondary generalized epilepsy had an increased risk of mortality.

Treatments administered to patients can also modify outcomes and thus may be considered when adjusting for prognostic indicators. Although interventions are not considered to be prognostic factors *per se*, differential application or receipt of treatments in patients may influence outcomes.[1]

In their analyses, Bedford *et al.*[5] included age at onset of infection (neonatal period or later), organism associated with the infection, birth weight, and gestational age as prognostic factors.

What are the results?

The results of a prognosis study have to do with quantification of the number of events that occur over a period of time.[2] This result can be expressed in different ways, which are described below.

How large is the likelihood of the outcome event(s) in a specified period of time?

Most simply, the outcome of a prognosis study can be expressed as a percentage.[1] For example, a study of infants born with HIV infection found that 26% had died at a median follow-up of 5.8 years.[8] Thus, one could say that an infant born with HIV infection has a 26% chance of dying at 5.8 years.

We know, however, that the risk of a particular outcome may vary in patients with different prognostic factors. Estimates of risk in patients with different prognostic factors are often presented as relative risks or odds ratios. The *relative risk (RR)* is the risk of patients with a specific prognostic factor experiencing the outcome divided by the risk of patients without the specific prognostic factor experiencing the outcome. An RR also can be used to represent the risk of patients with the disease experiencing the outcome divided by the risk of patients without the disease (control group) experiencing the outcome. If the risk of the outcome is the same in patients with and without the prognostic factor, the RR will be 1.0. If the RR is less than 1.0, the risk of the outcome is reduced in patients with the specific prognostic factor compared with patients without the prognostic factor. If the RR is greater than 1.0, the risk of the outcome is increased in patients with the prognostic factor compared with those without the prognostic factor. The further away the RR is from 1.0, the greater the strength of the association between the prognostic factor and the outcome (see Chapter 11). For various statistical reasons, some studies will express the outcome as the odds of the event rather than the risk of the event. The *odds ratio (OR)* is the odds of the outcome in the patients with a specific prognostic factor divided by the odds of the outcome in patients without the prognostic factor (see Chapter 11). The interpretation of ORs of 1, less than 1, and greater than 1 is similar to that for RRs.

Sometimes, we will be interested in determining whether the risk of a particular outcome changes over time. For example, we know that the risk of death after an MI is highest immediately after the event and decreases thereafter.[2] To address changes in the risk of a particular outcome over time, authors often use survival analysis and represent the results as a survival curve or Kaplan Meier curve.[2] A *survival curve* is a graph of the number of events (or freedom from events) over time.

In the study by Bedford *et al.*[5] we find that 247 children (16%) who had meningitis had severe or moderate disabilities at 5 years of age, whereas only 21 children in the control group (1.5%) had such disabilities. The RR of 10.33 means that children who had meningitis in their first year of life were over 10 times more likely to have moderate or severe disabilities by age 5 years than children who did not have meningitis. You will recall that the authors considered age at infection, organism, birth weight, and gestational age as prognostic factors. Bedford *et al.*[5] found that children who had meningitis within the first month of life were more likely to have moderate disabilities at 5 years than those who had meningitis after the first month; the percentage of children with severe disabilities did not differ by age of onset. As well, rates of severe or moderate disability differed by the type of infecting organism. After controlling for birth weight and gestational age, children who had had meningitis still had a 7-fold increase in the risk of severe or moderate disability (weighted RRs of 7.11 and 7.64, respectively). From these data, you discern that Amy's parents' concerns about subsequent developmental disabilities seem warranted.

How precise are the estimates of likelihood?

Studies can only provide *estimates* of the true risk of an outcome.[1] Thus, it is important to determine the precision of estimates of risk. An RR provides an estimate of the risk of a given outcome for the study sample. Readers, however, need to be fairly certain that the estimated RR is close to the true population RR. Confidence intervals (CIs) are the most accurate means of showing precision.[1] The *95% CI* is the range of risks within which we can be 95% sure that the true value for the whole population lies.[2] In everyday terms, this means that the CI helps clinicians to know how close the findings of the study are to what they may experience.

Returning to the study by Bedford *et al.*[5] we see that the RR of 10.33 for moderate or severe disability at 5 years had a 95% CI of 6.60 to 16.0. This means that we can be 95% certain that the true population RR is between 6.6% and 16% and that Amy may have that same RR. The weighted RRs and 95% CIs for severe or moderate disability after controlling for birth weight and gestational age were 7.11 (4.30 to 11.7) and 7.64 (4.56 to 12.79), respectively. Thus, we see that the RRs are associated with a moderate degree of precision.

Can I apply the results in practice?

Were the study patients similar to my own?

Generalizability of findings is a primary concern for researchers and users of evidence. In a study report, the sample must be described in sufficient detail so that clinicians can compare the sample to their own patients. As with any research, the more similar the study sample is to a clinician's patients, the more certain she can be about applying the findings in clinical decisions.

Based on the study report by Bedford *et al.*[5] we don't know much about the demographic characteristics of the sample. Information relating to the age, sex and perhaps economic background of the sample might have been helpful for readers attempting to discern similarities or differences with their own patients. We do know, however, that this was a national study done in England and Wales. Readers from other countries should consider whether differences in their own settings could substantially alter the findings (e.g. differences in health care or disease rates). We also know that the children with meningitis and those in the control group were followed up through their general practitioners, a context similar to the primary care setting in which you see Amy as a patient.

Will the results lead directly to selecting or avoiding therapy?

The study by Bedford *et al.*[5] found that children with meningitis were over 10 times more likely to have moderate to severe disabilities by age 5 years than children who did not have meningitis. We also know that prognostic factors such as age of onset, birth weight and gestational age do not really differentiate between children who are more or less likely to develop these disabilities. Type of infecting organism was, however, associated with the likelihood of moderate to severe disability. Obviously, none of this information will provide you, or Amy's parents, with a definitive answer about what to do. Together, you will need to decide how to deal with the increased risk of disability. Decisions may relate to assessment, that is, what types of assessment can help to identify disabilities, and when (and how frequently) should these assessments be done? You will likely need to gather more information on the specific types of disabilities that may occur and whether any treatments are effective in preventing, delaying or overcoming these disabilities.

Are the results useful for reassuring or counselling patients?

As suggested previously, treating a patient is not always the desired goal. Sometimes, evidence from a prognostic study can assist practitioners or families to determine whether interventions should be initiated, especially if the likelihood of adverse outcomes is high. Similarly, some diseases have good prognoses, and patients and families may decide to forgo treatment because a positive outcome is likely. Patients and families should be involved in clinical decisions and provide their views on the risks and benefits of any assessments or treatments given the likelihood of the outcomes of interest. Your interpretation of the results of the study by Bedford et al.[5] suggests that the risk of disability, while increased, does not preclude consideration of assessment or other intervention. With this in mind, you discuss with Amy's parents their views about the value of assessing Amy over the next couple of years or doing nothing.

Resolution of clinical scenario

You meet with Amy's parents to discuss what you have learned from the study by Bedford et al.[5] You note that you do not know much about the demographics of the study sample or how meningitis was treated. You also note that the authors followed up over 90% of children up to 5 years of age, which increases your confidence in the findings. It is clear that about 1 in 6 children who have meningitis in the first year of life (i.e. 16%) will have moderate to severe developmental disabilities at 5 years of age. The risk is about 10 times that of children generally but differs depending on the type of infective agent. In Amy's case, the infective agent was Neisseria meningitidis, which is associated with 9.4% risk of severe to moderate disability. This risk is about six times that of children generally. If Amy had been infected by Group B streptococcus, a somewhat rarer infective agent, she would have had a 30% risk of moderate to severe disability, which is about 20 times that of children generally. Based on this information, you and Amy's parents begin to discuss Amy's likely needs.

Summary

Studies of prognosis can provide clinicians with useful information about the expected outcomes of a disease or condition and the probability at which they are likely to occur. Assessment of relevant prognostic factors can help to identify which patients are more or less likely to experience a given outcome and can serve as a basis for clinical decisions about treatment. Some key considerations when appraising studies of prognosis include the sample (an inception cohort, where patients have a similar prognostic risk), inclusion of relevant prognostic factors in data collection and analysis, sufficient length of follow-up with respect to the outcomes of interest, percentage of patients followed up (higher percentages help to minimize bias), and objectivity of outcomes (more objective outcomes and blinding of outcome assessors help to minimize bias).

LEARNING EXERCISES

1. Practise formulating clinical questions around issues of prognosis relevant to your area of expertise. Search for relevant research in PubMed using the Clinical Queries function.
2. You work in diabetes care and are planning a foot-care educational programme in which you want to provide some evidence-based estimates of the likelihood of foot infection in people with diabetes and known risk factors.
   (a) Focus your uncertainty into a searchable question.
   (b) Search for relevant research using the Clinical Queries function in PubMed.

Solutions to learning exercises
2a. The focused questions would be:

- *What proportion of people with diabetes develop an infected foot lesion?*
- *Which factors increase the probability of foot infection in people with diabetes?*

2b. Searching PubMed using Clinical Queries and the terms 'foot infection diabetes' for a narrow, spe-
cific search identified 46 papers (PubMed accessed 11 December 2006), including the following:
Lavery LA, Armstrong DG, Wunderlich RP, Mohler MJ, Wendel CS, Lipski BA. Risk factors for foot
infections in individuals with diabetes. Diabetes Care *2006;**29**:128–93. The paper reports on a*
cohort study and, therefore, is worthy of further scrutiny. You can now apply the appraisal crite-
ria in Box 22.1 to assess the validity of the study results.

References

1 Laupacis A, Wells G, Richardson WS, Tugwell P. Users' guides to the medical literature. V. How to use an article about prognosis. Evidence-Based Medicine Working Group. *JAMA* 1994;**272**:234–7.

2 Randolph A, Bucher H, Richardson WS, Wells G, Tugwell P, Guyatt G. Prognosis. In: Guyatt G, Rennie D (editors). *Users' Guides to the Medical Literature. A Manual for Evidence-Based Clinical Practice.* Chicago: American Medical Association, 2002:141–54.

3 Hardie K, Jamrozik K, Hankey GJ, Broadhurst RJ, Anderson C. Trends in five-year survival and risk of recurrent stroke after first-ever stroke in the Perth Community Stroke Study. *Cerebrovasc Dis* 2005;**19**:179–85.

4 Children infected with meningitis before 1 year of age were at increased risk of disability at 5 years of age. *Evid Based Nurs* 2002;**5**:59. Abstract of: Bedford H, de Louvois J, Halket S, Peckham C, Hurley R, Harvey D. Meningitis in infancy in England and Wales: follow up at age 5 years. *BMJ* 2001;**323**:533–6.

5 Bedford H, de Louvois J, Halket S, Peckham C, Hurley R, Harvey D. Meningitis in infancy in England and Wales: follow up at age 5 years. *BMJ* 2001;**323**:533–6.

6 de Louvois J, Blackbourn J, Hurley R, Harvey D. Infantile meningitis in England and Wales: a two year study. *Arch Dis Child* 1991;**66**:603–7.

7 Camfield CS, Camfield PR, Veugelers PJ. Death in children with epilepsy: a population-based study. *Lancet* 2002;**359**:1891–5.

8 Gray L, Newell ML, Thorne C, Peckham C, Levy J, for the European Collaborative Study. European Collaborative Study. Fluctuations in symptoms in human immunodeficiency virus-infected children: the first 10 years of life. *Pediatrics* 2001;**108**:116–22.

Additional resources

Online critical appraisal checklists

University of Toronto Centre for Evidence-Based Medicine http://www.cebm.utoronto.ca/practise/ca/prognosis/
University of Alberta http://www.med.ualberta.ca/ebm/prognosisworksheet.htm

Online exercises

ScHARR, University of Sheffield http://www.shef.ac.uk/scharr/ir/adept/prognosis/contents.htm

Chapter 23

EVALUATION OF STUDIES OF CAUSATION (AETIOLOGY)

Joy Adamson

Clinical scenario

You have been appointed as the Nurse Manager of a nursing home that provides long-term care for older people and have become aware that a large proportion of residents have pressure ulcers. You know that many preventive measures, such as special beds and mattresses, are promoted, but feel unsure as to which residents are most at risk and which characteristics predict those most likely to develop pressure ulcers. Although you know there are some pressure ulcer risk prediction tools available, you are not sure that these would apply to your residents and so would like to read some original research on the topic. Your long-term goal is to ensure that care is targeted at those residents at highest risk so that preventable ulcers are avoided. Your focused clinical question is *Which characteristics of nursing home residents place them at high risk of pressure ulcer development?*

The search

You begin by searching *Evidence-Based Nursing* online (www.evidencebasednursing. com) using the search term 'pressure ulcer*'. This search (undertaken 23 July 2007) identifies eleven abstracts, none of which addresses questions of risk factors. Similarly, a search of *Evidence-Based Medicine* finds no relevant studies. You try PubMed (http://www.ncbi.nlm.nih.gov/entrez/query.fcgi), which is freely available online. You select the 'Clinical Queries' search option and the 'Etiology' search because you are looking for articles concerned with the causation of pressure ulcers. You decide that your search should emphasize sensitivity over specificity so that you can minimize the risk of missing relevant articles (see Chapter 6). Your search terms are 'pressure ulcer*' AND 'nursing home*'. This search identifies 139 abstracts, one of which, 'A longitudinal study of risk factors associated with the formation of pressure ulcers in nursing homes', sounds particularly relevant.[1]

Types of research studies

Studies that consider risk factors (often referred to as exposures) for certain diseases (often referred to as outcomes) are generally called *analytical observational studies*.

They are distinct from randomized controlled trials because the researcher does not manipulate the exposure; rather, the exposure is merely measured, and its association with the outcome is calculated. With respect to the clinical scenario, you are interested in the effect of patient characteristics (the exposures) on the development of pressure ulcers (the outcome).

The most common types of observational studies to assess risk factors for disease are cross-sectional studies, case-control studies, and cohort studies. Each has a distinctly different design and differs in its advantages and disadvantages. Each of the study types will be described briefly in terms of a study that seeks to determine whether low body mass index (BMI) (exposure) is a risk factor for pressure ulcers (outcome).

In a *cross-sectional study*, data on exposure and outcome are measured at the same point in time, on the same individuals. For example, data may be collected from a sample of residents from five nursing homes. Care providers would complete a questionnaire about each resident that would include information on weight and height (to calculate BMI), some measure of the number, and perhaps severity, of pressure ulcers, as well as other factors that might be linked to pressure ulcers, such as age, recent hospital stay, chronic conditions, and mobility. These data would then be analysed to see if residents with low BMI were more or less likely to also have at least one pressure ulcer.

In a *case-control study*, researchers would identify a group of nursing home residents with pressure ulcers, the *cases*. They would also identify a group of nursing home residents who did not have pressure ulcers, the *controls*. The researchers would then collect information on previous exposures (e.g. BMI on entry into the nursing home) for each case and control patient. The difference in the prevalence of the exposure (BMI) between the case and control patients would then be compared. Case-control studies look back in time to measure exposures and are therefore called *retrospective* studies. Case-control studies can also be 'nested' within an existing cohort study.

In a *cohort study*, the researcher identifies a group of nursing home residents who do not have pressure ulcers and measures their BMIs. This group is then followed up over time to determine how many, and which, residents develop pressure ulcers.

The study we identified from our literature search is a prospective cohort study. Brandeis et al.[1] followed up a cohort of all new residents of 78 nursing homes over a 1-year period. Residents included in the study did not have pressure ulcers at the time of nursing home admission or 3 months later when baseline measurements were done. This time delay was to ensure that risk factors external to the nursing home would not influence the study findings. All residents were then followed up for a further 3 months.

Measures of effect in studies of causation

In studies of causation, we are interested in the relation between certain patient risk factors (exposures) and a particular condition or disease (the outcome). The relation between risk factors and outcomes is usually presented in terms of *relative risk*, that is, how much more (or less) risk do people with a particular characteristic have of developing the condition. Depending on the type of study and analysis, these relative risks are usually *risk ratios*, *relative risks* or *odds ratios*. Let us return to the

Table 23.1 Body mass index and pressure ulcers in a hypothetical sample of 3000 nursing home residents

		Pressure ulcers		
		Yes	No	Total
Body mass index	Low (<20 kg/m²)	116	1484	1600
	High (≥20 kg/m²)	74	1326	1400
	Total	190	2810	3000

example of the relation between BMI and pressure ulcers. Hypothetical data are used in Table 23.1 to show how results might be presented and the relative measures calculated.

We generally start by measuring the risk of having the outcome in the exposed group. In this case, we look at the first row of data in the table. The risk of having a pressure ulcer among those with low BMI is calculated by dividing the number of people who have pressure ulcers by the total number who have low BMI. Therefore, the risk of having the outcome in the exposed group is 116/1600 = 0.073. We can multiply this number by 100, so that it becomes a percentage (7.3%). We then repeat this process for people without the exposure, those with high BMI (second row of data in the table). The risk of having the outcome among those without the exposure is 74/1400 = 0.053 or 5.3%.

In order to calculate the *risk ratio*, we divide the risk of pressure ulcers among those with the exposure by the risk among those without the exposure. In this case, the risk ratio would be 0.073/0.053 = 1.37. A risk ratio of 1.37 indicates that those with low BMI are at 1.37 times (or 37%) greater risk of having the outcome than those with high BMI.

In case-control studies, because we begin with people with and without the disease, we generally cannot measure disease incidence. In this instance, we use the *odds ratio* as the measure of the size of the effect of the exposure on the outcome. However, the calculation of odds ratios is not confined to case-control studies.

We calculate the odds in the exposed group by dividing the number of people with low BMI who have pressure ulcers by the number of people with low BMI who do not have pressure ulcers (first row of data in table). We then repeat this calculation for those without the exposure.

Odds in the exposed group = 116/1484 = 0.078
Odds in the unexposed group = 74/1326 = 0.056

We obtain the ratio by dividing the odds of having a pressure ulcer among exposed people (low BMI) by the odds of having a pressure ulcer among unexposed people (high BMI).

Odds ratio = 0.078/0.056 = 1.39

Risk ratios and odds ratios are interpreted in largely the same way; that is, those with the exposure have 1.39 times the odds of having the outcome. The odds ratio and risk ratio are similar when the frequency of the outcome is low, but they become increasingly divergent as the outcome becomes more frequent. In this example, because the risk of pressure ulcers is quite low overall (190/3000 = 0.06 or 6%), the risk ratio (1.37) and the odds ratio (1.39) are very similar.

Are the results valid?

In order to assess the validity of a study of risk factors (or causation) of a particular condition, we need to assess the extent to which three factors, namely chance, bias and confounding, may have affected the study findings. The questions to guide this assessment are summarized in Box 23.1.

Magnitude of associations and the role of chance

Were there clearly stated, justified, *a priori* hypotheses?
Although cross-sectional, case-control, and cohort studies allow us to assess the effects of several exposure variables at the same time, such *multiple hypothesis testing* can pose problems. That is, the greater the number of statistical tests we perform

Box 23.1 Critical appraisal questions for studies of causation

Are the results valid?

Magnitude of associations and the role of chance

- Were there clearly stated, justified, *a priori* hypotheses?
- Was there evidence to reject the null hypothesis (presentation of p-values and 95% confidence intervals)?
- Was there evidence that the study was sufficiently powered?

Bias

- What was the study design? Cross-sectional study, case-control study, or cohort study?
- In a case-control study, how was the sample selected? Is this likely to be associated with the exposure?
- In a cohort study, how were participants allocated to exposure status? Is this likely to be associated with the outcome?
- Where possible, were objective or valid and reliable measurements used?
- In a case-control study, were the assessors of exposure blinded to outcome status?
- In a cohort study, were the outcome assessors blinded to exposure status?
- In a cohort study, was there substantial loss to follow-up? What were the characteristics of those who left the study?

Confounding

- Did the authors consider possible confounding factors? Were they accurately measured?
- Did the authors analyse the data to take into consideration the effects of these potential confounders (restriction, stratification, or statistical analysis)?
- If matching was used, did the authors perform a matched analysis?

What are the results?

Can I apply the results in practice?

within a single study, the more likely we are to obtain false-positive results. We can minimize this risk by clearly stating, at the beginning of a study, which hypotheses we intend to test, with accompanying justification. Justification would generally come from previous research studies.

The study by Brandeis et al.[1] followed from previous research that had examined risk factors for pressure ulcers, albeit using different study designs. Therefore, the risk factors that were considered in their study were justified on the basis of previous literature suggesting that these variables were clinically related to pressure ulcer formation.

Was there evidence to reject the null hypothesis (presentation of p-values and 95% confidence intervals)?

In most studies of causation, we use statistical methods to assess the *role of chance*. We are interested in whether residents with a specific characteristic (e.g. low BMI) are more likely to develop an outcome (e.g. pressure ulcers) than residents without the characteristic. Statistical tests would test the *null hypothesis* that BMI is not a risk factor for pressure ulcer development in nursing home residents. The results of these statistical tests are commonly presented as p-values and 95% confidence intervals (95% CIs).

By convention, the cut-off point for statistical significance for a p-value is usually 0.05. This value indicates that it is only 5% likely that the observed relation is because of chance. Obviously, the smaller the p-value, the less likely that an observed association between an exposure and outcome has occurred by chance. However, it is important to note that there is no clinical reason for assigning this level of significance. Therefore, it is generally no longer seen as good practice to simply report a finding as 'significant' or 'not significant' or to indicate $p < 0.05$ for significant findings. Instead, actual p-values and 95% CIs are preferred because they provide more detailed information about the strength of the evidence for rejecting or accepting the null hypothesis. It is important to note that p-values do not provide information about the strength of the association between the exposure and outcome; this information is provided by risk ratios or odds ratios. p-values simply provide us with evidence to make a judgement about how likely it is that a finding may have occurred by chance alone. Statistical significance does not, therefore, relate to clinical importance. In some instances, we may interpret a statistically significant difference between groups as a clinically unimportant difference based on our clinical experience.

In the study by Brandeis et al.[1] the authors generally presented 95% CIs around the estimates of effect but did not always present exact p-values. However, they did correctly interpret the CIs as evidence to accept or reject the null hypothesis.

Was there evidence that the study was sufficiently powered?

Statistical significance is related to the *power* of a study, which is linked to sample size. If the sample size is not large enough to detect an effect of an exposure on an outcome, then there is a risk that we may calculate a false-negative result. We might conclude, based on this false-negative result, that an exposure (e.g. BMI) is not related to an outcome (e.g. pressure ulcer development) when it may simply be that the study was not large enough to demonstrate such a relation. Readers of study reports should look for a *sample size calculation* to indicate that the study population was large enough to minimize the likelihood of false-negative results.

Although the study had a large sample size ($n = 4232$), the authors did not report whether the study was sufficiently powered. This is an important consideration in this study because the sample was drawn from 78 nursing homes. Individuals living in the same nursing home are more likely to have similar characteristics and therefore cannot be assumed to be completely independent for the purposes of statistical analysis. A larger sample size would be required to investigate this type of 'clustered' population than for a random population.

Bias

Readers always need to know whether a study measured what it set out to measure; this is an issue of *internal validity*. In an epidemiological study, *bias* refers to any systematic error that results in an incorrect estimate of the association between an exposure and outcome.[2] Bias is a concept that is sometimes difficult to grasp because the ways in which it can occur and its effects on study findings can be difficult to interpret.

Let us return to our example of the relation between BMI and pressure ulcer development. In a cohort study of all nursing home patients in a given area, we collect self-reported data on patient weight and height and then follow up patients for 6 months to see if they develop ulcers. From our data on exposures (BMI), we are able to divide the cohort by exposure status into those with high (H) and low (L) BMI as represented in Figure 23.1. However, in some cases, it was too difficult to measure the weight and height of residents, and the nursing staff made estimates. Where these estimates are inaccurate, nursing home residents have been assigned to the wrong exposure category. The actual distribution of exposure status is represented in Figure 23.2.

The error in the information collected is an example of *information bias*. More specifically, this bias is referred to as *misclassification bias* because some patients have been misclassified as having a high BMI when in fact they have low BMI, and vice versa. The effect of this type of bias on the results of a study depends on whether the misclassification is dependent on the outcome. Our example used a cohort study design, which means that we did not know the outcomes of patients at the time the exposures were measured. Therefore, it is unlikely that knowledge of the outcome could have influenced the measurement of BMI. It is more likely that residents for whom we have incorrect BMI information were randomly distributed among those

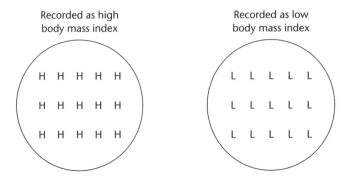

Figure 23.1 Data as measured.

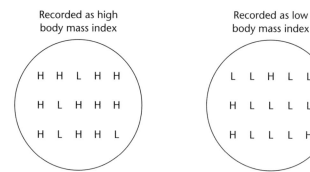

Recorded as high
body mass index

H H L H H

H L H H H

H L H H L

Recorded as low
body mass index

L L H L L

H L L L L

H L L L H

Figure 23.2   True data.

who developed pressure ulcers and those who did not. Therefore, this type of mis-classification is known as *random* or *non-differential*. This has the effect of moving the size of the association between the exposure and the outcome towards the null: that is, the study is less likely to show a relation between BMI and risk of pressure ulcer development.

Let us consider a hypothetical case-control study of residents with and without pressure ulcers who are asked about previous exposures, including recent hospital stays. When asked to remember how many days they had been in hospital, some patients report this information slightly incorrectly. As before, this is a form of information bias. The fact that some patients had developed pressure ulcers made them think more about what had happened to them recently. Thus, residents with pressure ulcers were more likely to accurately report the length of hospital stay, whereas those without pressure ulcers tended to underestimate their length of stay. Because the misclassi-fication of the exposure information is dependent on the outcome, this is known as *non-random differential misclassification*. It is also known as *recall bias* because the misclassification is based on memory. Residents without pressure ulcers would be more likely to underestimate their length of hospital stay, and therefore any association between increased length of stay and risk of developing pressure ulcers would be overestimated, as shown in Table 23.2.

Table 23.2   Self-reported length of previous hospital stay (exposure) and pressure ulcer development (outcome)

		Pressure ulcers	
		Cases	Controls
Long hospital stay (>10 days)	Yes	15	10
	No	5	10

Odds in the exposed group (long hospital stay = yes) = 15/10 = 1.5.
Odds in the unexposed group (long hospital stay = no) = 5/10 = 0.5.
Odds ratio = odds in exposed group/odds in unexposed group = 3.0.

Table 23.3 Length of previous hospital stay based on hospital records (exposure) and pressure ulcer development (outcome)

		Pressure ulcers	
		Cases	Controls
Long hospital stay (>10 days)	Yes	15	13
	No	5	7

Odds in the exposed group (long hospital stay = yes) = 15/13 = 1.15.
Odds in the unexposed group (long hospital stay = no) = 5/7 = 0.71.
Odds ratio = odds in exposed group / odds in unexposed group = 1.62.

We decide to check if the self-reported number of days in hospital matched what was reported in hospital records. We do indeed find that residents with pressure ulcers (cases) accurately reported their length of stay, whereas those without pressure ulcers (controls) tended to underestimate their length of stay. This is an example of *differential misclassification*. Data from the hospital records and the resulting calculations are summarized in Table 23.3.

Using the 'true' data on hospital stay (from hospital records) showed that the original calculation *overestimated* the size of the association between longer hospital stays and pressure ulcer development. When the data from hospital records were used, the numbers in the exposed group (i.e. long hospital stay = yes) were more similar between the cases and controls than when self-report data were used.

The other main category of bias is *selection bias*, which refers to errors in the process of identifying the study population. For example, in a case-control study, are exposed cases more (or less) likely to be selected than unexposed cases? In a cohort study, is allocation of exposure status related to development of the outcome? In most cohort studies, the outcome status of participants is unknown at the time the exposure data are collected. For this reason, cohort studies are generally thought to be less prone to bias than case-control or cross-sectional studies. Therefore, the findings of cohort studies are generally thought to be more credible than the findings of case-control or cross-sectional studies. However, cohort studies are not feasible for all questions of causation. For example, a study of a rare condition would require an impractically large sample size to ensure that an adequate number of people would develop the outcome. Similarly, conditions with long latency periods would require impractically long follow-up periods.

What was the study design? Cross-sectional study, case-control study, or cohort study?
Brandeis et al.[1] describe a longitudinal cohort study.

In a case-control study, how was the sample selected? Is this likely to be associated with the exposure?

In a cohort study, how were participants allocated to exposure status? Is this likely to be associated with the outcome?
In the Brandeis et al.[1] paper, the population was all new admissions to nursing homes during a 2-year period. All participants were free from pressure ulcers at the start of

the study, therefore selection of participants could not have been influenced by the outcome.

In effect, when we consider the role of bias, we are looking for alternative explanations for the study findings. Is there really a relation between BMI and pressure ulcers, or could the observed finding be explained by some error in the measurement of BMI or pressure ulcers? Bias can be a major problem in observational studies but can be minimized through good planning at the start of a study to ensure the sample is unbiased and by using the most objective outcome measures. These could include standardized instruments and questionnaires, validated for the relevant populations. This does not mean that objective measures are free of bias. A researcher who believes that BMI may be a cause of pressure ulcers may tend to round up the weights of participants known to have the outcome. More objective outcome measures can reduce opportunities for information bias. The risk of information bias can also be reduced by ensuring that outcome assessors are unaware of the exposure status of participants.

Unfortunately, once a study is biased, there is nothing a researcher can do about it. Thus, it is important to consider the potential role of bias at the planning stage of a study and to ensure that selection of participants and collection of data are done in ways that minimize bias.

Where possible, were objective or valid and reliable measurements used?

The study by Brandeis et al.[1] was based on computerized data, routinely collected from all nursing home residents. These data were collected during assessments by trained nurses and were shown to be 90% reliable. The study used strict criteria for diagnosis of the outcome and did not include Stage I pressure ulcers in the analysis because of the potential difficulty of reliable identification.

In a case-control study, were the assessors of exposure blinded to outcome status?

In a cohort study, were the outcome assessors blinded to exposure status?

It was unclear who did the outcome assessments and whether they were blinded to participants' exposure status in the Brandeis et al.[1] paper.

In a cohort study, was there substantial loss to follow-up? What were the characteristics of those who left the study?

A further issue for cohort studies relates to the follow-up of participants over time to see if they develop the outcome of interest. Readers need to consider whether there has been substantial loss to follow-up and, in particular, if those who dropped out differ according to the exposure, the outcome, or both. The length of the follow-up period is related to the latency period of the outcome of interest. For chronic diseases, it may be necessary to follow up participants for several years before sufficient numbers develop the outcome. However, the longer the period of follow-up, the more difficult it will be to ensure complete, or near complete, collection of outcome data. In the Brandeis et al.[1] study no participants were lost to follow-up, probably because they tended to remain living in the nursing home.

Confounding

Confounding is another form of alternative explanation for the findings of observational studies. A classic example of confounding is provided by studies that show a

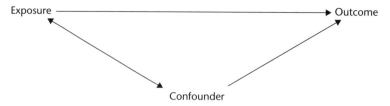

Figure 23.3 Confounding.

strong relation between coffee consumption and lung cancer. Does coffee drinking cause lung cancer? It is more likely that the relation between coffee drinking (the exposure), and lung cancer (the outcome) is confounded by smoking patterns: people who drink more coffee are also more likely to smoke, which is related to lung cancer. In the assessment of confounding, we are interested in whether a third variable, which is associated with both the exposure and the outcome, could explain any observed relation between these factors. Confounding is represented diagrammatically in Figure 23.3.

Did the authors consider possible confounding factors? Were they accurately measured?

Did the authors analyse the data to take into consideration the effects of these potential confounders (restriction, stratification, or statistical analysis)?

Unlike bias, if the effects of possible confounding factors are anticipated, they can be corrected during the analysis phase of a study. The simplest way to control for confounding is *restriction*. For example, in the example of coffee drinking and lung cancer, the effects of confounding could be controlled by restricting study participants to people who do not smoke. Unfortunately, many studies are affected by more than one confounding factor, which can make the application of restrictions difficult.

Stratification is another technique to examine the possible effects of a third variable on an outcome. Rather than restricting the sample (e.g. excluding people who smoke), stratification allows researchers to examine separately the relation between coffee drinking and lung cancer in smokers and non-smokers and then compare the two results. This provides us with an idea of the effect of coffee drinking on lung cancer, independent of smoking.

Several statistical techniques can be used to account for the possible effects of confounding factors. The benefit of such techniques, the most common of which are *regression* techniques (e.g. logistic regression), is that several potential confounding factors can be considered simultaneously; we call this *adjusting* for each of the confounders. For example, Margolis et al.[4] were interested in whether men were at increased risk of developing pressure ulcers compared with women. The unadjusted rate ratio for this relation was 0.78, which means that men were 22% ([1.00 − 0.78] × 100) less likely to develop pressure ulcers than women; the 95% CI of 0.70 to 0.88 (which does not cross 1) suggests that this finding is unlikely to be the result of chance. However, when potential confounding factors, including age and other medical conditions, were taken into account, the adjusted rate ratio for pressure ulcers in men compared with women was 1.01 – that is, towards the null – with a 95% CI of 0.89 to 1.15. When age and medical conditions were taken into account, the data no longer provided evidence of a relation between sex and pressure ulcers. These statistical techniques are also referred to as *multivariable* techniques because they consider the effects of several variables at the same time, each taking the others into account.

Brandeis *et al.*[1] used a mixed approach to deal with confounding. Although the authors did not discuss the variable incidence of pressure ulcers across nursing homes in terms of confounding, they did, in a sense, attempt to account for these effects through stratification. The authors divided the data according to homes with high and low incidences of pressure ulcers and examined the variables associated with pressure ulcers for each group separately. However, they did not attempt to adjust for other potential confounding factors, such as number of chronic conditions or nutritional intake. The authors did mention in their discussion the possible effect of burden of disease as a way of explaining the observed sex differences in pressure ulcer risk. Although they did logistic regression analysis, they did not include these potential confounding factors in their regression model.

If matching was used, did the authors perform a matched analysis?

Case-control studies more commonly use *matching* as a technique to control for confounding factors. That is, controls are selected to ensure that the distribution of potential confounders is similar to that among the cases. Cases can be individually matched, for example, on age group and sex, or matched across the entire group of cases and controls. Although matching can improve the efficiency of a study, matching on too many factors is inadvisable as it may introduce selection bias, and, of course, it would not be possible to determine the effects of matched variables on outcome. If matching is part of the study design, then this must be taken into account in the data analysis. For further information on matching, readers can refer to Rothman and Greenland.[3]

What are the results?

Table 23.4 shows selected results from the study by Brandeis *et al.*[1] Several risk factors were identified as being related to the development of pressure ulcers in 'high-incidence' homes. For example, the odds ratio for the relation between

Table 23.4 Patient risk factors associated with pressure ulcer incidence

Risk factor	Odds ratio (95% CI)	p-Value
Homes with a high incidence of pressure ulcers		
Ambulatory difficulty	3.3 (2.0 to 5.3)	<0.001
Faecal incontinence	2.5 (1.6 to 4.0)	<0.001
Diabetes mellitus	1.7 (1.2 to 2.5)	<0.006
Difficulty feeding oneself	2.2 (1.5 to 3.3)	<0.001
Homes with a low incidence of pressure ulcers		
Male	1.9 (1.2 to 3.6)	<0.007
Ambulation difficulty	3.6 (1.7 to 7.4)	<0.001
Difficulty feeding oneself	3.5 (2.0 to 6.3)	<0.001

ambulatory difficulty and pressure ulcers was greater than 1.0; that is, residents with ambulatory difficulties had a greater risk of developing pressure ulcers than residents without ambulatory difficulties. In fact, they were three times as likely to develop pressure ulcers. The 95% CI of 2.0 to 5.3 around this odds ratio does not include 1 (the null), and therefore we have evidence to reject the null hypothesis.

Can I apply the results in practice?

The study by Brandeis et al.[1] suggests several possible risk factors for the onset of pressure ulcers in a nursing home setting. Two risk factors were found for both high- and low-incidence nursing homes: ambulatory difficulty and difficulty feeding oneself. These two factors had relatively strong associations with pressure ulcer development: residents with either of these characteristics were at least 2.2 times more likely to develop pressure ulcers than those without these characteristics. Other risk factors were faecal incontinence and diabetes mellitus for high-incidence nursing homes and male sex in low-incidence homes. The study was a longitudinal cohort study, and therefore we know that the outcome developed after the exposures and not the other way round (referred to as *reverse causality*). Because the outcome was not known at the time the exposures were measured, it is unlikely that there was any differential misclassification dependent on the outcome. Any misclassification of the exposures or the outcome is likely to have been random, which would have moved any observed associations towards the null. Nevertheless, the observed associations were quite strong. The study was perhaps weakest in terms of the way in which it dealt with confounding. For example, some of the observed associations may have been attenuated if the authors had controlled for the burden of disease among nursing home residents. However, it is unlikely that this would have explained all of the observed associations.

It is important to note that observational studies can only tell us about associations between exposures and outcomes. The findings do not necessarily tell us whether an exposure actually *causes* an outcome. In order to be more confident of the causes of an outcome, we generally depend on summaries of evidence from several studies.

Resolution of the clinical scenario

Based on the findings of Brandeis et al.[1] you suggest that residents with ambulatory difficulties be prioritized for the use of pressure-relieving mattresses.[5] You also decide to continue your research by identifying other studies (with various study designs) to see if they identify similar risk factors or perhaps suggest other high-risk groups.

LEARNING EXERCISE

Use PubMed's Clinical Queries feature to identify aetiological studies in your area of interest. Use the critical appraisal checklist in this chapter as an aid to appraising the validity of the most relevant articles identified.

References

1 Brandeis GH, Ooi WL, Hossain M, Morris JN, Lipsitz LA. A longitudinal study of risk factors associated with the formation of pressure ulcers in nursing homes. *J Am Geriatr Soc* 1994;42:388–93.
2 Unwin N, Carr SM, Leeson J, Pless-Mulloli T. *An Introductory Study Guide to Public Health Epidemiology.* Buckingham: Open University Press, 1997.
3 Rothman KJ, Greenland S, editors. *Modern Epidemiology.* Second edition. Philadelphia: Lippincott-Raven, 1998.
4 Margolis DJ, Knauss J, Bilker W, Baumgarten M. Medical conditions as risk factors for pressure ulcers in an outpatient setting. *Age Ageing* 2003;32:259–64.
5 Cullum N, McInnes E, Bell-Syer SE, Legood R. Support surfaces for pressure ulcer prevention. *Cochrane Database Syst Rev* 2004;(3):CD001735.

Chapter 24

EVALUATION OF STUDIES OF TREATMENT HARM

Susan Marks, Donna Ciliska and Andrew Jull

Previous chapters have described the evaluation of studies of the effectiveness of a treatment or intervention (Chapter 15) and studies of causation or aetiology (i.e. studies assessing the relation between certain exposures and the development of a specific disease or condition) (Chapter 23). This chapter will focus on related questions of the harmful effects of interventions or treatments, i.e. the undesirable outcomes of treatments prescribed by health care providers. The criteria (Box 24.1) are those identified in the original JAMA users' guide by Levine *et al.*[1]

Before we get started, a few preliminary notes. The concepts and criteria used to evaluate observational studies of treatment harm are similar to those used to assess

Box 24.1 Critical appraisal questions for studies of treatment harm

---

Are the results of the study valid?

- Were there clearly identified comparison groups that were similar with respect to important determinants of outcome other than the one of interest?
- Were the exposures and outcomes measured in the same way in the groups being compared?
- Was follow-up sufficiently long and complete?

What are the results?

- How strong is the association between the exposure and outcome?
- How precise is the estimate of risk?

Can I apply the results in practice?

- Are the results applicable to my patient(s)?
- What is the magnitude of the risk?
- Should I attempt to stop the exposure?
  - What is the strength of the study design?
  - What is the magnitude of effect if the exposure continues?
  - What are the potential adverse consequences of reducing or eliminating the exposure?
  - Is an acceptable alternative available?

---

studies of causation or aetiology. For example, an observational study may be conducted to determine the effects of second-hand smoke in the home on the development of asthma in children. In such a study, children exposed to second-hand smoke would be compared with those who were not exposed to see if the exposed and unexposed groups differed in terms of developing asthma. In this chapter, we will be focusing on the harms of a treatment or intervention. For example, a study by Madsen et al.[2] assessed whether children who received mumps, measles and rubella (MMR) vaccinations (intervention group) were more likely to develop autism than those who did not receive vaccinations (control group). In this chapter, we will primarily refer to the 'intervention group' (the equivalent of the exposed group) and the 'control group' (the unexposed group).

When considering studies of treatment harm, readers may encounter various terms used to refer to 'harm': studies may refer to risks, adverse events, side effects (often in relation to drugs), or the safety of an intervention.

Clinical scenario

You are a Nurse Practitioner working in a paediatric primary care clinic. Your patient is a 6-month-old infant presenting with recurrent otitis media. You feel that an antibiotic prescription is warranted but have recently heard concerns that use of antibiotics before the age of 1 year can lead to development of asthma. Thus, in addition to your concerns about the development of antibiotic resistance related to inappropriate use of antibiotics, you feel that you must also consider this potential risk when weighing the pros and cons of antibiotic treatment.

The search

You first define your clinical question: *Do antibiotics given to infants under 1 year of age increase the risk of subsequently developing asthma?* You decide to do a quick search on PubMed using the terms 'antibiotic and asthma and infant'. You find a meta-analysis by Marra et al.[3] on antibiotic exposure during infancy and development of asthma. Although you are familiar with the criteria for critically appraising the quality of a systematic review (see Chapter 19), you want to learn more about how primary studies approach questions of harm and how you can judge the validity and clinical usefulness of these studies. The review identified eight observational studies: four retrospective and four prospective studies. You know that a prospective study is a stronger design (see Chapter 7), so you retrieve a cohort study by Celedón et al.[4] that examined the relation between oral antibiotic use during the first year of life and development of asthma in early childhood. You systematically assess the study using the criteria summarized in Box 24.1.

Study designs for assessing questions of treatment harm

Questions of treatment harm can be assessed using different types of study designs.

Randomized controlled trials

The preferred study design for assessing questions of treatment harm is the randomized controlled trial (RCT). Some RCTs specifically focus on the adverse effects of a treatment (e.g. *Which of three techniques for giving intramuscular thigh vaccinations to infants and toddlers results in the fewest adverse reactions?*[5]), whereas others consider both the effectiveness (i.e. potential benefits to patients) and potential harms of an intervention (e.g. *What is the effectiveness and safety [i.e. adverse effects] of pressure bandages compared with no pressure bandages applied immediately after coronary angiography?*[6]). If you are able to identify an RCT examining the adverse effects of a treatment, you could proceed with assessing its validity and relevance using the criteria for evaluating studies of treatment or prevention outlined in Chapter 15.

Unfortunately, RCTs on the adverse effects of a treatment often are not available or are inadequate for several reasons. In some cases, particularly where the suspected adverse effects are severe and there is already some evidence of harm, it would be unethical to conduct an RCT. This could apply to our question about whether antibiotics given to infants increase the risk of developing asthma. Clearly, we have sufficient evidence that antibiotics are effective for treating many conditions. Thus, an RCT that compared the development of asthma in infants randomly allocated to receive antibiotics and those allocated to placebo would not be ethical as we would be withholding a treatment that we know to be effective from infants in the placebo group. Alternatively, for some conditions, it might be possible to design an RCT that compared antibiotics with some other active treatment.

An RCT is not feasible if an adverse outcome occurs very rarely because a very large sample size would be required to ensure sufficient power to detect differences between treatment groups in the rare event.[7] If the sample is too small, and the study has insufficient power, the chances of concluding that an intervention does not cause harm when it truly does (i.e. a *type II error*) are increased.

A second feasibility consideration is that some adverse effects develop many years after treatment. Lengthy follow-up in an RCT may be unfeasible because of the costs of following up participants and also the loss to follow-up that is likely to occur over time (again, decreasing the power of the study to detect significant differences in adverse effects if they do exist). As well, the length of follow-up needed to detect important adverse events related to an intervention may be unknown initially. For example, the development of specific types of cancer associated with some drugs may occur over many years. A classic example is the development of vaginal adenocarcinoma in the daughters of women who received diethylstilbestrol (DES) during their pregnancies. Exposure to the drug *in utero* was associated with the development of cancer many years later.[8]

Cohort studies

If an RCT is not available or has an inadequate sample size or length of follow-up, then a cohort study design is the next choice. In a *cohort study*, a group of people are followed up over time (i.e. prospectively) to see if they develop the outcome of interest. The cohort must include some people who received the intervention as well as a comparison group of people who did not receive the intervention; however, the 'exposure' to the intervention is not randomly allocated by the researcher as in an RCT. Rather, receipt or non-receipt of the intervention could be determined by clinicians or patients, with various factors contributing to the decision; studies such as these are often referred to as *natural experiments*.

Cohort studies are useful when a potential adverse event occurs infrequently.[1, 7] For example, cohort studies using large administrative databases could generate samples of hundreds of thousands of people and thus have sufficient power to detect differences between groups. The cohort study by Madsen *et al.* on the association between MMR vaccination and autism obtained vaccination data on 537 303 children from the Danish National Board of Health.[2] Database linkage with the Danish Psychiatric Central Register identified 738 children with autism or autism spectrum disorders (0.14%).[2]

Nested case-control studies are a variation of cohort studies, whereby cases and controls are identified within the context of a cohort study; thus, unlike most case-control studies, the direction of data collection is prospective rather than retrospective.

Case-control studies

In a *case-control study*, the investigators identify a group of people who have the outcome of interest (i.e. cases) as well as a group of people who do not have the outcome of interest (i.e. controls) and then 'look back' in time to determine whether the people in each group were exposed to the putative causative factor. In this respect, they differ from RCTs and cohort studies in that data are collected on the exposure (i.e. whether a patient received the intervention) *retrospectively*. Case-control studies may be useful when RCTs or cohort studies are not available or feasible: that is, when outcomes are very rare or take a long time to develop. The example of the effects of DES exposure *in utero* and later development of vaginal adenocarcinoma is a good example. An RCT or cohort study of this effect would have required follow-up of approximately 20 years to observe the outcome and very large sample sizes because of the rarity of the outcome, vaginal adenocarcinoma. Alternatively, a case-control study by Herbst *et al.*[8] compared eight women diagnosed with adenocarcinoma with 32 matched controls (born within 5 days of the cases) in terms of their mothers' use of DES during pregnancy (data collected retrospectively). They found a strong association between vaginal adenocarcinoma and *in utero* exposure to DES.

Case reports, case series and cross-sectional studies

These are the weakest types of studies for assessing harm associated with an intervention. A *case report* is a description of a single patient, whereas a *case series* is a description of several patients. No comparison or control groups are assessed, and as such we cannot be sure if an adverse outcome is related to the intervention, the disease or condition being treated, or some other related characteristic. Such studies are considered preliminary and may be used as a basis for planning further prospective studies. *Cross-sectional studies* examine a group of people and consider exposures and outcomes at a single point in time. Thus, it is not possible to determine the temporal relation between the exposure and the outcome (i.e. which came first: the exposure, or intervention, or the adverse outcome?). For example, in a cross-sectional study, Droste *et al.* administered questionnaires to the parents of 6- to 7-year-old children in Antwerp; questions addressed the use of antibiotics in the first year of life (e.g. *Did your child receive antibiotics in the first year of life?*) and the presence of asthma (e.g. *Has your child ever had asthma?*) and allergy symptoms (e.g. *Has your child ever had hayfever?*).[9]

Returning to our clinical scenario, we note that the study by Celedón *et al.*[4] was a prospective cohort study that followed up 4408 children enrolled in a health maintenance organization from birth to 5 years of age. Over the first year of life, data on antibiotic prescriptions were collected through the use of automated pharmacy records. As well, at 1, 2, 3, 4 and 5 years, data were collected on the presence of asthma from automated medical records of ambulatory care.

Are the results of the study valid?

Were there clearly identified comparison groups that were similar with respect to important determinants of outcome other than the one of interest?

It is important to determine whether patients who received the intervention and those who did not were similar at the beginning of the study in terms of important determinants (e.g. *confounders*) that might influence the likelihood of the adverse outcome. If important group differences exist at the beginning of a study, differences in adverse outcome could be attributed to these differences in prognostic factors rather than exposure to the intervention.

In our clinical question about the relation between early antibiotic use and development of asthma in children, one possible confounder could be the number of respiratory infections a child had during the first year of life. A *confounder* is a variable that is related to both the exposure and the outcome (see Chapter 23). It is possible that children who have multiple respiratory infections in the first year of life may be more likely to develop asthma than other children; it is also likely that these children would receive more antibiotic prescriptions (for these infections) than other children. Thus, an increased risk of asthma could be a result of the respiratory infections rather than, or in addition to, antibiotic use.

In an RCT, random allocation of participants to intervention and control groups allows us to be confident that groups were similar with respect to known and unknown characteristics related to outcome.[1] In a cohort study, there is no reason to believe that intervention and control groups would be similar to each other with respect to potential confounders, and group differences in confounding variables could be responsible for observed differences in outcome.[1] Similarly, *case-control studies* are also susceptible to the effects of group differences in confounding variables.[1] In fact, the potential for confounding is even greater than in cohort studies because the samples are already highly selected.[10]

In all study designs, it is important for authors to document the characteristics of patients who received and did not receive the intervention and to demonstrate comparability between groups in these characteristics or, if differences exist, to adjust for them using statistical techniques.

In the cohort study by Celedón *et al.*[4] the authors did not provide detailed data on baseline similarities or differences in the intervention and control groups in potential confounders. However, they did report that they did a multivariate analysis to assess the relation between antibiotic use in the first year of life and asthma at ages

2 and 5 years, adjusting for confounders such as respiratory illnesses in the first year of life. Respiratory illness is a potential confounder because it is related to antibiotic use and to development of asthma. The authors also note that they did not have data on parental history of asthma and allergies, another potential confounder.

Were the exposures and outcomes measured in the same way in the groups being compared?

Application of this criterion depends on the study design. In RCTs and cohort studies, attempts to minimize bias focus on 'outcome assessment'. If assessors of adverse outcomes are aware of exposure status (and the possible increased risk of an adverse event), they might search more diligently and thus be more likely to detect the adverse event or detect it at an earlier point in time. This is referred to as *surveillance bias* (also known as *information bias, detection bias, or ascertainment bias)*. Blinding of data collectors and outcome assessors to exposure status can help to minimize this bias.[1]

In case-control studies, you need to consider 'assessment of exposure'. Remember, data collection in a case-control study is retrospective. Those with the outcome of interest (cases) and those without the outcome (controls) are often asked to recall their exposure to suspected causative agents. Cases may be more likely to recall exposures to such causative agents than controls simply because they are sensitized or more interested in understanding the causes of their conditions. Differential recall of instances of exposure can lead to *recall bias*. Similarly, interviewers in case-control studies who are aware of the case/control status of participants might intentionally or unintentionally probe more or less deeply when asking about exposures. This is referred to as *interviewer bias*. Thus, case-control studies should attempt to blind those assessing exposure (treatment status) to the case or control status of patients; patients can be blinded to the purpose of the study.

The study by Celedón *et al.*[4] was a cohort study, and thus assessment of bias should focus on blinding of those assessing the adverse event (i.e. asthma at age 2 or 5). Data on asthma at 2 or 5 years of age was obtained from an automated medical record system for ambulatory care, a claims system for hospital admissions and emergency department visits, and a separate automated pharmacy system. The authors defined asthma as present if a child had ≥2 ambulatory visits or ≥1 emergency department visit or ≥1 hospital admission for asthma (all based on a specific ICD-9 code) or had received ≥2 dispensings of any asthma medication in the previous 12 months. The authors did not explicitly state that the outcome assessors (of asthma) did not have knowledge of antibiotic prescriptions. In fact, one of the definitions of asthma was based on dispensing of asthma medication. Thus, at the time that the outcome assessors reviewed the dispensing database to determine if asthma medication had been dispensed, they could also have seen the data on dispensing of antibiotics (the exposure). Such information could have led the outcome assessors to check the record more carefully (anticipating that a child would be more likely to have asthma) – that is, surveillance bias is a possibility. Often, authors collect exposure and outcome data from separate databases and use a computer program to link patient records in the two databases on the basis of a common identifier (e.g. patient number). In such an instance, a blinding statement would not be required because the automated linkage of exposure and outcome data would be considered objective.

Was follow-up sufficiently long and complete?

Patients who are unavailable for follow-up may have different outcomes than those who are available. The longer the follow-up period, the greater the possibility that follow-up will be incomplete.[1] As well, follow-up must be sufficiently long to observe the anticipated outcomes.

In the study by Celedón et al.[4] children were enrolled in the health maintenance organization database within 90 days of birth. Data collection was ongoing, and the presence of the adverse event (asthma) was assessed at ages 2 and 5 years. A total of 4672 infants were identified as members of the initial birth cohort; after excluding children who had no ambulatory visits during the first 2 years of life or were diagnosed with asthma before 1 year of age, 4408 eligible children were included in the study. This study used data from an existing health care database in which data collection occurred in a prospective manner. However, the same data were not prospectively collected for each child, and thus we are not able to assess loss to follow-up in the traditional way. That is, lack of data on primary care visits for asthma is not 'missing data': it is assumed to be the absence of the adverse event (no asthma).

Is follow-up to 2 years and 5 years sufficient to determine differences in the development of asthma? One would expect that 5 years after exposure is a reasonable length of time to observe the development of asthma in children.

What are the results?

How strong is the association between the exposure and outcome?

The data for a specific adverse outcome can be summarized in a simple 2×2 table (Figure 24.1). We can complete this table using data from table 1 in the original article by Celedón et al.[4] (Figure 24.2). Using the numbers in this table, we can calculate an estimate of the *strength of the association* between the exposure and the adverse event. The strength of the association between the intervention and the outcome is usually represented by relative risks or odds ratios (see Chapter 11).[1] The *relative risk (RR)* or *risk ratio* is the risk of people in the intervention group experiencing the adverse event divided by the risk of people in the control group experiencing the event. Using our 2×2 table, the RR is calculated as $[a/(a + b)]/[c/(c + d)]$. RRs are not applicable in case-control studies because they require samples of exposed and unexposed participants in which the proportion of participants with the adverse event can be calculated. In a case-control study, the proportion of patients with the adverse event (i.e. cases) is determined *a priori* by the investigator. Thus, the strength of association in case-control studies is represented as odds ratios; authors of RCTs and cohort studies may also choose to report the strength of association as odds ratios. The *odds ratio (OR)* is the odds of having the adverse event in the intervention group divided by the odds of having the adverse event in the control group[11] and is calculated as $(a/c)/(b/d)$.

RRs or ORs of 1 indicate that the intervention and control groups did not differ for the adverse event. RRs and ORs >1 indicate an increased risk of the adverse event among those in the intervention group, whereas estimates <1 indicate a decreased risk of the event in the intervention group. Generally, the further away the RR or

	Adverse event	No adverse event
Intervention (exposed)	*a*	*b*
Control (unexposed)	*c*	*d*

Figure 24.1 A 2 × 2 table summarizing data on adverse outcomes. a = the number of patients who received the intervention and experienced the adverse event; b = the number of patients who received the intervention and did *not* experience the adverse event, c = the number of patients who did not receive the intervention and experienced the adverse event, and d = the number of patients who did not receive the intervention and did *not* experience the adverse event.

	Asthma at 2 years	No asthma at 2 years	
Antibiotics during first year	$a = 280$	$b = 3012$	$a + b = 3292$
No antibiotics during first year	$c = 43$	$d = 1073$	$c + d = 1116$
	$a + c = 323$	$b + d = 4085$	$a + b + c + d = 4408$

Figure 24.2 A 2 × 2 table summarizing data from Celedón *et al.*[4]

OR is from 1.0, the greater the strength of the association between the intervention and the outcome.

Returning to the data above from the study by Celedón *et al.*[4] we can calculate both the RR and OR:

$$\text{RR} = \frac{a/(a+b)}{c/(c+d)} = \frac{280/3292}{43/1116} = 0.09/0.04 = 2.3$$

$$\text{OR} = \frac{a/c}{b/d} = \frac{280/43}{3012/1073} = 6.51/2.81 = 2.3$$

An RR of 2.3 means that children who received antibiotics during the first year of life were more than twice as likely to develop asthma by age 2 as children who received no antibiotics during the first year of life. An OR of 2.3 means that the odds of developing asthma in children who received antibiotics during the first year of life were more than twice that of those who did not receive antibiotics.

However, this is an unadjusted estimate of the strength of association. Recall our earlier discussion of potential confounders and the need to adjust analyses for these variables. At 2 years of age, the OR, adjusted for sex, primary care visits, and upper and lower respiratory tract infections, was 1.2. Thus, the strength of association was reduced from 2.0 to 1.2 after adjustment for confounders.

How precise is the estimate of risk?

You can determine the precision of the estimate of risk by looking at the 95% confidence interval (CI) around the estimate. The 95% CI is the range of values within which we can be 95% sure that the true value for the entire population lies. If the 95% CI around an RR or OR crosses 1, then the result is considered to be non-significant: that is, the range of values includes the possibility of both a decreased risk of the outcome (values <1) and an increased risk of the outcome (values >1), as well as the possibility of no effect (RR or OR = 1).

If there is an association between the intervention and the adverse event, the lower limit of the CI provides an estimate of the minimal strength of association.

Celedón et al.[4] reported the 2-year and 5-year results comparing children who received 1–2 antibiotic courses and those who received no antibiotics (Table 24.1). Note that, for the results at 1–2 years of age, none of the 95% CIs cross 1. Thus, each OR is statistically significant. On the other hand, at 2–5 years of age, each of the 95% CIs crosses 1. Thus, none of these ORs are statistically significant.

Looking at the results for 2–5 years, we see that when the analysis was adjusted only for sex, the CI around the OR of 1.1 was 0.8 to 1.5. This means that we can be 95% sure that the true OR for the population is between 0.8 and 1.5; that is, the odds of developing asthma in children who received 1–2 courses of antibiotics during their first year may be as low as 0.8 (i.e. a reduced risk) or as high as 1.5.

Can I apply the results in practice?

Are the results applicable to my patient(s?)

In determining whether your patients are similar to those in a particular study, you should consider similarities and differences in terms of exposures, as well as other potentially important factors such as sex, age and race.[1]

Table 24.1 Adjusted odds ratios for presence of asthma at 1–2 and 2–5 years of age in children who received antibiotics during the first year of life

Variables adjusted for	Odds ratios (95% CI)	
	1–2 years of age	2–5 years of age
Sex	2.0 (1.4 to 2.9)	1.1 (0.8 to 1.5)
Sex and office visits	1.8 (1.3 to 2.6)	0.9 (0.7 to 1.3)
Sex, office visits, and lower respiratory tract infections	1.9 (1.3 to 2.7)	1.1 (0.8 to 1.4)
Sex, office visits, and upper respiratory tract infections	1.2 (1.1 to 1.3)	1.0 (0.8 to 1.4)

Assessing the generalizability of the findings of studies of treatment harm can be complicated. The frequency and severity of adverse events depend on both the clinical setting and participants.[12] Often, studies of treatment harm include patients who have the disease of interest, but are otherwise healthy; in the 'real' world, many patients have comorbid conditions.[12]

The patient in our clinical scenario is a 6-month-old infant with recurrent otitis media, who is otherwise healthy. The clinical setting is a primary care clinic. Similarly, the study by Celedón et al.[4] included infants attending a health maintenance organization. The only exclusion criteria were a diagnosis of asthma before 1 year of age and lack of ambulatory visits during the first 2 years of life. Thus, our setting and patient are similar to those reported in the study by Celedón et al.

What is the magnitude of the risk?

As previously discussed, RRs and ORs tell us that a given outcome occurs more or less frequently in patients exposed or not exposed to an intervention. However, we are also interested in the magnitude of risk in the context of clinical importance. The number needed to treat (NNT), or number needed to harm (NNH) in the case of an adverse event, is one measure of clinical importance that can be calculated using data from RCTs or cohort studies. The *NNH* is the number of patients who would need to be exposed to the intervention to cause one additional adverse outcome. The NNH is the reciprocal of the difference in adverse events between the intervention and control groups. Usually, this would only be calculated if the study findings were significant. However, for illustrative purposes, we can use the 2×2 table in Table 24.1 to calculate the NNH as follows:

$$NNH = 1/[a/(a + b) - c/(c + d)]$$

Using the data from the study by Celedón et al. summarized in Table 23.2, we calculate the NNH as

$$1/[280/(280 + 3012) - 43/(43 + 1073)]$$
$$= 1/(0.085 - 0.039) = 1/0.046$$
$$= 21.7 = 22$$

Thus, we would need to expose 22 infants to antibiotics in the first year of life to cause one additional diagnosis of asthma at age 2 years. Of course, we would also want to calculate the 95% CIs so that we could assess the precision of our NNH estimate. However, the specifics of calculating the CI around this estimate are beyond the scope of this chapter.

The NNH could also be calculated from an adjusted OR and the control (unexposed) event rate using the following formula:

$$NNH = 1/(OR - 1) \times \text{control event rate} + 1/(OR/(OR - 1) \times (1 - \text{control event rate})$$

Should I attempt to stop the exposure?

This is often the core issue for both clinicians and patients: should these findings lead me to act differently? For nurse clinicians, the question may be whether or not to prescribe, deliver, or suggest a particular intervention to patients. Four factors should be considered: (a) What is the strength of the study design? (b) What is the magnitude of effect if the exposure continues? (c) What are the potential adverse consequences of reducing or eliminating the exposure? (d) Is an acceptable alternative available?

Returning to the clinical scenario, you are faced with the question of whether or not to prescribe antibiotics to the 6-month-old infant presenting with recurrent otitis media based on the findings of the study by Celedón et al.[4]

1. *Strength of the study design*: The study had a prospective cohort design. The authors did not state that outcome assessors were blinded, and the collection of some measures of both the intervention (antibiotic prescriptions) and the outcome (asthma defined by prescriptions for asthma medication) from the same source suggest that incomplete blinding of outcome assessors could have contributed bias. The analysis adjusted for sex, primary care visits, and respiratory illnesses in the first year of life; however, the authors stated that they did not have data on the indication for antibiotic use during the first year (i.e. antibiotics prescribed for respiratory illnesses) or parental history of asthma and allergies, which they identify as potential confounders.
2. *Magnitude of effect if exposure continues*: As previously discussed, at 5 years, the adjusted ORs indicated no significant association between antibiotic use during the first year of life and development of asthma at 2–5 years of age. As well, the adjusted OR for children receiving >4 courses of antibiotics in the first year of life was also non-significant (0.9, CI 0.6 to 1.3), suggesting that the risk of asthma did not increase with increased exposure to antibiotics. The existence of such a *dose–response relationship* (i.e. exposure to greater amounts of the intervention is associated with increased magnitude of the outcome, and vice versa) strengthens the likelihood that a causal relation exists between the intervention and the outcome
3. *Potential adverse consequences of reducing or eliminating the exposure*: The obvious consequence of not prescribing antibiotics to your patient for this episode of recurrent otitis media is that the illness episode may be prolonged. In a meta-analysis of individual patient data, Rovers et al.[13] showed that antibiotics reduced the risk of an extended course of acute otitis media by 16% (95% CI 11 to 22) compared with placebo or no treatment, along with reductions in pain and fever of 14% and 8%, respectively.
4. *Availability of acceptable alternatives*: A possible alternative would be to delay prescribing antibiotics for up to 72 hours. An RCT of 315 children with acute otitis media showed that delayed prescribing of antibiotics (for 72 h) did not differ from immediate prescribing for earaches at 3 months or 1 year.[14]

Resolution of the scenario

Although Celedón et al.[4] found a significant increase in the risk of a diagnosis of asthma at 1–2 years of age among infants who received antibiotics during the first year of life, the strength of association based on adjusted analysis was rather low (OR 1.2, CI 1.1 to 1.3). As well, antibiotic use during the first year was not associated with an increased risk of asthma at 2–5 years of age. You feel that there is insufficient evidence to avoid an antibiotic prescription and sufficient evidence to support the use of antibiotics for treating this episode of recurrent otitis media.

LEARNING EXERCISES

1. Identify a clinical question related to harm of treatment. For example, what are the harmful effects of chemotherapy or radiation for people with cancer? Is there a link between paracetamol (acetaminophen) use and liver disease?
2. Conduct a search to identify a relevant article to address the question identified above. Hint: use the 'Etiology' category in 'Clinical Queries' in PubMed.
3. In the identified article, find the odds ratio or relative risk. Interpret to a classmate or colleague, in your own words, the meaning of that result, and the confidence interval surrounding the odds ratio or relative risk.

References

1 Levine M, Walter S, Lee H, Haines T, Holbrook A, Moyer V, for the Evidence-Based Medicine Working Group. Users' guides to the medical literature. IV. How to use an article about harm. *JAMA* 1994;**271**:1615–19.
2 Madsen KM, Hviid A, Vestergaard M, Schendel D, Wohlfarht J, Thorsen P, Olsen J, Melbye M. A population-based study of measles, mumps, and rubella vaccination and autism. *N Engl J Med* 2002;**347**:1477–82.
3 Marra F, Lynd L, Coombes M, Richardson K, Legal M, Fitzgerald JM, Marra CA. Does antibiotic exposure during infancy lead to development of asthma? A systematic review and metaanalysis. *Chest* 2006;**129**:610–18.
4 Celedón JC, Fuhlbrigge A, Rifas-Shiman S, Weiss ST, Finkelstein JA. Antibiotic use in the first year of life and asthma in early childhood. *Clin Exp Allergy* 2004;**34**:1011–16.
5 Cook IF, Murtagh J. Optimal technique for intramuscular injection of infants and toddlers: a randomised trial. *Med J Aust* 2005;**183**:60–3.
6 Botti M, Williamson B, Steen K, McTaggart J, Reid E. The effect of pressure bandaging on complications and comfort in patients undergoing coronary angiography: a multicenter randomized trial. *Heart Lung* 1998;**27**:360–73.
7 Cullum N, Guyatt C. Harm. In: DiCenso A, Guyatt G, Ciliska D (editors). *Evidence-Based Nursing. A Guide to Clinical Practice.* St Louis: Elsevier Mosby, 2005:71–86.
8 Herbst AL, Ulfelder H, Poskanzer DC. Adenocarcinoma of the vagina. Association of maternal stilbestrol therapy with tumor appearance in young women. *N Engl J Med* 1971;**284**:878–81.
9 Droste JH, Wieringa MH, Weyler JJ, Nelen VJ, Vermeire PA, Van Bever HP. Does the use of antibiotics in early childhood increase the risk of asthma and allergic disease? *Clin Exp Allergy* 2000;**30**:1547–53.
10 Rothman KJ. *Epidemiology: an introduction.* Oxford: University Press, 2002.
11 Strauss SE, Richardson WS, Glasziou P, Haynes RB. *Evidence-Based Medicine: How to Practice and Teach EBM.* Third edition. New York: Elsevier, 2005:177–97.
12 Ioannidis JP, Evans SJ, Gotzsche PC, O'Neill RT, Altman DG, Schulz K, Moher D, for the CONSORT Group. Better reporting of harms in randomized trials: an extension of the CONSORT statement. *Ann Intern Med* 2004;**141**:781–8.
13 Rovers MM, Glasziou P, Appelman CL, Burke P, McCormick DP, Damoiseaux RA, Gaboury I, Little P, Hoes AW. Antibiotics for acute otitis media: a meta-analysis with individual patient data. *Lancet* 2006;**368**:1429–35.
14 Little P, Moore M, Warner G, Dunleavy J, Williamson I. Longer term outcomes from a randomised trial of prescribing strategies in otitis media. *Br J Gen Pract* 2006;**56**:176–82.

Chapter 25

EVALUATION OF QUALITATIVE RESEARCH STUDIES

Cynthia K. Russell and David M. Gregory

Clinical scenario

You work on a palliative care unit where you have many opportunities to discuss end-of-life decisions with patients and their family members. In a recent team meeting of your unit's providers, the topic of 'appropriate' treatment choices for persons at end of life comes up. Some providers believe that they should counsel patients and their family members to 'help them make better end-of-life decisions so that they will have a good death'. There is, however, no consensus about how this should be done.

The search

You volunteer to see if any studies have been done on decision-making at the end of life. You remember that your institution has an online subscription to *Evidence-Based Nursing*. You sign in and go to the advanced search screen. In the field 'Word(s) Anywhere in Article' you type in 'end-of-life decisions' (in quotations because you are looking for articles that include all four words together). Nine matches are found. The first is an abstract entitled 'Providers tried to help patients and families make end of life decisions'.[1] You review the full text of the abstract, which describes a qualitative study by Norton and Bowers[2] that seems to address the issues of interest. You get a copy of the full article from the library so that you can more fully assess the usefulness of this study for your team.

Many authors have proposed criteria for appraising qualitative research (see Table 25.1).[3–12] Some question the appraisal process because of a lack of consensus among qualitative researchers on quality criteria.[6–8, 10] Despite this controversy, and while recognizing that criteria will continue to evolve, we provide a set of guidelines to help nurses identify methodologically sound qualitative research studies that can inform their practice. Our standard approach to appraising an article from the health care literature is readily applicable (see Box 25.1).

Table 25.1 Qualitative authors' conceptualizations of quality criteria for qualitative reports

Miles & Huberman, 1994[11]	Thorne, 1997[5]	Sandelowski & Barroso, 2002[6]	Morse et al. 2002[7]	Holliday, 2002[12]
These authors offer minimum guidelines for the report structure of qualitative studies. The report should: 1. Tell what the study was about or came to be about 2. Communicate a clear sense of the social and historical context of the settings where data were collected 3. Provide detail of the inquiry process 4. Provide basic data in a focused form so that readers can, in parallel with the researcher, draw warranted conclusions 5. Articulate the researchers' conclusions and describe their broader meaning	Thorne describes four evaluation criteria that cross the spectrum of qualitative research: 1. Epistemological integrity 2. Representative credibility 3. Analytic logic 4. Interpretive authority Thorne goes on to describe five additional areas of critique that relate to disciplinary knowledge: 1. Moral defensibility 2. Disciplinary relevance 3. Pragmatic obligation 4. Contextual awareness 5. Probable truth	According to the authors, most readers in health-related disciplines want and/or expect information in 13 categories: 1. Research problem 2. Research purpose(s)/question(s) 3. Literature review 4. Orientation to the target phenomenon 5. Method 6. Sampling 7. Sample 8. Data collection 9. Data management 10. Validity 11. Findings 12. Discussion 13. Ethics The authors added a 14th category to the list: Form	The authors advocate for attention to six strategies that are meant to ensure rigour: 1. Investigator responsiveness 2. Methodological coherence 3. Sampling sufficiency 4. Developing a dynamic relationship between data collection and analysis 5. Thinking theoretically 6. Theory development	Holliday writes about the role of the following strategies for 'making appropriate claims': 1. Allowing ordinary voice: non-exploitative; not distorting the voices of participants 2. Cautious detachment: hedging; setting a cautious scene; making restrained sense; being careful with people's words 3. Suspending judgement: avoiding meaningless labels and easy answers 4. Placing people in relationships: organizing thoughts and experiences to discover what is going on

Box 25.1 Questions to help critically appraise qualitative research

Are the findings valid?

- Is the research question clear and adequately substantiated?
- Is the design appropriate for the research question?
- Was the method of sampling appropriate for the research question and design?
- Were data collected and managed systematically?
- Were the data analysed appropriately?

What are the findings?

- Is the description of findings thorough?

How can I apply the findings to patient care?

- What meaning and relevance does the study have for my practice?
- Does the study help me understand the context of my practice?
- Does the study enhance my knowledge about my practice?

Are the findings of the study valid?

Qualitative researchers do not speak about validity in the same terms as quantitative researchers. In keeping with the world views and paradigms from which qualitative research arises, validity, or whether the research reflects best standards of qualitative science, is described in terms of rigour, credibility, trustworthiness, and believability. Numerous articles and books focus on validity issues for qualitative research.[13–18] Similarly, there are several qualitative research designs, and each has slightly different conventions for their appropriate conduct. This chapter provides an overview of the critical appraisal of qualitative research, but, as with various quantitative research designs, there are variations in how rigour and validity are addressed in specific designs.

Is the research question clear and adequately substantiated?

Before proceeding with a fully fledged review of the study, readers should look for the precise question the study sought to answer and consider its relevance to their own clinical questions. The study report should clearly document what is already known about the phenomenon of interest.

Norton and Bowers[2] explored how providers described their work in changing patients' and families' treatment decisions at end of life from what providers deemed curative to palliative (unrealistic to more realistic). The stated purpose of the study was 'to develop a grounded theory of how decisions were negotiated among providers and family members near the end of a patient's life'. During the development of the grounded theory, the authors described how they identified 'several strategies providers used to assist patients and families to shift from curative to palliative treatment choices and goals'. The study report focused on those strategies. The authors clearly stated that this report focused on one portion of a larger grounded theory that was derived from the main study.

Norton and Bowers[2] discussed background literature on patient self-determination, advance directives, level of treatment received, beliefs about prognosis, changes of patient treatment decisions over time, and how individuals, families, and providers achieve agreement on treatment decisions.

Is the design appropriate for the research question?

More than 40 unique approaches to qualitative research methods have been identified.[19] As noted by Ploeg in Chapter 8, common approaches in published health care research include ethnography, grounded theory, and phenomenology. Other approaches include case studies, narrative research, and historical research. Traditional ethnography seeks to learn about culture from the people who actually live in that culture.[20] A grounded theory approach is used to discover the social-psychological processes inherent in a phenomenon,[21] whereas a phenomenological approach is used to gain a deeper understanding of the nature or meaning of the everyday 'lived' experiences of people.[22]

Qualitative approaches arise from specific disciplines and are influenced by theoretical perspectives within those disciplines. A critical analysis of a qualitative study considers the 'fit' of the research question with the qualitative method used in the study.[23] Although the specific criteria for proper application of each methodological approach vary somewhat, there are sufficient similarities among the approaches to discuss them in general.

The use of a grounded theory method was appropriate for the study by Norton and Bowers,[2] given that the authors were interested in the meanings that providers attributed to end of life treatment choices of patients and their families and how providers attempted to shift patients' and families' understandings of the 'big picture' to influence their treatment decisions. Thus, meanings and processes are central to the grounded theory method.

Was the method of sampling appropriate for the research question and design?

The emergent nature of qualitative research that results from the interaction between data collection and data analysis requires that investigators do not rigidly pre-specify a sample for data collection in strict terms, lest important data sources be overlooked. In quantitative studies, the ideal sampling standard is random sampling. Most qualitative studies use *purposeful (or purposive) sampling*, that is, the conscious selection of a small number of data sources that meet particular criteria. The logic and power of purposeful sampling lie in selecting information-rich cases (participants or settings) for in-depth study to illuminate the questions of interest.[16] This type of sampling usually aims to cover a range of potentially relevant social phenomena and perspectives from an appropriate array of data sources. Selection criteria often evolve over the course of analysis, and investigators return repeatedly to the data to explore new cases or new perspectives.

Readers of qualitative studies should look for sound reasoning in the description and justification of the strategies for selecting data sources. Patton[16] offers a succinct, clear and comprehensive discussion of the various sampling strategies used in qualitative research. Convenience sampling is one of the most commonly used, yet one of the least appropriate, sampling strategies. In *convenience sampling*, participants are selected primarily on the basis of ease of access to the researcher and, secondarily, for their knowledge of the subject matter. Purposive non-probability sampling strategies include the following:

1. *Judgemental sampling*, where theory or knowledge points the researcher to select specific cases.
   (a) *maximum variation sampling*, to document range or diversity;
   (b) *extreme or deviant case sampling*, where it is necessary to select cases that are unusual or special in some way;
   (c) *typical* or *representative case sampling*, to describe and illustrate what is typical and common in terms of the phenomenon of interest;
   (d) *critical cases*, to make a point dramatically;
   (e) *criterion sampling*, where all cases that meet some predetermined criteria are studied (this sampling strategy is commonly used in quality improvement).
2. *Opportunistic sampling*, where availability of participants guides on-the-spot sampling decisions.
3. *Snowball, network*, or *chain sampling*, where people nominate others for participation.
4. Theory-based *operational construct sampling*, where incidents, time periods, people, or other data sources are sampled on the basis of their potential manifestation or representation of important theoretical constructs.

Participant observation studies typically use opportunistic sampling strategies, whereas grounded theory studies use theory-based operational construct sampling.

Sample size is a critical question for all research studies. A study that uses a sample that is too small may have unique and particular findings such that its qualitative transferability or quantitative generalizability becomes questionable. In qualitative research, however, even studies with small samples may help to identify theoretically provocative ideas that merit further exploration. Studies with samples that are too large are equally problematic. Whereas quantitative research has specific guidelines that frame researchers' decisions about adequate sample size, there are only general principles, reflective of judgement and negotiation, for qualitative researchers. Examination of several areas will help readers to identify the adequacy of sample size in qualitative studies. First, references about the specific method used may offer some guidance. For example, sample sizes in phenomenological studies are typically smaller than those in grounded theory and ethnographic studies. Secondly, the trade-off between breadth and depth in the research affects sample size. Studies with smaller samples can more fully explore a broader range of participants' experiences, whereas studies with larger samples typically focus on a more narrow range of experiences. Thirdly, readers can review published studies that used similar methods and focused on similar phenomena for guidance about sample size adequacy. Qualitative researchers judge the adequacy of a sample for a given study by how comprehensively and completely the research questions were answered. Readers of qualitative studies are encouraged to review the researcher's documentation of sample size and selection throughout the course of the study.

Norton and Bowers[2] interviewed 15 health care providers. Given that theoretical sampling is a key sampling strategy in grounded theory research, the authors discussed how they altered the design of the interviews to identify whether providers assessed patients' and families' understanding, whether they used strategies to help patients and their families come to a more realistic understanding of their situations, and how providers understood their actions and what they were trying to accomplish. As the research progressed, Norton and Bowers[2] described theoretical sampling of types of providers (nurses and physicians), work settings (home health, family practice, oncology, and intensive care), and work experience (experienced or novice, in terms of number of years of experience as a health care provider and experience with persons who were dying). The authors clearly indicate the hypotheses (or 'hunches') that stimulated their explorations of particular types of participants. Recruitment was conducted through letters of invitation, with a 60% response rate, which means the researchers would have sent out approximately 25 letters of invitation. The types of provider who decided not to participate were unclear from the report. Often it is useful to determine why participants refuse to enrol in a study, as their decisions may inform researchers about the phenomenon of interest.

Were data collected and managed systematically?

Qualitative researchers commonly use one or more of three basic strategies for collecting data. One strategy is to witness events and record them as they occur (*field observation*). Another strategy is to question participants directly about their experience (*interviews*). Finally, researchers may review written material (*document analysis*). Readers should consider which data collection strategies researchers used and whether these strategies would be expected to offer the most complete and accurate understanding of the phenomenon.

Regardless of the strategy, the approach to data collection must be comprehensive to avoid focusing on particular, potentially misleading, aspects of the data. Several aspects of a qualitative report indicate how extensively the investigators collected data: the number of observations, interviews, or documents; the duration of the observations and interviews; the duration of the study period; the diversity of units of analysis and data collection techniques; the number of investigators involved in data collection and analysis; and the degree of investigators' involvement in data collection and analysis notes.[24–27] Taping and transcribing interviews (or other dialogue) is often desirable but is not necessary for all qualitative studies.

All participants were interviewed once, and three providers were interviewed a second time. Initial interviews were completed using open-ended questions and lasted 60–90 minutes. Later interviews lasted 30–60 minutes as the questions became more focused. The authors included a table in their article that provided examples of changes in interview questions for participants 1–5, 6–10, and 11–15.

Although Norton and Bowers[2] note that fieldwork was part of 'member checking', they did not fully describe the inclusion of a participant observation component in their research. When the grounded theory method was initially developed by Glaser and Strauss,[28] they included participant observation and interviews as data collection methods. At this time, most grounded theory studies only use interviews for data generation.

The authors did not incorporate an examination of records. A chart review might have illuminated what providers wrote about patient and family treatment choices and providers' documentations of their attempts to influence those choices. The omission of such data does not weaken the study but might have offered additional perspectives on the research question.

The study was conducted in a mid-size mid-western city in the United States (US). Participating providers were recruited from home health and family practice, oncology practice, and intensive care units. The study was published in 2001, and the research was likely done approximately 2–5 years before that date. Although the authors did not clearly indicate the date of the study, a quick look at the references reveals that Norton completed her dissertation in 1999, and these data were collected during her dissertation. Some peer-reviewed journals have policies that specify that research data may not be older than 5 years in order to ensure currency, relevance, and contemporary understanding of phenomena. The Norton and Bowers data were collected and published within the standard time frame for data freshness.

Interviews were audiotaped, transcribed verbatim, and checked for accuracy before data were entered into a computer qualitative data management system. Norton and Bowers[2] used QSR NUD*IST 4 to assist in qualitative data management. Other procedures used to enhance the credibility of the findings reveal the authors' attention to the analysis process. As principal investigator, Norton wrote that she was engaged in the collection and analysis of data for a period of 22 months, during which time she met weekly with a multidisciplinary, grounded theory, dimensional analysis group. Members of this group would have offered critique and commentary of the ongoing analysis based on their disciplinary perspectives, thus enlarging on those of Norton. Group members focused on the type of analysis used, thereby helping to ensure that the analysis procedures were rigorous and adhered to the tenets of the method. Weekly meetings meant that the researcher remained immersed in the data and thinking about the data, which increased the likelihood that she would not arrive at premature closure in her analysis. It is unclear if Norton was the sole data collector. The authors described the memos and matrices used to track methodological decisions and the development of the grounded theory.

Were the data analysed appropriately?

In Chapter 13, Thorne described the inductive reasoning process as one which qualitative researchers rely on to interpret and structure meanings derived from the data. Qualitative researchers often begin with a general exploratory question and preliminary concepts. They then collect relevant data, observe patterns in the data, organize these into a conceptual framework, and resume data collection to both explore and challenge their developing conceptualizations. This cycle may be repeated several times. The iterations among data collection and data interpretation continue until the analysis is well developed and further observations yield redundant, minimal or no new information to further challenge or elaborate the conceptual framework or in-depth descriptions of the phenomenon (a point often referred to as *saturation*[28] or *informational redundancy*[29]). This 'analysis-stopping' criterion is so integral to qualitative analysis that authors seldom declare that they have reached this point; they assume readers will understand.

In the course of analysis, key findings may also be corroborated using several information sources, a process called *data triangulation*. Triangulation is a metaphor and does not mean literally that three or more sources are required. The appropriate number of sources depends on the importance of the findings, their implications for theory, and the investigators' confidence in their validity. Because no two qualitative data sources will generate exactly the same interpretation, much of the art of qualitative interpretation involves exploring why and how different information sources yield slightly different results.[30] Readers may encounter several useful triangulation techniques for validating qualitative data and their interpretation in analysis.[31, 32] *Investigator triangulation* requires that more than one investigator collect and analyse the data, such that the findings emerge through consensus between or among investigators. This is typically accomplished by an investigative team. Inclusion of team members from different disciplines helps to prevent personal or disciplinary biases of a single researcher from excessively influencing the findings. *Theory triangulation* is a process whereby emergent findings are examined in relation to existing social science theories.[31, 33] It is conventional for authors to report how their qualitative findings relate to prevailing social theory, although some qualitative researchers suggest that such theories should not be used to guide the research design or analysis.

Some researchers seek clarification and further explanation of their developing analytic framework from study participants, a step known as *member checking*. Most commonly, researchers specify that member checking was done to inquire whether participants' viewpoints were faithfully interpreted, to determine whether there are gross errors of fact, and to ascertain whether the account makes sense to participants with different perspectives.

Qualitative research reports may describe the use of qualitative analysis software packages.[34–36] Readers should not equate the use of computers with analytic rigour. Such software is merely a data management tool for efficiently storing, organizing, and retrieving qualitative data. These programs do not perform analyses. However, the manner in which data are organized may assist the researcher with analysis and interpretation. Fundamentally, the investigators do the analysis as they create the keywords, categories, and logical relations used to organize and interpret the electronic data. The soundness of qualitative study findings depends on investigator judgements, which cannot, as yet, be programmed into software packages.

We indicated earlier that qualitative data collection must be comprehensive (i.e. adequate in its breadth and depth) to yield a meaningful description. The closely related criterion for judging whether data were analysed appropriately is whether this comprehensiveness was determined, in part, by the research findings, with the aims of challenging, elaborating and corroborating the findings. This is most apparent when researchers state that they alternated between data collection and analysis, collected data with the purpose of elucidating the 'analysis in progress', collected data until analytic saturation or redundancy was reached, or triangulated findings using any of the methods mentioned.

Norton and Bowers[2] note that member checking was ongoing throughout the study, with fieldwork and second interviews of three providers. They also described member checks with 'small groups of providers similar to those who participated' when they conducted interactive presentations of their findings.

Breadth in qualitative inquiry is enhanced by the researcher's attention to multiple perspectives and vantage points in relation to the area of inquiry. In the study by Norton and Bowers,[2] breadth was evidenced by their purposeful sampling of different types of health care providers (registered nurses and physicians) who worked in various practice areas (home health, family practice, oncology, and intensive care). They also noted that the three providers who participated in second interviews were purposefully chosen for the depth and breadth of their experiences as related to the study question. In Norton's larger study, perspectives of family members' were also obtained.

Depth, in qualitative research, is enhanced by the number and type of data collection points within the inquiry. Norton and Bowers[2] interviewed 12 providers once and three providers a second time. Consistent with grounded theory procedures, interviews done early in the research lasted longer than later interviews, when questions became more focused. Another strategy by which Norton and Bowers attained depth in their research was to follow grounded theory procedures for *constant comparative analysis*, whereby analysis of data occurred simultaneously with collection of new data. This strategy facilitates early identification of 'thin' analysis and provides opportunities for immediate correction through asking questions to obtain more data.

What are the findings?

Is the description of findings thorough?

Qualitative researchers are challenged to make sense of massive amounts of data and transform their understandings to a written form. The written report is often a barrier to qualitative research use because of its lack of clarity and relevance, except to a limited audience.[37] Sandelowski[37] describes the challenges facing authors, as they make decisions in balancing description (the facts of the cases observed) with analysis (the breakdown and recombining of data) and interpretation (the new meanings created from this process).

Good research often involves 'messiness', raising as many questions as it purports to answer. Holliday[18] describes the appropriate role of 'cautious detachment' in qualitative research. The 'truths' of qualitative research are relative to the research setting. Therefore, it is important that authors not overstep the interpretive boundaries of their study by making it seem as if all their questions were answered with certainty and without raising additional questions. A comparison of the findings and discussion sections of a study report is helpful for judging whether authors are truthful to the data and the local context of a given qualitative study.

Norton and Bowers[2] used clearly understood and consistent terminology, as well as a figure, to help readers situate specific findings within the more comprehensive research question. Their use of participants' terminology, identified with quotation marks or block quotes, facilitates readers' understanding of important ideas. There is a mix of abstract conceptualizations (i.e. laying the groundwork) with concrete descriptions of conceptualizations and strategies used by providers (e.g. teaching, planting seeds).

Throughout their article, Norton and Bowers[2] provided data that showed the varying attitudes, beliefs and actions of providers. They documented various strategies used by providers to shift patients from curative to palliative treatment choices. Importantly, they noted how most strategies were used for more than one purpose. In presenting the number of strategies, the varying purposes of enacting a given strategy, and different interpretations of incorporating the strategies, the authors showed respect for the participants and were true to their purpose of examining the various ways that providers worked with patients and families at the end of life.

Norton and Bowers[2] situated their findings within the literature they reviewed as background, using statements such as 'Consistent with the findings from previous research studies . . .' and then listing those studies. Readers will sometimes find phrases such as 'the results extend what was found by' and 'in contrast to the findings of [reference], the results of this study suggest'. The referent for such phrases will logically be found in the background section of the article.

Norton and Bowers[2] consistently discussed decision-making, treatment preferences, choices, and health care providers' interactions with patients and families, all of which were areas explored in the results section. The authors clearly articulated that future research is needed to explore patients' and family members' understandings of their conditions and decision-making.

Can I apply the findings in practice?

What meaning and relevance does the study have for my practice?

Thorne[5] suggests that critiquing qualitative research in health sciences disciplines demands not only a focus on traditional appraisal criteria, but also an examination of the more complex question of what meaning can be made of the findings. The moral question of how research findings may be used in ways not intended and not benefiting health science disciplines and persons who require health care is an important one, given that 'health science disciplines exist because of a social mandate that entails a moral obligation toward benefiting individuals and the collective'.[5] Thorne describes five criteria for appraising the disciplinary relevance and usefulness of a study:

1. Are there convincing claims about why this knowledge is needed (moral defensibility)?
2. Is the knowledge appropriate to the development of the discipline (disciplinary relevance)?
3. Does the study produce usable knowledge (pragmatic obligation)?
4. Is the study situated in a historical context and within a disciplinary perspective (contextual awareness)?
5. Is there evidence of ambiguity and creation of meaning (probable truth)?

The study by Norton and Bowers[2] met Thorne's five criteria for appraising the disciplinary relevance and usefulness of a study.[5] The authors clearly articulated the need for this research. Given that nurses and other health care professionals interact with patients and families as they make end-of-life treatment decisions, the topic is relevant to health care disciplines. The description of strategies that providers used in shifting patients and their families from curative to palliative treatment decisions is illuminating for health care professionals who work in palliative care settings as well as for providers who work with patients and families around other important life decisions. The study situates itself within the historical context of advances in technology, complex end-of-life decisions, persons' rights to self-determination, and advance directives. The authors concluded the article by noting that only providers' perspectives were presented, and, even within that unique group, there was no one 'right' or consistent way that providers engaged with patients and their families. They also rightly pointed out what their study did not explore.

Does the study help me understand the context of my practice?

The context in which a study is conducted influences the findings of all research, but it is particularly important in qualitative research. Readers of qualitative research must determine the potential applicability of the findings to their own contexts. Inadequate reporting of the social and historical context of a study makes it difficult for readers to determine if a study's results can be 'transferred' with any legitimacy to their situation.

Norton and Bowers[2] provided an adequate description of the context and setting of their study. The findings can sensitize providers to some of the implicit and unspoken ideas they may have and enact as they work with patients and families at the end of life. Framing their efforts as 'work' legitimates the energy and time expended by providers.

Does the study enhance my knowledge about my practice?

One criterion for the transferability of a qualitative study is whether it provides a useful map for readers to understand and navigate in similar social settings themselves. Readers need to consider the similarity of the patients and setting of a given study to their own.

The findings of Norton and Bowers[2] suggest the potential for exploring providers' strategies for shifting patients' and families' treatment-related decisions in other contexts unrelated to palliative care and end of life.

Resolution of the clinical scenario

After appraising the article, you return to your next team meeting to lead a discussion on counselling patients and their family members on appropriate end-of-life treatment choices. You point out that patient, family and provider decisions have been individually explored in various contexts. Limited research, however, has focused on understanding the intersection of patient, family-member and provider decision-making about decisions for end-of-life or other treatments. You observe that even though the study by Norton and Bowers[2] has important information about how providers used various strategies to shift patients' treatment decisions, there was no consistent picture of how this was done, or even if it should be done. You note that the researchers pointed out that some people might interpret providers' use of strategies as paternalistic and possibly coercive. Given that this was a preliminary study, you caution your colleagues to avoid implementing the strategies in such a way as to influence the treatment decisions of patients and their family members. Rather, you emphasize that one of the finer points of clinical applicability of this study is that of sensitizing providers to the ways in which they may consciously or unconsciously act to influence patients' and family members' treatment decisions. Furthermore, providers can reflect on their own practice in light of the findings. Such reflection offers the opportunity for comparing and contrasting one's current practice and provides new possibilities for re-envisaging one's future practice. You recommend that this topic be explored further on your unit.

LEARNING EXERCISES

1. Use the database of your choice and a search strategy from Chapters 5 and 6 to find a research report for each the following types of qualitative research: grounded theory, phenomenology and ethnography.

Table 25.2 Worksheet for determining whether a qualitative article is appropriate for critique

Question	Yes	No	Rationale
1. Is the article solely a qualitative article that uses only one qualitative method?			An article that reports on a study conducted using mixed methods (qualitative and quantitative methods) will have irrelevant information for a qualitative critique, whereas an article that reports on a study conducted using multiple qualitative methods will likely have insufficient information for the critique
2. Does the article report on a synthesis or review of several different studies?			Articles that report a synthesis of several studies typically are constrained in the amount of information included about each individual study
3. Does the article report on a single qualitative study?			If an article reports on two or more qualitative studies, even if they were focused on the same subject matter, there will be insufficient information provided for you to do a thorough review of each of the studies. Published articles must be quite brief, and inclusion of two studies in one article means that some important information for your evaluation will be left out
4. Does the article report on a secondary analysis or a re-examination of a prior study?			The critique process for an article that is conducted using secondary analysis is different from the evaluation of a traditional qualitative research study
5. Does the article have the following sections: (a) abstract, (b) introduction, (c) methods/procedures, (d) findings/results, (e) discussion/conclusions, and (f) practical applications / clinical relevance?			Although the titles of the sections of a research article will vary among journals, most articles that report on research will include most of these sections
6. Does the article include statements such as (a) 'the research question was . . .', (b) 'the research method was . . .', and (c) 'the findings/results were . . .'?			These statements, or some version of them, are commonly seen whether an article is reporting qualitative or quantitative research. They should be easy to find at the beginning or end of major sections of the article
7. Does the article use the term 'hypothesis' in the introduction, methods/procedures, or findings/results sections?			Although some qualitative research ends by generating hypotheses, most qualitative research does not begin with a hypothesis. When finding the term 'hypothesis' in an article, ensure that the article is reporting on a qualitative, rather than quantitative, study
8. From a quick scan of the article, are you able to find information relevant to each of the sections in the evaluation guide?			If you are unable to find information that would provide answers to the areas addressed in the critique criteria, then you should look for a different article to critique.

2. After you locate an article, use the guide outlined in Table 25.2 to help ensure you have an appropriate article for critique. For each question, a tick in the shaded box makes it more likely that you have identified an appropriate article.
3. Once you have decided that the article is useful for critique, use the questions in Box 25.1 to critique the study.

References

1 Providers tried to help patients and families make realistic end of life decisions. *Evid Based Nurs* 2002;5:64. Abstract of: Norton SA, Bowers BJ. Working toward consensus: providers' strategies to shift patients from curative to palliative treatment choices. *Res Nurs Health* 2001;24:258–69.
2 Norton SA, Bowers BJ. Working toward consensus: providers' strategies to shift patients from curative to palliative treatment choices. *Res Nurs Health* 2001;24:258–69.
3 Giacomini MK, Cook DJ. Users' guides to the medical literature: XXIII. Qualitative research in health care. A. Are the results of the study valid? *JAMA* 2000;284:357–62.
4 Giacomini MK, Cook DJ. Users' guides to the medical literature: XXIII. Qualitative research in health care. B. What are the results and how do they help me care for my patients? *JAMA* 2000;284:478–82.
5 Thorne S. The art (and science) of critiquing qualitative research. In: Morse JM, editor. *Completing a Qualitative Project: Details and Dialogue*. Thousand Oaks, CA: Sage, 1997:117–32.
6 Sandelowski M, Barroso J. Reading qualitative studies. *International Journal of Qualitative Methods* 2002;1(1):Article 5. http://www.ualberta.ca/~ijqm/ (accessed 11 December 2006).
7 Morse JM, Barrett M, Mayan M, Olson K, Spiers J. Verification strategies for establishing reliability and validity in qualitative research. *International Journal of Qualitative Methods* 2002;1(2):Article 2. http://www.ualberta.ca/~ijqm/ (accessed 11 December 2006).
8 Barbour RS. Checklists for improving rigour in qualitative research: a case of the tail wagging the dog? *BMJ* 2001;322:1115–17.
9 Forchuk C, Roberts J. How to critique qualitative research articles. *Can J Nurs Res* 1993;25:47–55.
10 Chapple A, Rogers A. Explicit guidelines for qualitative research: a step in the right direction, a defence of the 'soft' option, or a form of sociological imperialism? *Fam Prac* 1998;15:556–61.
11 Miles MB Huberman M. *Qualitative Data Analysis: An Expanded Sourcebook*. Second edition. Thousand Oaks: Sage, 1994.
12 Holliday A. *Doing and Writing Qualitative Research*. Thousand Oaks: Sage, 2002.
13 Denzin NK, Lincoln YS, editors. *Handbook of Qualitative Research*. Second edition. Newbury Park: Sage, 2000.
14 Grbich C. *Qualitative Research in Health: An Introduction*. St Leonards, Australia: Allen and Unwin Publishers, 1998.
15 Munhall P, Oiler-Boyd C. *Nursing Research: A Qualitative Perspective*. Third edition. New York: National League for Nursing, 2001.
16 Patton MQ. *Qualitative Research and Evaluation Methods*. Third edition. Newbury Park: Sage, 2002.
17 Taylor SJ, Bogdan R. *Introduction to Qualitative Research Methods*. Third edition. New York: John Wiley and Sons, 1998.
18 Holliday A. *Doing and Writing Qualitative Research*. Thousand Oaks: Sage, 2001.
19 Tesch R. *Qualitative Research: Analysis Types and Software Tools*. Bristol: Falmer Press, 1990.

20 Atkinson PA, Coffey AJ, Delamont S, Lofland J, Lofland LH, editors. *Handbook of Ethnography*. London: Sage, 2001.
21 Strauss A, Corbin JM. *Basics of Qualitative Research: Grounded Theory Procedures and Techniques*. Newbury Park: Sage, 1990.
22 van Manen M. *Researching Lived Experience: Human Science for an Action Sensitive Pedagogy*. London: Althouse Press, 1990.
23 Crotty M. *The Foundations of Social Research: Meaning and Perspective in the Research Process*. St Leonards, Australia: Allen and Unwin Publishers, 1998.
24 Kirk J, Miller ML. *Reliability and Validity in Qualitative Research*. London: Sage, 1986.
25 Schatzman L, Strauss AL. *Field Research: Strategies for a Natural Sociology*. Englewood Cliffs: Prentice-Hall, 1973:94–107.
26 Lincoln YS, Guba EG. *Naturalistic Inquiry*. London: Sage, 1985:250–88.
27 Patton MQ. *Qualitative Research and Evaluation Methods*. Third edition. Newbury Park: Sage, 2002:199–276.
28 Glaser BG, Strauss AL. *Discovery of Grounded Theory*. New York: Aldine de Gruyter, 1967:101–16.
29 Lincoln YS, Guba EG. *Naturalistic Inquiry*. London: Sage, 1985:221–49.
30 Stake RE. *The Art of Case Study Research*. London: Sage, 1995:107–20.
31 Lincoln YS, Guba EG. *Naturalistic Inquiry*. London: Sage, 1985:289–331.
32 Patton MQ. *Qualitative Research and Evaluation Methods*. Third edition. Newbury Park: Sage, 2002:460–506.
33 Denzin NK. *Sociological Methods*. New York: McGraw Hill, 1978.
34 Russell CK, Gregory DM. Issues for consideration when choosing a qualitative data management system. *J Adv Nurs* 1993;**18**:1806–16.
35 Richards L, Richards T. Computing in qualitative analysis: a healthy development? *Qual Health Res* 1991;**1**:234–62.
36 Weitzman EA. Software and qualitative research. In: Denzin NK, Lincoln YS, editors. *Handbook of Qualitative Research*. Second edition. Newbury Park: Sage, 2000:803–20.
37 Sandelowski M. Writing a good read: strategies for re-presenting qualitative data. *Res Nurs Health* 1998;**21**:375–82.

Additional resources

Useful websites

Caelli K, Ray L, Mill J. 'Clear as mud': toward greater clarity in generic qualitative research. *International Journal of Qualitative Methods* 2003;2(2):Article 1. http://www.ualberta.ca/~ijqm/english/engframeset.html (accessed 23 July 2007).
Fossey E, Harvey C, McDermott F, Davidson L. Understanding and evaluating qualitative research. *Aust NZ J Psychiatry* 2002;36:717–32. http://www.ruralhealth.utas.edu.au/gr/resources/docs/fossey-et-al-evaluating-qual-research.pdf (accessed 11 December 2006).
Giacomini M, Cook DJ, for the Evidence-Based Medicine Workgroup. A user's guide to qualitative research in health care. Centre for Health Evidence. http://www.cche.net/usersguides/qualitative.asp (accessed 11 December 2006).
Law M, Stewart D, Letts L, Pollock N, Bosch J, Westmorland M. Guidelines for critical review form – qualitative studies. 1998. http://www.fhs.mcmaster.ca/rehab/ebp/pdf/qualguidelines.pdf (accessed 11 December 2006).
Law M, Stewart D, Letts L, Pollock N, Bosch J, Westmorland M. Critical review form – qualitative studies. 1998. http://www.fhs.mcmaster.ca/rehab/ebp/pdf/qualreview.pdf (accessed 11 December 2006).

Appraising qualitative research: health care references

1 Barbour RS. Checklists for improving rigour in qualitative research: a case of the tail wagging the dog? *BMJ* 2001;**322**:1115–17.

2 Giacomini MK, Cook DJ. Users' guides to the medical literature: XXIII. Qualitative research in health care. A. Are the results of the study valid? *JAMA* 2000;**284**:357–62.

3 Giacomini MK, Cook DJ. Users' guides to the medical literature: XXIII. Qualitative research in health care. B. What are the results and how do they help me care for my patients? *JAMA* 2000;**284**:478–82.

4 Hoddinott P, Pill R. A review of recently published qualitative research in general practice. More methodological questions than answers? *Fam Prac* 1997;**14**:313–19.

5 Mays N, Pope C. Qualitative research in health care. Assessing quality in qualitative research. *BMJ* 2000;**320**:50–2.

6 Morse JM, Barrett M, Mayan M, Olson K, Spiers J. Verification strategies for establishing reliability and validity in qualitative research. *International Journal of Qualitative Methods* 2002;**1**(2):Article 2. http://www.ualberta.ca/~ijqm/ (accessed 11 December 2006).

7 Sandelowski M, Barroso J. Reading qualitative studies. *International Journal of Qualitative Methods* 2002;**1**(1):Article 5. http://www.ualberta.ca/~ijqm/ (accessed 11 December 2006).

Chapter 26

APPRAISING AND ADAPTING CLINICAL PRACTICE GUIDELINES

Ian D. Graham and Margaret B. Harrison

Clinical practice guidelines are 'systematically developed statements to assist practitioner and patient decisions about appropriate health care for specific clinical circumstances'.[1] They are intended to offer concise instructions on how to provide health care services.[2] The most important benefit of clinical practice guidelines is their potential to improve both the quality or process of care and patient outcomes.[3] Increasingly, clinicians and clinical managers must choose from numerous, sometimes inconsistent and occasionally contradictory, guidelines.[4] This situation is further complicated by concerns about the quality of available guidelines.[5–11] Indeed, adoption of guidelines of questionable validity can lead to the use of ineffective interventions, inefficient use of scarce resources, and, perhaps most importantly, harm to patients.[12, 13] Determining which guidelines are high-quality products worthy of adoption can be daunting. Every effort should be made to identify existing guidelines that have been rigorously developed and to adopt or adapt them for local use.[12] However, organizations and clinicians should scrutinize the methods by which the guidelines were developed, as well as the content and utility of the recommendations. Even guidelines developed by prominent professional groups or government bodies should not be exempt from this scrutiny as it has been shown that these guidelines may be of substandard quality.[10]

The Practice Guideline Evaluation and Adaptation Cycle[14–16] is a framework for organizing and making decisions about which high quality guidelines to adopt (Figure 26.1). Although the cycle was originally intended for use by organizations and groups wanting to implement best practice, most of the steps are also helpful in guiding evaluation of guidelines by individual clinicians. This chapter will describe strategies for identifying, critically appraising, and adopting or adapting guidelines for local use based on the Practice Guideline Evaluation and Adaptation Cycle.

1. Identify a clinical area in which to promote best practice

The first step is to select an area in which to promote best practice. Reasons for selecting a particular area can include the prevalence of the condition or its associated burden, concerns about large variations in practice or care gaps, costs associated with different practice options, the likelihood that a guideline will be effective in

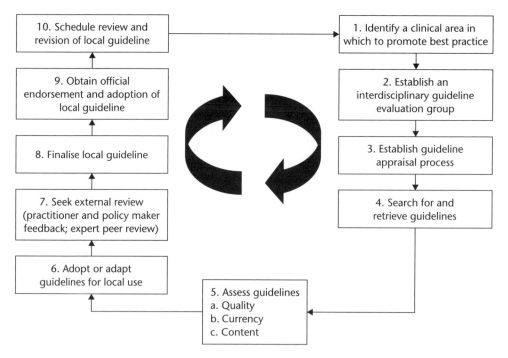

Figure 26.1 Practice guidelines evaluation and adaptation cycle. Adapted from Graham ID, Harrison MB, Brouwers M. Evaluating and adapting practice guidelines for local use: a conceptual framework. In: Pickering S, Thompson J, editors. *Clinical Governance in Practice.* London: Harcourt, 2003:213–29.

influencing practice, a desire to keep practice up to date or evidence-based, or awareness of the existence of relevant evidence-based guidelines.

2. Establish an interdisciplinary guideline evaluation group

3. Establish a guideline appraisal process

When an organization or group is interested in providing best practice, a local interdisciplinary guideline evaluation group should be established comprising key stakeholders, including patients or individuals from the community, who will be affected by the selection of guideline recommendations.[14] The advantages of using a group to evaluate guidelines include sharing of work among group members, reduced potential for bias in the evaluation process, and increased awareness of guidelines and opportunities for group members to develop ownership of the resulting decisions.

It is important to select an appraisal process. Guideline appraisal instruments are intended to be used to systematically assess and compare guidelines using the same criteria. They typically consist of a several quality criteria or items that assess the extent to which each guideline meets these criteria. To date, many appraisal instruments have been developed.[17] The Appraisal of Guidelines Research and Evaluation

(AGREE) Instrument (http://www.agreetrust.org)[18] is rapidly becoming accepted as the gold standard for guideline appraisal. The AGREE instrument has been tested in 11 countries on more than 100 guidelines and more than 200 appraisers.[18] It is endorsed by the World Health Organization, the Council of Europe, and the Guidelines International Network (http://www.g-i-n.net).

The AGREE instrument was designed to assess the process of guideline development and the extent to which the process is reported. It consists of 23 Likert scale items organized into six domains (see Box 26.1). Each domain is intended to capture a separate dimension of guideline quality. Each guideline assessed is assigned a standardized dimensional score ranging from 0 to 100. AGREE also includes a question to

Box 26.1 AGREE quality criteria[18]

Scope and purpose

1. The overall objective(s) of the guideline is (are) specifically described.
2. The clinical question(s) covered by the guideline is (are) specifically described.
3. The patients to whom the guideline is meant to apply are specifically described.

Stakeholder involvement

4. The guideline development group includes individuals from all the relevant professional groups.
5. The patients' views and preferences have been sought.
6. The target users of the guideline are clearly defined.
7. The guideline has been piloted among target users.

Rigour of development

8. Systematic methods were used to search for evidence.
9. The criteria for selecting the evidence are clearly described.
10. The methods used for formulating the recommendations are clearly described.
11. The health benefits, side effects and risks have been considered in formulating the recommendations.
12. There is an explicit link between the recommendations and the supporting evidence.
13. The guideline has been externally reviewed by an expert panel prior to publication.
14. A procedure for updating the guideline is provided.

Clarity and presentation

15. The recommendations are specific and unambiguous.
16. The different options for management of the condition are clearly presented.
17. Key recommendations are easily identifiable.
18. The guideline is supported with tools for application.

Applicability

19. The potential organizational barriers in applying the guideline have been discussed.
20. The potential cost implications of applying the recommendations have been considered.
21. The guideline presents key review criteria for monitoring and/or audit purposes.

Editorial independence

22. The guideline is editorially independent from the funding body.
23. Conflicts of interest of guideline development members have been recorded.

provide a global assessment of the overall quality of the guideline; that is, whether one would 'strongly recommend this guideline for use in practice without modifications', 'recommend this guideline for use in practice on condition of some alterations or with provisos', or 'not recommend this guideline (not suitable for use in practice)'. Complete information about the instrument can be found at www.agreetrust.org.

With the AGREE instrument, only domain scores can be calculated. The six domain scores cannot be combined into a total score because there is no way to weight the importance of each domain. Although some might want to view the results of this quantitative evaluation as an objective measure of guideline quality, it is important to remember that scores are influenced by the extent to which the guideline developers 'described' the methods used to develop the guideline and reached consensus on the recommendations. A rigorously developed guideline may score poorly if the process was not well described.

Clinical scenario

Nurses caring for patients post stroke wanted to provide best practice across the continuum of care in their community. A working group was formed, with nurses representing acute care, long-term care, and rehabilitation settings. The group identified the first clinical priority for nursing care as the development of a consistent, evidence-based approach for risk assessment in three key areas: risk of falling, skin breakdown, and swallowing problems. In reviewing current practices, they found that all settings had existing evidence-based policies for assessment of falls and pressure ulcers. Assessment of dysphagia, however, was an area of concern. The group invited a local speech and language pathologist and representatives from rehabilitation therapy and medicine to join the working group. The working group decided to actively engage each of their settings in the process and to use a transparent and rigorous approach in order to develop a solid foundation for future implementation of the risk assessment recommendations. Given its reputation, they decided to use the AGREE instrument to evaluate guidelines that included risk assessment recommendations for individuals with stroke.

4. Search for and retrieve guidelines

The next step is to clarify the issues of particular interest. The PICO approach involves considering the Population, Intervention, Control or context, and Outcomes of interest.[19, 20] (see Chapter 3). Based on the identified areas of interest, criteria for searching for and selecting guidelines for review are identified. Such criteria may include language of publication (e.g. English only) or date of publication (e.g. within the past 5 years). One study suggests that recommendations included in well developed guidelines (e.g. those produced by the US Agency for Healthcare Research and Quality) may become outdated within 3–4 years of release.[21] The same study, however, noted that wound care guidelines were still current up to 7 years after their release. Although the language and year of publication can be used to limit the search for guidelines, other criteria can only be applied once potentially relevant guidelines have been retrieved. For example, a group may only be interested in guidelines based on high-quality scientific literature and therefore exclude consensus documents. Alternatively, they may include only guidelines developed by credible professional organizations

and exclude those developed by one person. Regardless, the criteria should be determined before starting the search.

To ensure that high-quality guidelines are not inadvertently missed, a systematic
search for all relevant guidelines on the topic should be done (see Chapters 4, 5 and
6). Guidelines can be identified using a few simple strategies. Check the US National
Guideline Clearinghouse (http://www.guideline.gov), sponsored by the US Agency
for Health Care Research and Quality. Another guideline repository is the Guidelines
International Network (G-I-N) (http://www.g-i-n.net). G-I-N is an international not-
for-profit association of organizations and individuals involved in clinical practice guidelines. Although G-I-N membership is required to access guidelines compiled by the
network, non-members can access the websites of some of the guideline developers.
Another efficient strategy is to search the websites of known guideline developers (e.g.
Scottish Intercollegiate Guidelines Network or the Royal College of Nursing). To be
thorough, it is also important to search the National Library of Medicine, which can
be done for free using PubMed (http://www.ncbi.nlm.nih.gov/). Search terms known
as MeSH (Medical Search Headings) and text words that can be used are 'practice
guideline', 'practice guidelines', 'clinical practice guideline', 'clinical practice guidelines', 'standards', 'consensus statement', and 'consensus'.[10] 'Practice guidelines' can
also be used as a publication type (pt) in searching.[12]

Increasingly, guideline developers are posting their guidelines directly on the web.
This avoids delays in publication of guidelines by journals, permits rapid updating
of guidelines, and reduces dissemination costs. When guidelines are posted directly
to the web, there is a greater chance that they may not be indexed in commonly
consulted bibliographic databases such as MEDLINE. For this reason, it is prudent
to also search for guidelines on the Internet using a search engine such as Google
(http://www.google.com). One should not assume that guidelines found on the Internet
are poor quality or that those indexed in MEDLINE are necessarily high quality.[22]
All guidelines that meet the predetermined inclusion criteria should be retrieved. Because
the appraisal process is based on information reported by guideline developers, all
relevant documents related to the development process should be retrieved. In some
cases, the published guideline will have minimal information about the development
process because this information is presented elsewhere, perhaps in a technical
report. Efforts should be made to obtain such supplemental documents.

The working group began by identifying guidelines they were familiar with and
those currently used in their settings. The bibliographies of these guidelines were scanned
to identify additional guidelines. The working group decided to restrict the search to
guidelines published in English or French as the group did not have the capability
of reviewing documents in other languages and to restrict the search to documents
published in the past 6 years. Next, the group enlisted the help of a local hospital
librarian, who worked with them to develop a search strategy to identify general
guidelines about the care of individuals with stroke, with the expectation that many
of these might include recommendations about dysphagia. They also decided to search
specifically for guidelines about dysphagia. Databases searched were MEDLINE,
EMBASE/Excerpta Medica, CINAHL, and the US National Guideline Clearinghouse
database. Websites of known guideline developers were accessed, and a Google Internet
search was done. The following topic-related key words were used alone and in combination to identify general stroke guidelines: cerebrovascular accident, cerebrovascular disorders, stroke, rehabilitation, spasticity, electromyography, gait, assistive devices,
and equilibrium. The search for guidelines on assessment of dysphagia included all

guidelines for the elderly and was not limited to the stroke population. Key words included 'risk', 'dysphagia', 'swallow disorders', and 'deglutition disorder'.

All guidelines identified by the search strategy were retrieved and assessed based on the following predefined criteria: (a) produced by a group or organization (i.e. not authored by one person), (b) included a bibliography, and (c) made recommendations for bedside swallowing assessment/screening targeted at clinicians such as nurses, speech–language therapists, general practitioners, physiotherapists, or occupational therapists. Six guidelines included recommendations for the bedside assessment of dysphagia and were considered appropriate for appraisal using the AGREE instrument.[23–28]

5. Assess the guidelines

Determining whether a guideline is valid involves three separate but related steps: appraising the quality of the guideline as a whole, determining whether the recommendations are up to date, and assessing the content of the recommendations.

(a) Assess the quality of the guideline as a whole

Ideally, the AGREE instrument should be applied to all guidelines meeting the minimum inclusion criteria. However, this may not be practical or possible depending on the number of guidelines identified, the number of individuals who can participate in the appraisal, and time constraints. One strategy for quickly identifying the higher quality, evidence-based guidelines is to first screen the guidelines using the AGREE's 'rigour of development' domain. The seven items comprising this domain specifically focus on the degree to which the guideline development process was evidence-based and how evidence/research was incorporated into the recommendations. No universal agreement exists about specific cut-off scores to identify high-quality guidelines. Some domains (e.g. rigour of development) may be considered more important than others and thus have a higher benchmark. The group should identify the range of acceptable quality scores (e.g. at least 60/100 or greater than 80/100) and whether different domains should have different cut-offs. Guidelines meeting the benchmark for the 'rigour of development' domain can then be assessed using the other AGREE domains. Those scoring below the cut-off can be excluded at this point. Regardless, the developers of the AGREE instrument suggest that four or more appraisers should be used to ensure adequate inter-rater reliability.

(b) Is the guideline up to date?

Guidelines that meet minimum quality criteria must then be assessed to determine whether they are still current. Methods of checking the currency of guidelines include reviewing the date of release/publication; scanning the bibliography for the dates of the original studies cited; and checking with developers about whether they still consider the guideline to be current or have plans to update it. A quick MEDLINE search for systematic reviews published since the release of the guideline may also be useful. Other sources of high-quality systematic reviews include the Cochrane Database of Systematic Reviews and Cochrane Controlled Trials Register (http://www.cochrane.org), the Centre for Reviews and Dissemination (http://

www.york.ac.uk/inst/crd/crddatabases.htm), and the Database of Abstracts of Reviews of Effects (DARE) (http://www.york.ac.uk/inst/crd/crddatabases.htm).[28] 'Netting the Evidence' (www.shef.ac.uk/scharr/ir/netting/) and the Joanna Briggs Institute (www.joannabriggs.edu.au/about/home.php) are useful for locating databases of evidence.

Six group members appraised each guideline using the AGREE instrument. The results of the quality appraisal process revealed some unexpected findings. Quality scores for rigour of development ranged between 16% and 82%. The two guidelines with the lowest quality scores on this dimension were from regional organizations well known to the working group members. For these reasons, the group decided to not exclude these guidelines at this stage despite their poor quality scores. Scores on the domain of scope and purpose were more consistent and exceeded 60% for all guidelines. Scores on stakeholder involvement ranged from 33% to 90%. The lower scores on this dimension largely reflected the lack of inclusion of patient views and the lack of pilot testing of the guidelines. Scores on clarity and presentation, applicability, and editorial dependence were also variable. Examination of the global assessment by the appraisers revealed that no guideline was rejected by a majority of working group members. Three guidelines were strongly recommended 'as is' by two-thirds of the appraisers. More than half rated the other three guidelines as being 'in need of modifications' or were unsure about whether to recommend them for use. All guidelines were produced since December 2000, suggesting that the recommendations were fairly current. The librarian also did a literature search for meta-analyses, reviews and primary studies on the assessment of dysphagia that could be used as supplementary material.

(c) Systematically assess the clinical content of guideline recommendations

Guideline appraisal instruments provide little detailed information on the actual recommendations being advanced in specific guidelines. Thus, if more than one guideline is being considered, the next step is to conduct a 'content analysis' of the recommendations in each guideline. It is useful to have one or two clinicians experienced in the content area produce a table comparing each guideline in terms of the specific recommendations made and the level of evidence supporting each recommendation (if such information is provided). Such a table, or *recommendations matrix*,[14] can be the focus of the group's discussion or an individual clinician's deliberations about the content of the recommendations from each guideline. The recommendations matrix facilitates identification of similar recommendations in different guidelines, as well as differences in recommendations between guidelines. The matrix also facilitates easy identification of recommendations supported by strong evidence. Often, guidelines include several recommendations supported by evidence of differing strengths. When this happens, a group may decide to select recommendations supported by the best evidence from the guidelines under consideration. A recommendations matrix also provides the basis for considering whether the recommendations will help in caring for individuals in the relevant settings.

To facilitate comparison of the recommendations among the six guidelines, a nurse and the speech–language pathologist created a recommendations matrix that included the level of evidence supporting each recommendation.

6. Adopt or adapt guidelines for local use

At this point, the group must decide whether it will adopt one of the guidelines 'as is' or adapt one or more of the guidelines (i.e. select some, but not all, re-commendations from different guidelines). Recommendations must be considered in terms of whether they will be helpful for caring for individuals and whether they are appropriate and feasible to implement in the specific practice setting(s) (e.g. resources available to purchase special equipment needed to comply with guide-line recommendations).

The choices at this step are to *adopt* or *adapt* existing guidelines. *Adopting* a guide-line involves choosing the best guideline and accepting all recommendations as writ-ten. This may not be practical or feasible for many reasons, and the group may need to *adapt* or tailor one or more guidelines to their needs. Selection of this option may be appropriate if the recommendations are not a good fit with the practice setting (e.g. some recommendations may not apply to the types of individuals seen in the setting, or a practice group may be willing to accept only recommendations supported by strong evidence). As well, implementation issues, such as contextual factors or logistical or resource considerations, can make implementation of some recommen-dations impractical. Guideline adaptation essentially involves taking the best or most appropriate recommendations and repackaging them into a new local guideline.

Guideline developers are always concerned that local adaptation of guidelines will result in modifications to recommendations that ignore the evidence. Local adapta-tion of existing guidelines should never involve changing evidence-based recommen-dations unless the supporting evidence has changed since release of the guideline. If recommendations are modified in any way, the rationale for changes should be expli-citly stated in the resulting local guideline document. The group may also want to reconsider evidence that was located when conducting the search for systematic reviews as it could influence which recommendations are adapted.

After reviewing the recommendations and supporting evidence, the working group decided it would produce the local guideline for dysphagia risk assessment by adapting recommendations from existing guidelines. In some cases, the wording of existing recommendations was modified slightly to make them clearer. Caution was used when rewording recommendations to ensure that the intent of the original re-commendation was not altered. Their recommendations for dysphagia risk assessment were as follows:

(i) All patients should be kept NPO until their swallowing has been screened using a simple, valid, bedside testing protocol (adapted from Department of Veterans Affairs/Department of Defense,[23] Level B; Royal College of Physicians,[24] Level B).

(ii) The gag reflex alone is a poor predictor of swallowing function and should not be used for screening for dysphagia in stroke patients (Scottish Intercollegiate Guidelines Network – Dysphagia,[25] Level B).

(iii) Patients should be reviewed for dysphagia at least once a week after the initial assessment (adapted from Scottish Intercollegiate Guidelines Network – Dysphagia,[26] Level B).

The working group also decided to review the literature to identify a suitable valid bedside dysphagia testing protocol.

7. Seek external review of the proposed local guideline

When the guideline evaluation process is undertaken on behalf of a group, the resulting draft of local recommendations should be sent to local practitioners, other stakeholders, and organizational policy-makers for review and comment. This step should be done even if a single guideline is adopted in its entirety. Seeking feedback on the proposed guideline ensures that those intended to use the guideline have an opportunity to review the document and identify potential difficulties for implementation before the guideline is finalized. This step allows policy-makers to consider the organizational effects of implementing the recommendations and to begin preparing for its future adoption. It also serves as the first wave of dissemination of the guideline and provides the group with an opportunity to address the issues raised by reviewers before finalizing the local guideline.

Depending on the extensiveness of the adaptation process, it may also be reasonable to send the local guideline to external experts for review of its content validity, clarity, and applicability.[16] This can help to ensure that recommendations from existing guidelines have not been taken out of context or adapted inappropriately.

8. Finalize the local guideline

9. Obtain official endorsement and adoption of the guideline by the organization

The group should consider all feedback and, if necessary, modify the local guideline recommendations to address concerns. All changes made should be documented in the local guideline as well as reasons for not making suggested changes. Being explicit and transparent about the process should increase the credibility of the process among potential guideline users.

Once finalized, official endorsement of the guideline should be sought from policy-makers in settings where the guideline is intended to be implemented. This step involves review of the proposed guideline (which may have been modified based on feedback) by the organization, and formal adoption, with official status. This is done, for example, when an organization endorses a guideline as policy. This administrative step provides the organization with a final opportunity to consider the effects of the proposed guideline on its functioning. The formal decision-making and procedural process required to endorse a guideline needs to be explicit and documented by the organization. Once the organization provides its 'seal of approval', the guideline is ready for dissemination and implementation. If plans for dissemination and implementation of recommendations have not been considered, they should be at this point (see Chapters 27–29).

10. Schedule review and revision of the local guideline

The group should develop a plan for when and how the local guideline will be reviewed and updated (which will obviously depend on when the original guideline expires) or provide a guideline expiry date. Other criteria for determining when a guideline needs updating include changes in evidence on existing benefits or harms associated with recommendations, important outcomes, available interventions, evidence that current practice is optimal, values placed on outcomes, and resources available for health care.[29]

Depending on the extent of the changes to recommendations required by new evidence, the guideline evaluation group may want to simply seek practitioner or policy-maker feedback on the changes, or begin the entire guideline evaluation cycle over again. In any case, plans for reviewing and revising the guideline should be documented. Individual clinicians who make decisions about which guidelines or specific recommendations they will personally follow must also be aware of the currency of the guidelines and any new guidelines or evidence that may be more current.

Resolution of clinical scenario

The local guideline document was sent to the practice committees or councils in each of the settings involved for review and feedback. The working group reviewed the feedback from all sources. The feedback revealed that front-line nurses were positive about assessing individuals for swallowing problems but needed training and time to develop confidence in their assessment skills. The local guideline was finalized and sent to the regional stroke team as well as to the heads of programmes in each setting for official endorsement and adoption. Working with clinical managers, the working group developed a strategy to plan for staff education, phase-in of the recommendations, and enhancement of current documentation processes to capture dysphagia assessment. Furthermore, the working group, managers and librarian developed a strategy for periodically reviewing the literature for new guidelines on the topic or updates of existing guidelines in order to keep the local guideline current.

Summary

Practice guidelines have the potential to improve the process of care as well as patient outcomes. However, their beneficial effects are contingent on successful implementation.[30–32] Clinical settings can move towards explicit use of evidence in practice by adopting existing guidelines or by local adaptation of existing guidelines. Careful consideration of available guidelines using the process described above can inform clinical- and programme-level decision-making about which guidelines or recommendations are most suitable for their settings. Use of a rigorous and transparent process for identifying, appraising, and adopting/adapting guidelines is crucial as practice guidelines are essentially a multi-faceted intervention, and the decisions made affect both patients and providers.

LEARNING EXERCISES

1. Identify a clinical area in which to promote best practice. What are the reasons for selecting this particular area? What is the clinical question you would like addressed by a guideline?
2. If you were developing a group to evaluate and adapt practice guidelines for your clinical question, who would you ask to be a member of the group and why?

3. How would you go about searching for practice guidelines that might be relevant to your clinical question? Which databases would you search? Which search terms would you use? What other criteria would you use to restrict your searching and why (e.g. year of publication, language, etc.)?
4. Download the AGREE instrument from the web (www.agreetrust.org), and practise using it to appraise a guideline that you are familiar with. Although the AGREE instrument is easy to use, it does take some practice to become familiar with the quality items and how to score them. Have a colleague use the AGREE instrument to appraise the same guideline, and compare your responses. If you disagree on certain items, discuss the reasons for the disagreements.
5. Develop a strategy for how you would go about adopting/adapting practice guidelines in your setting. Think about how you might operationalize each step of the Practice Guideline Evaluation and Adaptation Cycle. Will some steps be particularly challenging to complete in your setting? Which ones? What will make it challenging, and what might you do to overcome these challenges?

References

1 Field MJ, Lohr KN, editors. Committee on Clinical Practice Guidelines. Institute of Medicine. *Guidelines for Clinical Practice: From Development to Use*. Washington: National Academy Press, 1992.
2 Woolf SH, Grol R, Hutchinson A, Eccles M, Grimshaw J. Clinical guidelines: potential benefits, limitations, and harms of clinical guidelines. *BMJ* 1999;**318**:527–30.
3 Grimshaw J, Freemantle N, Wallace S, Russell I, Hurwitz B, Watt I, Long A, Sheldon T. Developing and implementing clinical practice guidelines. *Qual Health Care* 1995;**4**:55–64.
4 Lewis SJ. Further disquiet on the guidelines front. *CMAJ* 2001;**165**:180–1.
5 Littlejohns P, Cluzeau F, Bale R, Grimshaw J, Feder G, Moran S. The quantity and quality of clinical practice guidelines for the management of depression in primary care in the UK. *Br J Gen Pract* 1999;**49**:205–10.
6 Sudlow M, Thomson R. Clinical guidelines: quantity without quality. *Qual Health Care* 1997;**6**:60–1.
7 Varonen H, Mäkelä M. Practice guidelines in Finland: availability and quality. *Qual Health Care* 1997;**6**:75–9.
8 Ward JE, Grieco V. Why we need guidelines for guidelines: a study of the quality of clinical practice guidelines in Australia. *Med J Aust* 1996;**165**:574–6.
9 Shaneyfelt TM, Mayo-Smith MF, Rothwangl J. Are guidelines following guidelines? The methodological quality of clinical practice guidelines in the peer-reviewed medical literature. *JAMA* 1999;**281**:1900–5.
10 Grilli R, Magrini N, Penna A, Mura G, Liberati A. Practice guidelines developed by specialty societies: the need for a critical appraisal. *Lancet* 2000;**355**:103–6.
11 Graham ID, Beardall S, Carter AO, Glennie J, Hebert PC, Tetroe JM, McAlister FA, Visentin S, Anderson GM. What is the quality of drug therapy clinical practice guidelines in Canada? *CMAJ* 2001;**165**:157–63.
12 Feder G, Eccles M, Grol R, Griffiths C, Grimshaw J. Clinical guidelines: using clinical guidelines. *BMJ* 1999;**318**:728–30.
13 Woolf SH, George JN. Evidence-based medicine. Interpreting studies and setting policy. *Hematol Oncol Clin North Am* 2000;**14**:761–84.
14 Graham ID, MB Harrison, Brouwers M. Evaluating and adapting practice guidelines for local use: a conceptual framework. In: Pickering S, Thompson J, editors. *Clinical Governance in Practice*. London: Harcourt, 2003:213–29.
15 Graham ID, Harrison MB, Brouwers M, Davies BL, Dunn S. Facilitating the use of evidence in practice: evaluating and adapting clinical practice guidelines for local use by health care organizations. *J Obstet Gynecol Neonatal Nurs* 2002;**31**:599–611.

16 Graham ID, Harrison MB, Lorimer K, Piercianowski T, Friedberg E, Buchanan M, Harris C. Adapting national and international leg ulcer practice guidelines for local use: the Ontario Leg Ulcer Community Care Protocol. *Adv Skin Wound Care* 2005;**18**:307–18.

17 Graham ID, Calder LA, Hébert PC, Carter AO, Tetroe JM. A comparison of clinical practice guideline appraisal instruments. *Int J Technol Assess Health Care* 2000;**16**:1024–38.

18 AGREE Collaboration. Development and validation of an international appraisal instrument for assessing the quality of clinical practice guidelines; the AGREE project. *Qual Saf Health Care* 2003;**12**:18–23.

19 Glasziou P, Del Mar C, Salisbury J. *Evidence-Based Medicine Workbook*. London: BMJ Books, 2003.

20 Badenoch D, Heneghan C. *Evidence-Based Medicine Toolkit*. London: BMJ Publishing Group, 2002.

21 Shekelle PG, Ortiz E, Rhodes S, Morton SC, Eccles MP, Grimshaw JM, Woolf SH. Validity of the Agency for Healthcare Research and Quality clinical practice guidelines: how quickly do guidelines become outdated? *JAMA* 2001;**286**:1461–7.

22 Hurdowar A, Graham ID, Bayley M, Harrison MB, Wood-Dauphinee S, Bhogal S. Quality of stroke rehabilitation clinical practice guidelines. *Journal of Evaluation in Clinical Practice*. In press.

23 Veterans Health Administration, Department of Defense. VA/DoD clinical practice guideline for management of stroke rehabilitation. Washington, DC: Department of Veteran Affairs, 2003. http://www.oqp.med.va.gov/cpg/STR/STR_GOL.htm (accessed 16 April 2006).

24 Royal College of Physicians. *National Clinical Guidelines for Stroke*. Update 2002. London: Royal College of Physicians, 2002. http://www.rcplondon.ac.uk/pubs/books/stroke/ (accessed 16 April 2006).

25 Scottish Intercollegiate Guidelines Network. *Management of Patients with Stroke. Rehabilitation, Prevention and Management of Complications, and Discharge Planning.* Guideline No. 64. Edinburgh: SIGN, 2002. http://www.sign.ac.uk/guidelines/fulltext/64/index.html (accessed 16 April 2006).

26 Scottish Intercollegiate Guidelines Network. *Management of Patients with Stroke: Identification and Management of Dysphagia*. Guideline No. 78. Edinburgh: SIGN, 2004. http://www.sign.ac.uk/pdf/sign78.pdf (accessed 16 April 2006).

27 Heart and Stroke Foundation of Ontario. *Improving Recognition and Management of Dysphagia in Acute Stroke*. Heart and Stroke Foundation of Ontario: Toronto, 2002. http://209.5.25.171/ClientImages/1/DysphagiaBooklet2002Final.pdf (accessed 16 April 2006).

28 College of Audiologists and Speech and Language Pathologists of Ontario. Preferred practice guideline for dysphagia. Toronto: CASLPO, 2000. http://www.caslpo.com/english_site/DysphagiaPPGFinal.doc (accessed 16 April 2006).

29 Shekelle P, Eccles MP, Grimshaw JM, Woolf SH. When should clinical guidelines be updated? *BMJ* 2001;**323**:155–7.

30 Grimshaw JM, Russell IT. Effect of clinical guidelines on medical practice: a systematic review of rigorous evaluations. *Lancet* 1993;**342**:1317–22.

31 Worrall G, Chaulk P, Freake D. The effects of clinical practice guidelines on patient outcomes in primary care: a systematic review. *CMAJ* 1997;**156**:1705–12.

32 Thomas LH, McColl E, Cullum N, Rousseau N, Soutter J. Clinical guidelines in nursing, midwifery and the therapies: a systematic review. *J Adv Nurs* 1999;**30**:40–50.

Chapter 27

MODELS OF IMPLEMENTATION IN NURSING

Ian D. Graham, Jo Logan, Jacqueline Tetroe, Nicole Robinson and Margaret B. Harrison

Considerable resources are devoted to clinical and health services research and the production of new knowledge that could contribute to effective and efficient patient care. However, new research evidence will not benefit individuals and populations unless health care systems, organizations and professionals apply it in practice.[1, 2] Unfortunately, one of the most consistent findings in health services research is that the transfer of research findings into practice is unpredictable and can be a slow and haphazard process.[3] Nursing research has shown repeatedly that there are many barriers to nurses implementing research knowledge in practice.[4–6] When the transfer of knowledge to practice is inappropriately long, users of health services are denied treatments of proven benefit, and policy-makers are left uninformed about results that could affect their decision-making.

Clinical scenario

A director at a tertiary hospital is concerned about the occurrence of pressure ulcers in her area and wants to strengthen the quality of skin care provided to patients. She decides to implement some evidence-based clinical practice guidelines. One of the nurse managers volunteers to take the lead. He forms a task force with an Advanced Practice Nurse, two senior and two junior Registered Nurses and two student nurses who are enthusiastic about the project. Because the implementation of clinical practice guidelines on all 60 nursing units of the hospital seems a daunting task, members of the task force decide to brainstorm ideas. The student nurses and recent graduates had learned about nursing theory in school and how such theory was useful in complex situations. They knew that they would have to find a different type of theory or conceptual model to help with this effort to change practice relating to skin care. They agreed to review the literature on change and to see if they could find models for change. But, where to start?

Changing clinical practice is complex and challenging. Factors known to influence the uptake of practice guidelines include characteristics of the practice guideline, potential adopters, and aspects of the practice setting or organizational context in which the change is to occur.[7–9] Given the complexity of behaviour change and the multiple factors that can influence it in positive and negative ways, there is growing recognition that implementation efforts should be guided by conceptual models or frameworks.[10]

Conceptual models and theories of implementation

The terms 'conceptual models', 'conceptual frameworks' and 'conceptual systems' are often used synonymously and represent global ideas about a phenomenon. They are used to clarify, describe and organize.[11] *Conceptual models* have the basic purpose of focusing, ruling in things that are relevant and ruling out things that have less importance. The usefulness of conceptual models comes from the organization they provide for thinking, observing, and interpreting what is seen. They provide a systematic structure and a rationale for activities. In general, conceptual models are made up of concepts and propositions designed to focus users on what is important to the issue.

There is often confusion or disagreement about the terms 'conceptual model' and 'theory'. A *theory* is an organized, heuristic, coherent and systematic articulation of a set of statements related to significant questions that are communicated in a meaningful whole.[12] It describes observations, summarizes current evidence, proposes explanations, and yields testable hypotheses. It is a symbolic depiction of aspects of reality that are discovered or invented for describing, explaining, predicting and controlling a phenomenon.[11, 12] Differences relate to the level of abstraction or the degree of evidence to support the development of the concepts and relationships proposed.[13] This chapter will focus on conceptual models or frameworks, which is how most developers refer to their proposals for planned implementation of research findings in practice.

The field of implementing research in practice is relatively new compared with clinical fields, such as surgical or maternal–child nursing. The idea of using conceptual models to help nurses implement research evidence gained strength in the 1970s and 1980s when several models were tried.[14–16] Conceptual models of implementation are essentially models or theories of change. Change models/theories fall into two basic types: classical and planned.[11] *Classical model/theories of change* (sometimes referred to as *descriptive* or *normative theories*) are passive; they explain or describe how change occurs. An example of a classical theory of change is Rogers' diffusion theory[9, 17] or Kuhn's conceptualization of scientific revolutions.[18] These theories describe change but were not specifically designed to be used to cause change. Other implementation models or theories in this category are those that have been proposed as ways of thinking about or researching knowledge translation, such as Lomas's Coordinated Implementation Model[19, 20] or the multidimensional framework proposed by Kitson *et al.*[21] Although classical models/theories of change can be informative and helpful for identifying determinants of change, researchers, policy makers and change agents tend to be more interested in planned change models/theories that are specifically intended to be used to guide or cause change.[11]

A *planned change model/theory* is a set of logically interrelated concepts that explain, in a systematic way, the means by which planned change occurs, that predict how various forces in an environment will react in specified change situations, and that help planners or change agents control variables that increase or decrease the likelihood of the occurrence of change.[22, 23] *Planned change*, in this context, refers to deliberately engineering change that occurs in groups that vary in size and setting. Those who use planned change models/theories may work with individuals, but their objective is to alter ways of doing things in social systems.

Some members of the task force attended a conference on research utilization, and one of the presentations provided a review of some nursing and interdisciplinary planned action models/theories. The task force members reported the results of that presentation to the group.

A review by Graham et al. sought to identify and analyse planned action models/theories. They conducted a focused literature search of the social science, education, management, and health sciences literature. They searched the following electronic bibliographic databases from 1980 to May 2005: Sociological Abstracts, SOCIOFILE, Applied Social Science Index and Abstracts (ASSIA), Bath Information and Data Services – Social Science Citations (BIDS), PsycInfo, International Public Affairs Information Service (PAIS), Education Resource Information Center (ERIC), MEDLINE, Cumulative Index to Nursing and Allied Health Literature (CINAHL), and Dissertation Abstracts. Search terms included combinations of knowledge implementation (and other related terms such as translation, transfer, mobilization, exchange, utilization, diffusion), innovation and implementation (plus the related terms above), translation and research or results, diffusion of innovation, theoretical models, concept formation, and nursing models. An information specialist designed and performed the searches. All searches were restricted to literature published in English or French because team members had fluency in these languages. They also used Google to search the Internet for models/theories and searched sites of journal publishing companies (e.g. Blackwell Synergy). Search terms included combinations of diffusion, dissemination, evidence, implementation, innovation, knowledge, practice, research, transfer, translation, and utilization. The journal Science Communication *(formerly* Knowledge: Creation, Diffusion, Utilization*) was hand searched. References of retrieved documents were also scanned for other potentially relevant citations. At least two co-investigators from two different disciplines initially screened the results of all searches to identify potentially relevant hits. The electronic searches yielded 3840 articles and 144 dissertation references. The Internet search identified 103 additional documents. Hand searches of the references of relevant articles and key journals identified an additional 142 papers of potential interest. Two individuals reviewed each potentially relevant abstract and decided whether the article was worth retrieving in full. In total, the literature search yielded 78 articles that were subject to data abstraction by two individuals. This involved abstracting the key or core concepts of each model/theory, determining the action phases, and deciding whether each fit the inclusion/exclusion criteria related to being a planned action theory/model/framework.*

Graham et al. identified seven nursing and 12 interdisciplinary planned action models/theories published after 1980 (Table 27.1).[24] The theories/frameworks had many commonalities in the steps or phases of a planned action model/theory:

- Identify a problem that needs addressing
- Identify the need for change
- Identify the change agents
- Identify the target audience
- Identify, review and select and/or adapt the knowledge/research relevant to the problem and local context (e.g. practice guidelines or research findings)
- Assess barriers to using the knowledge
- Select and tailor interventions to promote the use of the knowledge
- Implement or pilot implement the knowledge

Table 27.1 Models and theories of knowledge utilization relevant to nursing and published since 1980

	Nursing								Interdisciplinary												
	Dufault[27]	Benefield[28]	Stetler[29]	Pape[30]	DiCenso/RNAO[31]	Hickey[32]	Titler[33]	Total/7	Lavis[34]	Rosswurm[35]	Graham[36]	Ashford[37]	Dearing[38]	NHMRC[40]	Hyde[39]	Motwani[41]	Doyle[42]	Fooks[43]	Grol/Wensing[44]	Grol/Grimshaw[45]	Total/12
Identify the problem	1	1	1	1	1	1	1	7		1	1	1		1	1		1	1		1	8
Identify the need for change	1	1	1			1		4	1	1		1	1	1	1			1	1	1	9
Identify the change agents				1	1	1	1	4	1		1	1	1	1	1			1			7
Identify the target audience				1	1	1		3		1	1	1	1	1	1	1		1			8
Assess barriers	1	1	1	1	1	1	1	6	1	1	1			1	1		1	1			7
Review evidence/literature or develop/adapt knowledge	1	1	1	1	1	1	1	7		1		1	1	1	1	1	1	1	1		9
Tailor/develop implementation intervention	1	1	1	1	1	1	1	7	1	1	1	1	1	1	1	1	1	1	1	1	12
Link(age)	1	1	1				1	2	1	1	1	1		1	1						6
Pilot test / implement the knowledge	1	1	1	1	1	1		6	1			1	1	1	1	1	1	1	1	1	10
Develop evaluation plan			1	1	1	1	1	5	1		1			1	1	1	1	1	1	1	9
Evaluate the process/outcomes of using the knowledge	1	1	1		1	1	1	6	1	1	1	1	1	1	1	1	1	1		1	11
Sustain use of the knowledge	1		1				1	3		1	1								1		3
Disseminate results of implementation process	1	1			1	1		4			1	1					1				3
Total number of elements /13	8	9	9	8	10	11	9	9.1	8	9	10	10	7	11	11	6	8	10	6	6	8.5

- Link to appropriate individuals or groups who have vested interests in the project
- Develop a plan to evaluate use of the knowledge
- Evaluate the process and outcomes of using the knowledge
- Sustain ongoing knowledge use
- Disseminate results of the implementation process

The task force now had 19 models/theories from which to choose one to guide their implementation project. They also found some articles and book chapters on clinical practice guidelines and how to evaluate and adapt guidelines for local use (see Chapter 26).[7, 25] The next question was how to choose between the models? One of the students suggested a theory analysis.

A *theory analysis* is a useful process for determining the strengths and limitations of theories and to identify similarities and differences between theories. The following are the steps in a theory analysis:[26]

1. Determine the origins of the theory. The 'origins of a theory' refers to the original development of the theory. Who developed it? Where are they from (institution, discipline)? What prompted the originator to develop it? Is the theory inductive or deductive in form? Does evidence exist to support or refute the development of the theory?
2. Examine the meaning of the theory. The meaning of a theory has to do with the concepts of the theory and how they relate to each other. What are the concepts or main ideas comprising the theory? How are the concepts defined? What is the relationship between or among concepts?
3. Analyse the logical consistency of the theory. The logical adequacy of a theory is the logical structure of the concepts and statements. Are there any logical fallacies in the structure of the theory?
4. Define the degree of generalizability and parsimony of the theory. *Generalizability* refers to the extent to which the theory may be extended to other situations. *Parsimony* refers to how simply and briefly a theory can be stated and still be complete in its explanation of the phenomenon in question.
5. Determine the testability of the theory. *Testability* refers to whether a theory can be supported with empirical data. A theory that cannot generate hypotheses that can be tested empirically through research is not testable.
6. Determine the usefulness of the theory. Usefulness of a theory is about how practical and helpful the theory is to the discipline in providing a sense of understanding and/or predictable outcomes.

Resolution of the clinical scenario

Realizing that they had insufficient resources or time to submit all 19 models[27–45] to a theory analysis, the task force decided that the most prudent approach would be to have each member read a couple of models. They then met to compare their impressions of the models and narrowed the field to two or three models, which they then submitted to a theory analysis. The short list was comprised of the Iowa[33] and Registered Nurses Association of Ontario (RNAO)[31] models and the Ottawa Model of Research Use.[36] For each of these papers, two nurses independently abstracted data for the theory analysis. The task force developed a grid to summarize the main features of a theory analysis to permit more careful comparison of the various models. Table 27.2 presents the results of the

Table 27.2 Comparison of the IOWA model, RNAO model, and Ottawa Model of Research Use (OMRU)

	Titler/IOWA[33]	DiCenso/RNAO[31]	Graham and Logan/OMRU[36]
1(a) Originator		Registered Nurses' Association of Ontario (RNAO)	
1(b) Originator's affiliations	Department of Nursing Services and Patient Care (Titler MG, Kleiber C, Steelman V, Rakel BA, Budreau G, Everett LQ); University of Iowa Hospitals and Clinics, Office of the Provost (Buckwalter KC); University of Iowa College of Nursing (Tripp-Reimer T); University of Colorado Hospital, Denver, Colorado (Goode CJ)	School of Nursing and Department of Clinical Epidemiology and Biostatistics, McMaster University (DiCenso A); Centre for Professional Nursing Excellence, RNAO (Bajnok I); Mount Sinai Hospital (Borycki E); School of Nursing, Ottawa University and Ontario Ministry of Health and Long-Term Care (Davies B); Clinical Epidemiology Unit, Ottawa Health Research Institute (OHRI) and School of Nursing, University of Ottawa (Graham I); School of Nursing, Queen's University, Ottawa Hospital and Clinical Epidemiology Unit, OHRI (Harrison M); School of Nursing, University of Ottawa (Logan J); Children's Hospital of Eastern Ontario Research Institute (McCleary L); Northwestern Regional Cancer Clinic (Power M); RNAO (Scott J)	School of Nursing, University of Ottawa (Graham I, Logan J); Clinical Epidemiology Unit, OHRI (Graham I)
1(c) Original theory's publication date and date of most recent version	1994, 2001	2002	1998, 2004

Origins of theory

Origins of theory	**1(d) What prompted originator to develop the theory? (motivation)**	The IOWA model was developed and originally implemented at the University of IOWA Hospitals and Clinics to guide the use of research findings for improvement of patient care	The RNAO develops nursing best practices. They wanted to ensure the use of best practices and saw the need for an implementation toolkit. The goal of the toolkit was to provide clear direction to organizations and their leaders about how best to ready a setting for change and how to plan and implement a carefully crafted set of strategies to achieve success	Model development was prompted by the lack of practical models to promote research, especially models adopting a parsimonious, holistic approach that considered all aspects of the process of research use that could be helpful to organizational and clinical policy makers for selecting research use strategies and resources needed to support these *'Impetus for developing the model derived not only from our intellectual curiosity about research use but from our desire to support the multifaceted work on research transfer taking place academically and clinically at the University of Ottawa and the Clinical Epidemiology unit of the Loeb Research Institute.'*[8]
	1(e) How was the theory derived?	Literature	Literature, experience	Literature and personal experience
	1(f) Is there evidence to support development?	Yes	Yes	Yes

Table 27.2 (Continued)

	Titler/IOWA[33]	DiCenso/RNAO[31]	Graham and Logan/OMRU[36]
2(a) Meaning of the theory: what are the concepts comprising the theory?	The elements of the model are 1(a) Problem-focused triggers 1(b) Knowledge-focused triggers 2(a) Determine priority of topic 2(b) Consider other triggers 3 Form a team 4 Assemble relevant research 5 Critique and synthesize research for use in practice 6 Determine sufficiency of research 7 If insufficient, conduct own research or use other evidence 8 Select outcomes to be achieved 9 Collect baseline data 10 Design the guideline 11 Implement or pilot units 12 Evaluate process and outcomes 13 Modify the guideline 14 Is change appropriate for adoption in practice? 15 Continue to evaluate quality of core and new knowledge 16 Institute the change in practice 17 Monitor and analyse structure, process, and outcome data 18 Disseminate results	The model consists of six components: 1 Identify clinical practice guideline to implement 2 Identify stakeholders 3 Determine environmental readiness for change 4 Select implementation strategies 5 Evaluation 6 Resources	The model consists of six key elements: 1 The evidence-based innovation 2 Potential adopters 3 The practice environment 4 Implementation interventions 5 Adoption of the innovation 6 Outcomes of adoption And three action phases: 1 Assess the evidence-based innovation, potential adopters, and practice environment for barriers and supports 2 Monitor the implementation interventions and adoption 3 Evaluate the outcomes

Meaning of theory

Meaning of theory

2(b) How are the concepts defined?

Problem-focused triggers (risk management data, process improvement data, internal/external benchmarking data, financial data, identification of clinical problem)

Knowledge-focused triggers (new research or other literature, standards or guidelines, philosophies of care, questions from institutional standards committee)

Is the topic a priority? (decide where the project fits into organizational, department, or unit specific priorities)

Form a team (responsible for development, implementation and evaluation of the EBP)

Assemble relevant research and literature

Critique and synthesize research

Is there sufficient research base to guide practice?

Pilot the change (select outcomes, collect baseline data, develop a written evidence-based practice guideline, try the guideline on one or more units with a small number of patients, evaluate process and outcomes, modify guideline based on data)

Is change appropriate?

Institute change (practice is adopted and integrated into practice throughout a patient population or organization)

Monitor and analyse (structure, process, outcome data)

Disseminate results

Identify clinical practice guideline: systematic approach for identifying a well developed, evidence-based guideline using the AGREE instrument

Stakeholders: identify stakeholders, their interests, support, and influence.

Environmental readiness: assess structure, culture, communication, leadership, knowledge/skills/attitude, commitment, resources, and interdisciplinary relations.

Implementation strategies: users provided with specific strategies to consider

Evaluation: develop plan to evaluate implementation based on structure, process, outcomes

Resources: identify all resources required and develop implementation budget (pp. 56–8)

Evidence-based innovation: potential adopters' perceptions of the attributes or characteristics of both the process by which research evidence was translated into some evidence-based recommendations and the innovation itself

Potential adopters of the evidence: patients, clinicians, and other policy-makers are all potential adopters of research

Practice environment: directs attention to identifying, describing and assessing influences within the practice environment

Implementation: strategies for getting evidence-based innovations to potential adopters and encouraging them to use these strategies

Adoption: making full use of an innovation as the best course of action available and represents behavioural change

Outcomes: represents the impact of using the evidence-based innovation

Assess: the model directs change agents to conduct a barriers assessment of the innovation, potential adopters, and the practice environment in order to identify factors that might hinder or support uptake

Monitor: introduction of the intervention is monitored to ensure that all potential adopters learn about the innovation and what is expected of them

Evaluate: impact of the implementation process on outcomes is evaluated to determine whether the innovation is having the intended effect and whether it has any unintended consequences

Table 27.2 (Continued)

	Titler/IOWA[33]	DiCenso/RNAO[31]	Graham and Logan/OMRU[36]
2(c) What is the relationship between/among concepts?	Flow chart where users move through a number of decision points	Stakeholders and resources to be considered and reconsidered during stages 3–5 (p. 56), linear progression	The model is dynamic in that it considers research use to be an interactive synergistic process of interconnected decisions and actions by different individuals related to each of the model's elements; it is not a sequential stage model of change
3 Logical consistency	No logical fallacies	No logical fallacies	No logical fallacies
4 Generalizability	Yes, seems to be	Yes, seems to be	Yes, seems to be
5 Parsimony	Yes	Yes	Yes
5(a) Are hypotheses offered?	No	No	No
5(b) Can hypotheses be generated?	Yes	No	No
5(c) Has the model been tested?	Yes	Yes	Yes
5(d) Type of validity testing used		Content	Face, content
5(e) How was it tested?	Has been used in nursing institutions around the world in several different studies; implemented at University of Iowa Hospitals and Clinics	Potential users of the toolkit were surveyed[46]	Used with some success in several studies and implementation projects (p. 90).
6 How useful or helpful is the theory?	Gives a complete description of the process, including doing further research if not enough studies have been done on a topic; and it is parsimonious	Provides a complete description and provides many useful tools that can be accessed from the Internet	Provides an action sequence similar to the clinical process that nurses use and is familiar in that respect. A major strength is that it was designed for multidisciplinary use when the clinical topic involved professions other than nursing; it is a parsimonious but comprehensive description of the key ideas. The OMRU has also successfully been used to guide implementation of pressure ulcer guidelines in a tertiary hospital

Testability (spans rows 5(a)–5(e))

theory analysis. Each model had some similarities, and each had strengths and limitations. The theory analysis revealed that the Iowa model gave a complete description of the process, including doing further research if an insufficient number of studies had been done on a topic. It was also parsimonious. The RNAO model also provided a complete description and included many useful tools that could be accessed from the Internet. The Ottawa Model of Research Use provided an action sequence similar to the clinical process that nurses use and so was familiar in that respect. A major strength was that it was designed for multi-disciplinary use when the clinical topic involved more professions than nursing. It was parsimonious but provided a comprehensive description of the key ideas. The Ottawa Model of Research Use had also successfully been used to guide implementation of pressure ulcer guidelines in a tertiary hospital.[8, 47] *The task force agreed that one more meeting was necessary to review the results of the theory analysis and decide on which model to adopt for their project. Some physicians and two physiotherapists were invited to join their final meeting because skin care is a multidisciplinary topic.*

Summary

Implementation science is a relatively new and complex field of inquiry. There are many planned change models and frameworks that have many common elements and action categories. Most models have yet to be tested. Selection of a planned change model should be guided by careful review of the model elements and action categories and the needs of change agents after considering the context in which they are working. Implementation models are useful for planning and focusing implementation efforts and can provide all stakeholders with a common script or understanding of the action plan. More research is needed to confirm the advantages of using particular planned change models. When a planned change model is used, change agents should consider documenting their experiences with the model so as to advance understanding of the usefulness of the model and provide information to others who are attempting similar projects.

LEARNING EXERCISES

1. Think about the issues presented in the scenario and the information presented in Table 27.2. Which model would you choose, and what would be the reasons for your choice?
2. Think about a best practice that should be implemented in your setting. Is the topic a nursing issue only or are other professions involved? What are the implications if it is a nursing or interdisciplinary best practice?
3. Consider the action categories presented in Table 27.1. Which categories will be particularly challenging and why?
4. As a member of the task force, do you think that the implementation model you are using should be shared with all nurses and others who are expected to change practice, or should the task force use the model for organizing the project but focus on the skin care clinical practice guideline when interacting with the other nurses?

References

1 Grimshaw JM, Ward J, Eccles MP. Getting research into practice. In: Pencheon D, Gray MJA, Guest C, Melzer D, editors. *Oxford Handbook of Public Health.* Oxford: Oxford University Press, 2001.

2 Graham ID, Logan J, Harrison MB, Straus SE, Tetroe J, Caswell W, Robinson N. Lost in knowledge translation: time for a map? *J Contin Educ Health Prof* 2006;**26**:13–24.

3 Agency for Healthcare Research and Quality. *Translating Research Into Practice (TRIP)-II.* Washington, DC: Agency for Healthcare Research and Quality, 2001. http://www.ahrq.gov/research/trip2fac.htm (accessed 21 January 2007).

4 Horsley JA, Crane J. Factors associated with innovation in nursing practice. *Fam Community Health* 1986;**9**:1–11.

5 Funk SG, Tornquist EM, Champagne MT. Barriers and facilitators of research utilization. An integrative review. *Nurs Clin North Am* 1995;**30**:395–407.

6 Lekander BJ, Tracy MF, Linquist R. Overcoming the obstacles to research-based clinical practice. *AACN Clin Issues Crit Care Nurs* 1994;**5**:115–23.

7 Grol R, Wensing M, Eccles M. *Improving Patient Care. The Implementation of Change in Clinical Practice.* Toronto: Elsevier, 2005.

8 Logan J, Graham ID. Toward a comprehensive interdisciplinary model of health care research use. *Science Communication* 1998;**20**:227–46.

9 Rogers EM. *Diffusion of Innovations.* Fifth edition. New York: The Free Press, 2003.

10 McDonald KM, Graham ID, Grimshaw J. Toward a theoretic basis for quality improvement interventions. In: Shojania KG, McDonald KM, Wachter RM, Owens DK, editors. *Closing the Quality Gap: A Critical Analysis of Quality Improvement Practices. Volume 1. Series Overview and Method.* Rockville, MD: Agency for Healthcare Research and Quality, 2004.

11 Rimmer Tiffany C, Johnson Lutjens LR. *Planned Change Theories for Nursing: Review, Analysis, and Implications.* Thousand Oaks: Sage, 1998.

12 Meleis A. *Theoretical Nursing: Development and Progress.* Third edition. New York: Lippincott Williams & Wilkins, 1997.

13 Barnum BS. *Nursing Theory: Analysis, Application, Evaluation.* Fifth edition. Philadelphia: Lippincott Williams & Wilkins, 1998.

14 Krueger JC, Nelson AH, Wolanin MO. *Nursing Research: Development, Collaboration, and Utilization.* Germantown: Aspen Systems, 1978.

15 Horsely JA, Crane J, Bingle J. Research utilization as an organizational process. *J Nurs Admin* 1978;**8**:4–6.

16 Stetler CB, Marram G. Evaluating research findings for applicability in practice. *Nurs Outlook* 1976;**24**:559–63.

17 Rogers EM. *Diffusion of Innovations.* Fourth edition. New York: The Free Press, 1995.

18 Kuhn TS. *The Structure of Scientific Revolutions.* Second edition. Chicago: University of Chicago Press, 1970.

19 Lomas J. Retailing research: increasing the role of evidence in clinical services for childbirth. *Milbank Q* 1993;**71**:439–75.

20 Lomas J. Teaching old (and not so old) docs new tricks: effective ways to implement research findings. In: Dunn E, Norton PG, Stewart M, Tudiver F, Bass M, editors. *Disseminating Research/Changing Practice.* Thousand Oaks: Sage, 1994:1–18.

21 Kitson A, Harvey G, McCormack B. Enabling the implementation of evidence based practice: a conceptual framework. *Qual Health Care* 1998;**7**:149–58.

22 Tiffany CR. Analysis of planned change theories. *Nurs Manage* 1994;**25**:60–2.

23 Tiffany CR, Cheatham AB, Doornbos D, Loudermelt L, Momadi GG. Planned change theory: survey of nursing periodical literature. *Nurs Manage* 1994;**25**:54–9.

24 Graham ID, Logan J, the KT Theories Research Group. *A review and theory analysis of planned change (knowledge transfer) theories.* Fourth Annual Clinical Nursing Research Conference/ La quatrieme conference annuelle de recherche en sciences infirmieres: Knowledge transfer: sharing the knowledge – sharing the care. Transfert des connaissances: partager le savoir-partager le soin sante, University of Ottawa School of Nursing and Tau Gamma Chapter of Sigma Theta Tau International, Ottawa 2006.

25 Estabrooks CA, Thompson DS, Lovely JJ, Hofmeyer A. A guide to knowledge translation theory. *J Contin Educ Health Prof* 2006;**26**:25–36.

26 Walker LO, Avant KC. *Strategies for Theory Construction in Nursing.* Fourth edition. Upper Saddle River: Prentice Hall, 2005.

27 Dufault M. Testing a collaborative research utilization model to translate best practices in pain management. *Worldviews Evid Based Nurs* 2004;1:S26–32.

28 Benefield LE. Implementing evidence-based practice in home care. *Home Healthc Nurse* 2003;21:804–9.

29 Stetler CB. Updating the Stetler Model of research utilization to facilitate evidence-based practice. *Nurs Outlook* 2001;49:272–9.

30 Pape TM. Evidence-based nursing practice: to infinity and beyond. *J Contin Educ Nurs* 2003;34:154–61.

31 DiCenso A, Virani T, Bajnok I, Borycki E, Davies B, Graham I, Harrison M, Logan J, McCleary L, Power M, Scott J. A toolkit to facilitate the implementation of clinical practice guidelines in healthcare settings. *Hosp Q* 2002;5:55–60.

32 Hickey M. The role of the clinical nurse specialist in the research utilization process. *Clin Nurse Spec* 1990;4:93–6.

33 Titler MG, Kleiber C, Steelman V, Rakel B, Budreau G, Everett L, Buckwalter K, Tripp-Reimer T, Goode C. The IOWA Model of evidence based practice to promote quality – care. *Crit Care Nurs Clin of North Am* 2001;13(4):497–509.

34 Lavis JN, Robertson D, Woodside JM, McLeod CB, Abelson J, for the Knowledge Transfer Study Group. How can research organizations more effectively transfer research knowledge to decision makers? *Milbank Q* 2003;81:221–48.

35 Rosswurm MA, Larrabee JH. A model for change to evidence-based practice. *Image J Nurs Sch* 1999;31:317–22.

36 Graham ID, Logan J. Innovations in knowledge transfer and continuity of care. *Can J Nurs Res* 2004;36:89–103.

37 Ashford J, Eccles M, Bond S, Hall LA, Bond J. Improving health care through professional behaviour change: introducing a framework for identifying behaviour change strategies. *British Journal of Clinical Governance* 1999;4:14–23.

38 Dearing JW. Improving the state of health programming by using diffusion theory. *J Health Commun* 2004;9(S1):21–36.

39 Hyde PS, Falls K, Morris JA, Schoenwald SK. *Turning Knowledge into Practice.* Boston: The Technical Assistance Collaborative Inc., 2003.

40 National Health and Medical Research Council. *How to Put the Evidence into Practice: Implementation and Dissemination Strategies.* Canberra: Commonwealth of Australia, National Health and Medical Research Council, 2000.

41 Motwani J, Sower VE, Brashier LW. Implementing TQM in the health care sector. *Health Care Manage Rev* 1996;21:73–82.

42 Doyle DM, Dauterive R, Chuang KH, Ellrodt AG. Translating evidence into practice: pursuing perfection in pneumococcal vaccination in a rural community. *Respir Care* 2001;46:1258–72.

43 Fooks C, Cooper J, Bhatia V. Making research transfer work: Summary report from the 1st National Workshop on Research Transfer Issues, Methods and Experiences. Toronto: ICES, IWH, CHEPA, 1997.

44 Grol R, Wensing M. What drives change? Barriers to and incentives for achieving evidence-based practice. *Med J Aust* 2004;180:S57–60.

45 Grol R, Grimshaw J. Evidence-based implementation of evidence-based medicine. *Jt Comm J Qual Improv* 1999;25:503–13.

46 Dobbins M, Davies B, Donesco E, Edwards N, Virani T. Changing nursing practice: evaluating the usefulness of a best practice guideline implementation toolkit. *Nursing Leadership* 2005;18:34–46.

47 Graham K, Logan J. Using the Ottawa Model of Research Use to implement a skin care program. *J Nurs Care Qual* 2004;19:18–24.

Chapter 28

CLOSING THE GAP BETWEEN NURSING RESEARCH AND PRACTICE

Mary Ann O'Brien

The existence of a gap between valid research evidence and nursing practice is not a new observation.[1] Thirty years ago, Nancy Roper commented that the nursing profession needed to base practice on scientific research.[2] Despite an accumulating body of knowledge about the effectiveness of many nursing practices, a gap often exists between what is known and what is practised. For example, the effectiveness of hand washing to reduce the transmission of infections is well known. Yet, handwashing practices remain suboptimal among nurses and physicians.[3]

Continuing professional education has been promoted as a way to bridge the gap between research and practice so that patients may benefit.[4–6] Davis et al.[6] described continuing medical education as the longest educational phase in the career of a physician, and this view applies to other health professionals who aspire to life-long learning. The term 'continuing professional education', however, sometimes conjures up images of traditional lectures with boring slides by 'experts' in dark rooms. A more encompassing description might be 'any and all ways by which [health professionals] learn and change after formal training is completed'.[7]

The first section of this chapter will summarize what is known about the effectiveness of continuing professional education and behaviour change strategies in general, and the second section will provide suggestions for choosing appropriate activities. Some of the suggestions will apply to nurse educators or administrators, whereas others will apply to individual nurses, depending on the complexity of the intervention. Some interventions, such as audit and feedback, are complex to implement because the processes of auditing practice, creating summaries, and providing feedback to individuals need to be established. The implementation of such processes involves cooperation among departments such as information technology and nursing administration. Other interventions, such as attending interactive workshops or reading evidence-based guidelines, could be implemented by individual nurses. However, to achieve change, there needs to be a culture where evidence-based practice is valued, and the responsibility to achieve high-quality practice is found across the organization, including hospital governance, nursing administration and education, as well as individual nurses.[8] To place sole responsibility for achieving evidence-based practice on individual nurses is unlikely to result in success, but leaving nurses out of the planning process is equally doomed to failure.

Barriers to implementing evidence-based nursing practice have been widely reported in the literature. In a systematic review, Estabrooks et al.[9] identified 630 articles published between 1972 and 2001 about the utilization of research evidence in nursing practice. The authors concluded that, despite a growing interest in barriers and facilitators of research utilization, the field was relatively underdeveloped and lacked sufficient conceptual work and that more collaboration among scholars was needed. Interest in the area includes researchers in different countries, such as Australia,[10] Canada,[11] Denmark,[12, 13] Finland,[14, 15] Greece,[16] Iran,[17] Ireland,[18] and the United Kingdom,[19–21] and in different nursing specialities, such as community care,[22] critical care,[23] mental health,[24] and paediatrics.[25, 26] Some of the common barriers, such as lack of support, lack of time, and lack of individual responsibility for initiating evidence-based nursing practice, seem to be organizational. Other barriers, such as lack of understanding of research publications, are at the level of the individual. Collectively, these reports suggest that the process of adopting research findings in nursing practice is a complex phenomenon, and thus efforts to implement interventions to promote evidence-based practice must recognize this complexity from the outset. Some researchers have proposed models to implement evidence-based practice that recognize different levels of responsibility. For example, Dobbins et al.[27] described a framework of research dissemination and utilization that included individual, organizational, environmental, and innovation characteristics.[27] Thompson et al.[28] emphasized that a discussion of evidence-based nursing should include the clinical decision-making context to which research-based information will be applied, as well as the sources of information that will be accessed. The next section summarizes what is known about strategies or interventions to improve professional practice.

Evaluation of behaviour change strategies

Systematic reviews of strategies to improve health professional practice have been conducted in several ways. Some reviews have been designed to answer broad questions about interventions in general. A recent example is a review by Grimshaw et al.[29] that examined different guideline dissemination and implementation strategies across different health care problems and included different types of health professionals. Other reviews focus on specific interventions, such as audit and feedback.[30] Another approach is to include only certain types of health professionals and exclude others. For example, Thomas et al.[31] included interventions specifically targeted at health care professionals (nearly all nurses) but excluded physicians. Finally, some reviews are conducted to address specific problems, such as immunizations.[32]

Broad reviews such as the one by Grimshaw et al.[29] can help provide insights about the effectiveness of many different types of intervention. In their review they identified 235 studies of different guideline dissemination and implementation strategies, including fairly simple strategies such as the dissemination of educational materials, and more complex strategies such as reminders to prompt health professionals.[29] They concluded that it is possible to improve professional practice, but usually the effects are modest. Across all studies, the median improvement was 10%, which may, at first glance, seem underwhelming, but the authors indicate that these results could be important from a population perspective. For specific interventions, the median effect varied. For example, distribution of educational materials resulted in a median absolute improvement of 8.1%, whereas the use of reminders to prompt health professionals achieved a median absolute improvement of 14.1%. Surprisingly, studies of multifaceted interventions, in which several interventions were used, did not appear to be more effective than single interventions.[29] The modest effects of interventions to improve practice echo the findings of an earlier report in which the authors concluded that there were 'no magic bullets' for improving practice.[33]

Other reviews have focused on different types of intervention, such as audit and feedback,[30] educational outreach visiting,[34] educational meetings,[35] and tailored interventions.[36] Jamtvedt et al.[30] identified 118 randomized controlled trials (RCTs) of different types of audit and feedback. They concluded that audit and feedback can be effective in improving health professional practice, but the effects are small to moderate. They found that effects were larger when baseline compliance with desired practice was low and if the intensity of audit and feedback was high.[30] O'Brien et al.[34] reported small-to-moderate effects associated with educational visiting. With respect to the effectiveness of educational meetings, larger effects were reported if meetings were interactive, whereas didactic meetings had little effect in improving practice.[35] Tailored interventions are those that addressed identified barriers to

Table 28.1 Interventions to promote behavioural change in health professionals*

Intervention	Description
Audit and feedback	Any written or verbal summary of clinical performance of health care professionals over a specified period of time. The summary may also include recommendations for clinical action
Educational outreach visits	Use of a trained person who meets with professionals in their practice settings to provide information with the intent of improving practice
Educational materials	Distribution of published or printed recommendations for clinical care, including clinical practice guidelines, audiovisual materials, and electronic publications
Interactive educational meetings	Participation of professionals in workshops that include discussion
Local consensus process	Inclusion of participating professionals in discussion to ensure that they agree that the chosen clinical problem was important and the approach to managing the problem was appropriate
Local opinion leaders	Use of providers nominated by their colleagues as 'educationally influential'
Multifaceted interventions	A combination that includes two or more of audit and feedback, reminders, local consensus processes, and patient-mediated interventions
Reminders	Any intervention, manual or computerized, that prompts professionals to perform a clinical action
Tailoring	An intervention tailored to address prospectively identified barriers to change

* Adapted from the Cochrane Effective Practice and Organisation of Care Review Group.

change.[36] This approach is attractive because, as discussed earlier, various barriers to the utilization of research evidence have been proposed. The authors identified 15 RCTs of tailored strategies but reported mixed results. From their review, they were unable to determine whether the barriers were valid and if they were adequately addressed by the intervention.[36]

Another systematic review focused specifically on the effectiveness of guidelines in professions allied to medicine. Participants were nurses in 17 of 18 RCTs identified.[31] In three of five studies, nurses who received guidelines had improvements in processes of care compared with those who did not, and in six of eight studies outcomes were improved. An older review[37] included studies, with various designs, that assessed continuing nursing education; both complex interventions and traditional activities, such as lectures, were included. The author concluded that, overall, continuing education was effective in improving practice. More recently, Robertson et al.[38] conducted a review of 15 research syntheses of continuing professional education published since 1993. They concluded that continuing education that is ongoing, interactive, contextually relevant, and based on needs assessments can improve knowledge, skills, attitudes, behaviour, and health care outcomes.[38]

A taxonomy of interventions to improve practice (Table 28.1) has been developed by the Cochrane Effective Practice and Organisation of Care review group (EPOC). This international group of researchers is interested in preparing and maintaining systematic reviews of the effectiveness of interventions that influence professional practice. A complete description of the scope and methods of EPOC can be found at www.epoc.uottawa.ca.

Getting research into practice

The good news is that there are interventions that improve health professional practice. The bad news is that there don't appear to be interventions that work all the time, and when they work the effects are rather ordinary. Getting research into practice is not as simple as choosing an intervention and hoping for the best. Aside from the intervention itself, mediating factors include the characteristics of patients and practitioners and the desired behaviour change.[27, 39, 40] Getting practitioners to start doing something new, such as routinely asking patients if they smoke, may require a different strategy than that used to get practitioners to stop doing something they do frequently. Furthermore, as previously discussed, administrative or financial policies within organizations and settings may act as disincentives to improving the practice of individuals.

Interventions should ideally be tailored to an individual's needs and should address administrative barriers where appropriate. In discussing the problem of inadequate handwashing, Grol and Grimshaw[3] suggest that a comprehensive approach that targets barriers to change and uses interventions directed towards the individual, team, patient and organization is needed to achieve lasting changes. In earlier work, Grol[41] provided a five-step cyclical process to changing practice. The first step is to develop a change proposal that is based on evidence and consensus, is not overly complex, and is adapted to the local context. In the second step, barriers to change are identified at individual and organizational levels. Barriers should be identified in terms of stages of change. The third step is to link interventions to barriers to change, recognizing that some interventions are better suited to gaining knowledge, whereas

Table 28.2 Implementation strategies for different needs*

Implementation strategies	Improve knowledge or attitudes	Improve skills	Change practice
Audit and feedback	+	?	+/−
Educational materials	+	?	+/−
Educational outreach visits	+	?	+/−
Lectures	+	−	−
Local opinion leaders	+	?	+/−
Multifaceted approaches	+	?	+/−
Reminders	+	?	+/−
Tailoring	?	?	+/−

* Adapted from Davis and Thomson.[43] + = Improvement based on evidence from randomized controlled trials; ? = evidence is unclear or unavailable; − = no improvement based on evidence from randomized controlled trials.

others might help to reinforce a behaviour that is already known. In the fourth step, a plan is developed whereby intermediate and long-term goals are identified with an appropriate timeline. The fifth step involves a process of continuous quality improvement. The concept of matching an intervention to the stage of readiness to change has also been proposed.[42] For example, primary care nurses are likely aware of the benefits of cervical screening. Although they may not require more information, they might need a prompt located on a patient's chart. If, however, nurses lack information, awareness or skills, then strategies that involve a high degree of interaction (e.g. educational workshops) might be effective. Table 28.2 provides a summary of implementation strategies for different needs.

Planning for improving the practice of individual nurses

As noted in previous sections, there are strategies to improve practice. However, many strategies require collaboration among different groups of people, such as information technology, and the active involvement of nursing administration. Although this is a good thing, it doesn't provide much direction to the individual nurse who wants to learn more. This section will address how nurses can take steps to improve their practice. We will assume that high-quality evidence exists for the practice area that the nurse wants to address.

As professionals, we need to develop ways of scrutinizing our practice with a view to self-improvement. This means being open to the possibility that there may be better ways of doing things. An initial needs assessment can be accomplished using strategies such as self-reflection, reading, and discussion with respected peers. As part of a self-reflection process, nurses can determine what is needed to improve their practice. They can ask themselves if they have the necessary knowledge and skills. A caveat: two studies have shown less impact on performance if clinicians chose their own topics for further learning, and more impact if lower preference topics were studied.[44, 45]

It may be that practitioners tend to choose topics in which they have the greatest interest and are already quite knowledgeable.

The next step is to choose a learning activity. Individual nurses can choose strategies such as reading evidence-based guidelines, attending interactive workshops, or attending a journal club. Another caveat: there may be discrepancies between a nurse's preferred sources of information or style of continuing education and what is most effective for improving practice. In a Canadian study of staff nurses working in seven surgical units, nurses preferred personal or interpersonal sources of information for clinical practice, including their own experience and discussions with co-workers and patients, rather than print-based sources, such as journal articles or textbooks.[46] The authors indicated that there was a need to understand nurses' preferences for knowledge gained through personal experience or social interaction. If nurses prefer to gain knowledge through social interaction, clinical nurse educators may be well suited to act as sources of information, role models, and mentors for developing evidence-based practice because of their advanced training and collegial interactions with other nurses.[47] Other health professionals or nurses practising in other settings may have different preferred sources of information. Tassone and Speechley[48] found that Canadian physiotherapists preferred short courses, whereas Covell et al.[49] reported that physicians preferred reading. However, poorly designed courses and reading alone may have little impact on practice.

Reading materials can be useful if they are evidence-based. Secondary sources such as evidence-based journals are ideal because they present only high-quality research and provide a clinician's commentary on each abstract. The *Cochrane Library* (http://www.cochrane.co.uk/en/clibintro.htm) is another important evidence-based source of information and should be available in medical and nursing libraries. Although short courses are popular, practice is likely to improve if lectures are minimized and high levels of reflection and interaction are encouraged.[35]

Completion of formal or informal educational activities, although important, is probably insufficient to improve practice. Changing behaviour is a complex process, and nurses may revert back to usual practices unless new behaviours are reinforced.[41, 42] Individual nurses should attempt to identify practical barriers to change, which need administrative or organizational support, and then attempt to influence existing managerial or quality improvement structures to address these barriers.

The gap between research and practice is not merely a consequence of nurses failing to keep up to date.[8, 50] MacGuire[8] summarized the problem concisely: 'the integration of research and practice has to be addressed at all levels of an organisation; from policy statements to procedure manuals and from managers, educators and clinicians to support workers within the framework of the management of change'.

Implementing evidence-based practice involves many systems and is unlikely to be accomplished through the use of educational strategies only.[8, 27, 51] Other efforts, such as organizational supports and resources that encourage nurses to participate in research projects,[52–54] connect with larger networks,[55, 56] and gain experience with critical appraisal tools and journal clubs, are important considerations that should not be overlooked.[51, 57, 58]

LEARNING EXERCISES

Please assume that high-quality evidence exists for the problem that you want to address.

Continuing professional development plan

Step 1. Choose a practice problem of interest to you. Try to select a problem that has the potential to improve the care of many patients. It is usually better to start small.

Step 2. Enlist help. Talk with other nurses who are usually supportive of you. Do you know a clinical nurse specialist who can listen to your ideas? It is difficult to move ahead with improving a practice problem if you try to do it alone.

Step 3. Decide what is lacking in the practice area. Is there a knowledge gap? Are new skills needed? Is there a coordination problem between departments or care providers? If so, it may be worthwhile to involve other departments or areas.

Step 4. Develop a plan with specific goals that are do-able. Ask yourself how you will know if practice has improved.

Step 5. Consider how to improve knowledge and skills. Reviewing evidence-based guidelines is likely to be a good starting point. External continuing education sessions may or may not be helpful to improve knowledge and skills. Check to ensure that the information is evidence-based and that time is available to practise new skills, if relevant. Small-group learning tailored to your goals may be an appropriate choice.

References

1 DiCenso A, Cullum N, Ciliska D. Implementing evidence-based nursing: some misconceptions. *Evid Based Nurs* 1998;**1**:38–9.

2 Roper N. Justification and use of research in nursing. *J Adv Nurs* 1977;**2**:365–71.

3 Grol R, Grimshaw J. From best evidence to best practice: effective implementation of change in patients' care. *Lancet* 2003;**362**:1225–30.

4 Davis DA, Thomson MA, Oxman AD, Haynes RB. Changing physician performance. A systematic review of the effect of continuing medical education strategies. *JAMA* 1995;**274**:700–5.

5 Felch WC. Bridging the gap between research and practice. The role of continuing medical education. *JAMA* 1997;**277**:155–6.

6 Davis D, O'Brien MA, Freemantle N, Wolf FM, Mazmanian P, Taylor-Vaisey A. Impact of formal continuing medical education: do conferences, workshops, rounds, and other traditional continuing education activities change physician behavior or health care outcomes? *JAMA* 1999;**282**:867–74.

7 Davis DA, Fox RD, editors. *The Physician as Learner: Linking Research to Practice.* Chicago: American Medical Association, 1994.

8 MacGuire JM. Putting nursing research findings into practice: research utilization as an aspect of the management of change. *J Adv Nurs* 1990;**15**:614–20.

9 Estabrooks CA, Winther C, Derksen L. Mapping the field: a bibliometric analysis of the research utilization literature in nursing. *Nurs Res* 2004;**53**:293–303.

10 Hutchinson AM, Johnston L. Bridging the divide: a survey of nurses' opinions regarding barriers to, and facilitators of, research utilization in the practice setting. *J Clin Nurs* 2004;**13**:304–15.

11 Paramonczyk A. Barriers to implementing research in clinical practice. *Can Nurse* 2005;**101**:12–15.

12 Adamsen L, Larsen K, Bjerregaard L, Madsen JK. Danish research-active clinical nurses overcome barriers in research utilization. *Scand J Caring Sci* 2003;**17**:57–65.

13 Egerod I, Hansen GM. Evidence-based practice among Danish cardiac nurses: a national survey. *J Adv Nurs* 2005;**51**:465–73.

14 Oranta O, Routasalo P, Hupli M. Barriers to and facilitators of research utilization among Finnish registered nurses. *J Clin Nurs* 2002;**11**:205–13.

15 Kuuppelomaki M, Tuomi J. Finnish nurses' views on their research activities. *J Clin Nurs* 2003;**12**:589–600.

16 Patiraki E, Karlou C, Papadopoulou D, Spyridou A, Kouloukoura C, Bare E, Merkouris A. Barriers in implementing research findings in cancer care: the Greek registered nurses perceptions. *Eur J Oncol Nurs* 2004;**8**:245–56.

17 Valizadeh L, Zamanzadeh V. Research utilization and research attitudes among nurses working in teaching hospitals in Tabriz, Iran. *J Clin Nurs* 2003;**12**:928–30.

18 Brenner M. Children's nursing in Ireland: barriers to, and facilitators of, research utilisation. *Paediatr Nurs* 2005;**17**:40–5.

19 Bryar RM, Closs SJ, Baum G, Cooke J, Griffiths J, Hostick T, Kelly S, Knight S, Marshall K, Thompson DR. The Yorkshire BARRIERS project: diagnostic analysis of barrier to research utilisation. *Int J Nurs Stud* 2003;**40**:73–84.

20 McCaughan D, Thompson C, Cullum N, Sheldon TA, Thompson DR. Acute care nurses' perceptions of barriers to using research information in clinical decision-making. *J Adv Nurs* 2002;**39**:46–60.

21 Veeramah V. Utilization of research findings by graduate nurse and midwives. *J Adv Nurs* 2004;**47**:183–91.

22 Griffiths JM, Bryar RM, Closs SJ, Cooke J, Hostick T, Kelly S, Marshall K. Barriers to research implementation by community nurses. *Br J Community Nurs* 2001;**6**:501–10.

23 Hodge M, Kochie LD, Larsen L, Santiago M. Clinician-implemented research utilization in critical care. *Am J Crit Care* 2003;**12**:361–6.

24 Carrion M, Woods P, Norman I. Barriers to research utilisation among forensic mental health nurses. *Int J Nurs Stud* 2004;**41**:613–19.

25 McCleary L, Brown GT. Research utilization among pediatric health professionals. *Nurs Health Sci* 2002;**4**:163–71.

26 Niederhauser VP, Kohr L. Research endeavors among pediatric nurse practitioners (REAP) study. *J Pediatr Health Care* 2005;**19**:80–9.

27 Dobbins M, Ciliska D, Cockerill R, Barnsley J, DiCenso A. A framework for the dissemination and utilization of research for health-care policy and practice. *Online J Knowl Synth Nurs* 2002;**9**:document 7.

28 Thompson C, Cullum N, McCaughan D, Sheldon T, Raynor P. Nurses, information use, and clinical decision making – the real world potential for evidence-based decisions in nursing. *Evid Based Nurs* 2004;**7**:68–72.

29 Grimshaw JM, Thomas RE, MacLennan G, Fraser C, Ramsay CR, Vale L, Whitty P, Eccles MP, Matowe L, Shirran L, Wensing M, Dijkstra R, Donaldson C. Effectiveness and efficiency of guideline dissemination and implementation strategies. *Health Technol Assess* 2004;**8**(6):iii–iv, 1–72.

30 Jamtvedt G, Young JM, Kristoffersen DT, O'Brien MA, Oxman AD. Audit and feedback: effects on professional practice and health care outcomes. *Cochrane Database Syst Rev* 2006;(2):CD000259.

31 Thomas L, Cullum N, McColl E, Rousseau N, Soutter J, Steen N. Guidelines in professions allied to medicine. *Cochrane Database Syst Rev* 1999;(1):CD000349.

32 Gyorkos TW, Tannenbaum TN, Abrahamowicz M, Bedard L, Carsley J, Franco ED, Delage G, Miller MA, Lamping DL, Grover SA. Evaluation of the effectiveness of immunization delivery methods. *Can J Public Health* 1994;**85**:S14–30.

33 Oxman AD, Thomson MA, Davis DA, Haynes RB. No magic bullets: a systematic review of 102 trials of interventions to improve professional practice. *CMAJ* 1995;**153**:1423–31.

34 O'Brien MA, Oxman AD, Davis DA, Haynes RB, Freemantle N, Harvey EL. Educational outreach visits: effects on professional practice and health care outcomes. *Cochrane Database Syst Rev* 1997;(4):CD000409.

35 O'Brien MA, Freemantle N, Oxman AD, Wolf F, Davis DA, Herrin J. Continuing education meetings and workshops: effects on professional practice and health care outcomes. *Cochrane Database Syst Rev* 2001;(1):CD003030.

36 Shaw B, Cheater F, Baker R, Gillies C, Hearnshaw H, Flottorp S, Robertson N. Tailored interventions to overcome identified barriers to change: effects on professional practice and health care outcomes. *Cochrane Database Syst Rev* 2005;(3):CD005470.

37 Waddell DL. The effects of continuing education on nursing practice: a meta-analysis. *J Contin Educ Nurs* 1991;**22**:113–18.

38 Robertson MK, Umble KE, Cervero RM. Impact studies in continuing education for health professions: update. *J Contin Educ Health Prof* 2003;**23**:146–56.

39 Cervero RM. Continuing professional education and behavioural change: a model for research and evaluation. *J Contin Educ Nurs* 1985;**16**:85–8.

40 Lomas J, Haynes RB. A taxonomy and critical review of tested strategies for the application of clinical practice recommendations: from 'official' to 'individual' clinical policy. *Am J Prev Med* 1988;**4**(4 Suppl):77–94.

41 Grol R. Beliefs and evidence in changing clinical practice. *BMJ* 1997;**315**:418–21.

42 Prochaska JO, DiClemente CC, Norcross JC. In search of how people change. Applications to addictive behaviors. *Am Psychol* 1992;**47**:1102–14.

43 Davis DA, Thomson MA. Continuing medical education as a means of lifelong learning. In: Silagy C, Haines A, editors. *Evidence Based Practice in Primary Care*. Second edition. London: BMJ Publishing Group, 2001.

44 Palmer RH, Louis TA, Hsu LN, Peterson HF, Rothrock JK, Strain R, Thompson MS, Wright EA. A randomized controlled trial of quality assurance in sixteen ambulatory care practices. *Med Care* 1985;**23**:751–70.

45 Sibley JC, Sackett DL, Neufeld V, Gerrard B, Rudnick KV, Fraser W. A randomized trial of continuing medical education. *N Engl J Med* 1982;**306**:511–15.

46 Estabrooks CA, Chong H, Brigidear K, Profetto-McGrath J. Profiling Canadian nurses' preferred knowledge sources for clinical practice. *Can J Nurs Res* 2005;**37**:118–40.

47 Milner MF, Estabrooks CA, Humphrey C. Clinical nurse educators as agents for change: increasing research utilization. *Int J Nurs Stud* 2005;**42**:899–914.

48 Tassone MR, Speechley M. Geographical challenges for physical therapy continuing education: preferences and influences. *Phys Ther* 1997;**77**:285–95.

49 Covell DG, Uman GC, Manning PR. Information needs in office practice: are they being met? *Ann Intern Med* 1985;**103**:596–9.

50 Tornquist EM, Funk SG, Champagne MT. Research utilization: reconnecting research and practice. *AACN Clin Issues* 1995;**6**:105–9.

51 Ciliska DK, Pinelli J, DiCenso A, Cullum N. Resources to enhance evidence-based nursing practice. *AACN Clin Issues* 2001;**12**:520–8.

52 Ashcroft T, Kristjanson LJ. Research utilization in maternal-child nursing: application of the CURN model. *Can J Nurs Adm* 1994;**7**:90–102.

53 Kitson A, Ahmed LB, Harvey G, Seers K, Thompson DR. From research to practice: one organizational model for promoting research-based practice. *J Adv Nurs* 1996;**23**:430–40.

54 Rodgers S. An exploratory study of research utilization by nurses in general medical and surgical wards. *J Adv Nurs* 1994;**20**:904–11.

55 Kettles AM. Grampian mental health divisional research unit. *Nurs Stand* 1997;**11**:33–4.

56 Leighton-Beck L. Networking: putting research at the heart of professional practice. *Br J Nurs* 1997;**6**:120–2.

57 Fink R, Thompson CJ, Bonnes D. Overcoming barriers and promoting the use of research in practice. *J Nurs Adm* 2005;**35**:121–9.

58 Kirchhoff KT, Beck SL. Using the journal club as a component of the research utilization process. *Heart Lung* 1995;**24**:246–50.

Chapter 29

PROMOTING RESEARCH UTILIZATION IN NURSING: THE ROLE OF THE INDIVIDUAL, THE ORGANIZATION AND THE ENVIRONMENT

Joan Royle and Jennifer Blythe

The term 'information society' was introduced in the 1980s to describe the information explosion precipitated by new computer-based technologies.[1] Today, computer systems enable health care professionals to manage patient information, access clinical guidelines and protocols, retrieve research reports, and remain up to date on health care policy. The Internet has become a formidable medium for information provision, sharing and exchange. Current challenges for producers of nursing information include devising effective dissemination strategies. Challenges for consumers include locating timely, accurate, relevant data to address the problem at hand.

Contexts of research utilization

Since the 1980s, when research was first recognized as an integral part of professional nursing, researchers have expressed concern about the gap between research findings and practice.[2] The exponential growth of nursing research in recent years has made it increasingly important for nurses to integrate new knowledge into their practice. The ideal is to practise evidence-based decision-making, a process that involves integrating clinical expertise, patient preferences, research evidence, and available resources in the decision-making process.[3]

Numerous researchers have investigated the causes of the research–practice gap. Most surveyed nurses about their attitudes, resources and experiences related to research utilization.[4] Based on a review of the literature, Funk *et al.*[4] concluded that barriers to research utilization involve the individual nurse, the organization, the quality of research, and the way that research results are communicated. Surveys using Funk's Barrier Scale showed widespread recognition of these barriers.[5] A review on research utilization found that organizational factors explained 80–90% of the variance in research use, environmental factors explained 5–10%, and individual characteristics explained 1–3%.[6] Although organizational factors predominate, multifaceted interventions directed at the individual, the environment and the organization are considered most likely to change practice.[7]

The individual nurse

Early studies, usually based on self-report, noted that nurses varied in the extent to which they used research.[8] Investigators expressed concern that most nurses read clinical or technical journals rather than research journals and rarely visited libraries.[9–11] Reasons for limited use of research included time constraints, limited knowledge of literature and critical appraisal skills, and limited authority or support to change practice. Other constraints included lack of resources in the workplace and inability to visit libraries. The literature suggests that nurses' perceptions of barriers to research use are consistent internationally.[12] As the nursing profession and information science have evolved, incorporating research knowledge as a component of evidence-based nursing has become more feasible.

A systematic review of individual determinants of research utilization by Estabrooks et al.[13] found a positive association between individual beliefs and increased research utilization and little evidence for other individual determinants of research use. Nurses who participated in research-related projects were more likely than other nurses to apply research in practice,[14] and intervention studies indicated that nurses engaged in research or educational activities used information resources, including computerized resources, when they had access to them and were supported.[15]

We are just beginning to understand how nurses actually access and apply information in practice. Studies based on observation or objective measures of information access (e.g. computer logs) provide more detailed evidence on how nurses actually use information and relate their decision-making behaviour to the clinical context.[16] These studies emphasize the complex environments in which nurses make clinical judgements, the multifaceted nature of the issues, and the time constraints under which decisions are made. Because of this complexity, human resources, rather than print or electronic resources, are preferred sources of information.[10, 16] For this reason, it is important to provide access to educators and experts who have responsibility for identifying and disseminating information on best practices. However, the ability of nurses to use research also depends on reference resources available in the workplace. Patient-specific data and reference sources are increasingly available in hospital information systems. A study evaluating a new hospital information system found that nurses used computerized information to answer questions related to nursing diagnoses, prepare care plans, learn about drugs and disease processes, obtain information for patients, validate knowledge, investigate new interests, and promote professional development.[17] Drug databases and nursing texts were used most frequently. Nurses accessed other information, including research material, when they were not making time-sensitive decisions affecting patient well-being (e.g. during quiet times on night shifts).[17]

The way in which nurses use the Internet (at home or at work) as a resource for answering clinical questions has not been well studied. With the wealth of health care information currently available, the ability to discern the quality of information is increasingly important. Knowledge of search techniques, such as those described in Chapters 4, 5 and 6, can help nurses locate the best evidence with minimum time and effort. Nurses also need the skills to integrate research findings with other evidence to support clinical judgement. Some nurses have learned critical appraisal skills during their nursing education, and dissemination of these skills to peers who have not had such training can facilitate decision-making in the nursing team. Journal clubs (where colleagues get together informally to critique and discuss research papers) are another useful strategy for facilitating research utilization.[18]

The organization

Organizational factors have the strongest influence over the extent to which nurses use research. Investigators have used a variety of organizational variables to study diffusion of information throughout organizations and identify barriers to research utilization.[18–20] Size and location of the organization and centralization of decision-making have been associated with research utilization, but conclusions about the importance of specific variables are inconsistent.[6] Nurses' use of print and electronic information varies among institutions depending on the availability of library and computer resources. Use of both print and electronic information is limited in smaller hospitals and primary care settings.[9, 20, 21] One study found that hospitals with more than 500 beds were more likely than those with ≤500 beds to have nursing research coordinators, access to nursing research experts and nursing faculty, nursing research committees, and libraries with nursing research journals; they were also more likely to implement research utilization programmes for staff nurses.[9]

The literature includes descriptions of interventions intended to improve research use by nurses in various health care settings, as well as general recommendations and models for applying research findings in clinical contexts.[18, 22, 23] Models have been developed to improve knowledge dissemination within hospitals and other health care institutions.[23–26] For example, Dobbins et al.[27] developed a model for changing practice in groups, units, wards or organizations, which comprised five stages: knowledge, persuasion, decision, implementation, and confirmation.[27] Chapter 27 provides a more in-depth discussion of models of implementation.

Research utilization is most successful when administrative support is available.[15, 28] Evidence-based practice has been realized most completely in institutions that have adopted it as policy and integrated it at all organizational levels.[22, 23] At the University of Iowa Hospitals, an infrastructure supporting research use encompassed both high-level management and frontline nurses.[23] Duties relating to research utilization were included in job descriptions, evidence-based practice was linked to quality assurance, and appropriate education was provided. Staff members who used research to solve clinical problems were recognized and rewarded. The Iowa model used triggers to alert nurses to clinical problems in the workplace and specified processes for solving them. Clinical nurses were allocated time and resources to be involved in all aspects of research. Because the organization placed a high priority on research utilization, nurses were motivated to become involved.[23]

Given the extent of health care information readily available in today's information-rich environment and its potential impact on patient care, institutions have a duty to ensure that their protocols and policies are current, and their staff are educated in the responsible use of information.

The environment: research quality and dissemination strategies

Barriers and facilitators to research use relate to the nature of research literature and the means by which it is disseminated. With the electronic revolution, access to research literature has become less of a barrier. However, use of research information by clinicians, including nurses, remains limited partly due to its theoretical nature. Research results are not directly translatable into clinical strategies. Ultimately, information systems may become sufficiently sophisticated such that all relevant information will be linked electronically to patients' medical records. However, modern systems fall short of this ideal, and locating appropriate information remains a challenge.

Given the limitations of current information systems, it is important that nurses and organizations find strategies to mitigate these shortcomings. Research about medical education suggests that evidence-based practice skills are best acquired in clinical environments.[29] Continuing education can increase nurses' skills in identifying, appraising, and applying research information. Peer mentoring and coaching are also effective strategies for helping colleagues to search for, evaluate and apply information.[15]

Limited research is available about how nurses actually evaluate research for use in practice settings. A study by French[30] identified three sets of evaluative criteria: research information, the task to which the research refers, and the fit of the task within the nursing context. Nurses evaluated research in terms of relevance and quality, and applied the criteria of effectiveness and practicality (including impact, effort and consequences for staff) when assessing the task. Evaluation of research in relation to the nursing context included consideration of nursing control, feedback from practice, feasibility, and conformity with the status quo. The study results reflected the organizational and political contexts in which the nurses practised. They show that attempts to influence research uptake must consider how research is perceived and evaluated by practitioners and how it serves their purposes.

The development of tools for evidence-based nursing requires time and resources and is dependent on collaboration among health care organizations and academic institutions. As communication among the global health care community improves, pooling of expertise on national and international levels becomes increasingly feasible. Centres for evidence-based nursing have been established in several countries, and plans are under way to create an international centre with links to centres worldwide.[31] These centres will provide access to critically appraised materials for nurses and organizations.

Summary

Reports on programmes aimed at promoting research utilization suggest possible strategies to overcome various barriers to research use.[23] In the future, information systems will integrate clinical data about patient treatments and preferences, available resources, expert opinion, and research evidence to provide nurses with current, patient-specific information to address complex clinical issues. Nurses will be able to plan treatment with knowledgeable patients who will also have access to health-related resources. Improved organizational and environmental support will be critical for nurses as they work with increasingly sophisticated information systems.

LEARNING EXERCISES

1. Select a clinical practice in your setting that you believe could be improved. Assume that you have relevant research evidence/guidelines to support this change.
   (a) What would facilitate the implementation of this change in your practice setting?
   (b) What would pose challenges to implementing the change in your practice setting?
   In answering each of these questions, consider how individual nurses, the organization, and the environment would be implicated in making the change.
2. Select the three greatest challenges to the proposed change in practice identified in question 1. Provide a rationale for your selection, and suggest strategies for addressing these barriers.
3. Make an inventory of the information resources available to nurses in your practice setting. What changes or additions could be made to this inventory to improve access to evidence to enhance your practice?

References

1 Naisbitt J. *Megatrends: Ten New Directions Transforming Our Lives*. New York: Warner Books, 1982.

2 Mowry MM, Korpman RA. Evaluating automated information systems. *Nurs Econ* 1987;5:7–12.

3 DiCenso A, Cullum N, Ciliska D. Implementing evidence-based nursing: some misconceptions. *Evidence-Based Nursing* 1998;1:38–9.

4 Funk SG, Champagne MT, Weise RA, Tornquist EM. Barriers to using research findings in practice: the clinician's perspective. *Appl Nurs Res* 1991;4:90–5.

5 Funk SG, Champagne MT, Wiese R, Tornquist EM. BARRIERS: the barriers to research utilization scale. *Appl Nurs Res* 1991;4:39–45.

6 Funk SG, Tornquist EM, Champagne MT. Barriers and facilitators of research utilization. An integrative review. *Nurs Clin North Am* 1995;30:395–407.

7 Dobbins M, Ciliska D, DiCenso A. Dissemination and use of research evidence for policy and practice: a framework for developing, implementing, and evaluating strategies. A report prepared for the Dissemination and Utilization Model Advisory Committee of the Canadian Nurses Association and Health Canada, 1998.

8 Thomson MA. Closing the gap between nursing research and practice. *Evidence-Based Nursing* 1998;1:7–8.

9 Mitchell A, Janzen K, Pask E, Southwell D. Assessment of nursing research utilization needs in Ontario health agencies. *Can J Nurs Adm* 1995;8:77–91.

10 Blythe J, Royle JA. Assessing nurses' information needs in the work environment. *Bull Med Libr Assoc* 1993;81:433–5.

11 Stephens LC, Selig CL, Jones LC, Gaston-Johansson F. Research application: teaching staff nurses to use library search strategies. *J Contin Educ Nurs* 1992;23:24–8.

12 Hutchinson AM, Johnson L. Bridging the divide: a survey of nurses' opinions regarding barriers to, and facilitators of, research utilization in the practice setting. *J Clin Nurs* 2004;13:304–15.

13 Estabrooks CA, Floyd JA, Scott-Findlay S, O'Leary KA, Gushta M. Individual determinants of research utilization: a systematic review. *J Adv Nurs* 2003;43:506–20.

14 Bostrom J, Suter WN. Research utilization: making the link to practice. *J Nurs Staff Dev* 1993;9:28–34.

15 Royle JA, Blythe J, Boblin-Cummings SL, Deber R, DiCenso A, Hayward RSA, Wright J, Bernsley J, Bayley L, Gill-Morton P, Smith SD. Nursing for the twenty-first century: using information technology to enhance nursing practice. Hamilton, Ontario: McMaster University, 1997.

16 Thompson C, Cullum N, McCaughan D, Sheldon T, Raynor P. Nurses, information use, and clinical decision making – the real world potential for evidence-based decisions in nursing. *Evidence-Based Nursing* 2004;7:68–72.

17 Royle JA, Blythe J, Potvin C, Oolup P, Chan IM. Literature search and retrieval in the workplace. *Comput Nurs* 1995;13:25–31.

18 Fink R, Thompson CJ, Bonnes D. Overcoming barriers and promoting the use of research in practice. *J Nurs Admin* 2005;35:121–9.

19 Brett JL. Organizational integrative mechanisms and adoption of innovations by nurses. *Nurs Res* 1989;38:105–10.

20 Champion VL, Leach A. Variables related to research utilization in nursing: an empirical investigation. *J Adv Nurs* 1989;14:705–10.

21 Royle JA, Blythe J, DiCenso A, Baumann A, Fitzgerald D. Do nurses have the information resources and skills for research utilization? *Can J Nurs Adm* 1997;10:9–30.

22 Goode CJ, Lovett MK, Hayes JE, Butcher LA. Use of research-based knowledge in clinical practice. *J Nurs Adm* 1987;17:11–18.

23 Stetler CB. Updating the Stetler model of research utilization to facilitate evidence-based practice. *Nurs Outlook* 2001;49:272–9.

24 MacGuire JM. Putting nursing research findings into practice: research utilization as an aspect of the management of change. *J Adv Nurs* 1990;15:614–20.

25 Titler MG, Kleiber C, Steelman V, Goode C, Rakel B, Barry-Walker J, Small S, Buckwalter K. Infusing research into practice to promote quality care. *Nurs Res* 1994;43:307–13.

26 Rycroft-Malone J, Kitson A, Harvey G, McCormack B, Seers K, Titchen A, Estabrooks C. Ingredients for change: revisiting a conceptual framework. *Qual Saf Health Care* 2002;11:174–80.

27 Dobbins M, Ciliska D, Estabrooks C, and Hayward S. Changing nursing practice in an organization. In: DiCenso A, Guyatt G, Ciliska D. *Evidence-Based Nursing: A Guide to Clinical Practice.* St Louis: Elsevier Mosby, 2005:172–200.

28 Logan J, Davies B. The staff nurse as research facilitator. *Can J Nurs Adm* 1995;8:92–110.

29 Coomarasamy A, Khan KS. What is the evidence that postgraduate teaching in evidence based medicine changes anything? A systematic review. *BMJ* 2004;329(7473):1017.

30 French B. Evaluating research for use in practice: What criteria do specialist nurses use? *J Adv Nurs* 2005;50:235–43.

31 Ciliska D, DiCenso A, Cullum N. Centres of evidence based nursing: directions and challenges. *Evid Based Nurs* 1999;2:102–104.

Chapter 30

NURSES, INFORMATION USE, AND CLINICAL DECISION-MAKING: THE REAL-WORLD POTENTIAL FOR EVIDENCE-BASED DECISIONS IN NURSING

Carl Thompson, Nicky Cullum, Dorothy McCaughan, Trevor A. Sheldon and Pauline Raynor

Nurses have probably always known that their decisions have important implications for patient outcomes. Increasingly, however, they are being cast in the role of active decision-makers in health care by policy makers and other members of the health care team. In 2002, for example, the UK Chief Nursing Officer outlined 10 key tasks for nurses as part of the National Health Service's modernization agenda and the breaking down of artificial boundaries between medicine and nursing.[1] The UK Department of Health has also declared that nurses are expected to access, appraise and incorporate research evidence into their professional judgement and clinical decision-making.[2] This active engagement with research evidence is the focus of this chapter. We will explore why it is necessary to consider the clinical decision-making context when examining the ways in which nurses engage with research-based information. We will also consider the relation between the accessibility and usefulness of information from different sources and the decisions to which such information is applied. Finally, we will argue that, if we are to encourage nurses to actively engage with research evidence during clinical decision-making, we need to better understand the relation between the decisions that nurses make and the knowledge that informs them.

Methods underpinning this chapter

In this chapter, we draw heavily on the findings of two major studies conducted at the University of York between 1997 and 2002.[3–9] Two case studies (one of acute care nurses and one of primary care and community nurses) were conducted in three geographical areas with different hospital types, population characteristics, and levels of health service provision. We purposively sampled participants according to a sampling frame constructed around variables deemed to be theoretically significant for clinical decision-making.[7] Data collection comprised 200 in-depth interviews with nurses and managers; 400 hours of non-participant observation of 'decision making and information use in action'; 4000 practice-based documents audited for characteristics such as age, research basis, authorship, etc; and statistically modelled (using the Q methodology approach[10]) perspectives on the accessibility, usefulness, and barriers to use of information sources from 242 nurses.

Evidence-based decision-making involves actively using information

Evidence-based decision-making involves combining the knowledge arising from one's clinical expertise, patient preferences, and research evidence within the context of available resources.[11] Evidence-based decision-making – like all decision-making – involves choosing from a discrete range of options, which may include doing nothing or a 'wait and see' strategy. All such choices are informed by an evaluation of available information: the process of using clinical judgement. In making evidence-based decisions, research evidence should not be taken at face value and adhered to uncritically, but should be given an appropriate weight in a decision depending on its internal and external validity. Integrating research evidence into decision-making involves forming a focused clinical question in response to a recognized information need, searching for the most appropriate evidence to meet that need, critically appraising the retrieved evidence, incorporating the evidence into a strategy for action, and evaluating the effects of any decisions and actions taken. These steps are important components of the active process that is evidence-based decision-making.

Evidence-based decision-making is a prescriptive approach to making choices, which is based on ideas of how theory can be used to improve real-world decision-making. However, before we plan a strategy to attain this ideal, it is important to identify our starting point: how do nurses currently use (and view) research-based information in decision-making? Surprisingly, little research has been done on this topic, except for studies that use self-report data from nurses as a source of evidence. We rejected self-report as the main source of evidence for answering our questions in favour of 'real-time' clinical observation and in-depth interviews, which we feel better reflect actual types and frequencies of different decisions and observed information use.

Information need, 'information behaviour' and clinical decision-making

One of the challenges of researching how people respond to information deficits is that such deficits, or information needs, are unobservable. 'Information need' is a construct that exists only in the mind of the person 'in need'.[12] Researchers can only hypothesize about the likely needs of nurses based on what they say, what we can deduce from watching their behaviour, or preferably both. 'Need' cannot be separated from the motives of information-seeking behaviour. If an information need is to be converted into action (e.g. reading *Evidence-Based Nursing* or accessing the *Cochrane Library*), then individuals must have a motive for doing so. In developing motives, individuals draw on personal frameworks of beliefs and values, which contain objects that have satisfied information needs in the past. Some objects (e.g.

MEDLINE) may be valued less than others (e.g. knowledgeable colleagues) because they previously failed to satisfy information needs.[12]

For proponents of evidence-based decision-making, the primary motive for engaging with research-based information is to reduce clinical uncertainty; that is, finding relevant research will increase one's certainty that a particular course of action is most likely to lead to the desired outcomes.[13] However, new information can also elucidate and/or confirm existing information, beliefs and values. Nurses often report that their rationale for seeking research evidence is to support their existing practice. The processes of searching for, appraising and integrating research information with existing knowledge have been labelled *information behaviour* by some researchers in the field of information science.[14]

The types of clinical decisions that nurses actually make provide clues about how (and what types of) research information might assist in decision-making. Other authors have examined the clinical decisions of health care professionals (and the clinical questions arising from such decisions) as expressions of potential information need.[15] Thus, decisions are an important context for information use. We will show how understanding the structure and characteristics of the decisions nurses face is important for understanding the ways in which information is accessed and processed by nurses.

Nurses' clinical decisions: a typology

Table 30.1 provides a typology of clinical decisions, with examples that were derived from interviews with, and observation of, acute and primary care nurses.[3–9] These decisions represent core choices that are only part of the architecture of the decision-making context for applying research knowledge. Nurses described several other elements of their clinical decisions and decision-making processes.

Frequency of decision-making

The number and types of decisions faced by nurses are related to the work environment, perceptions of their clinical role, operational autonomy, and the degree to which they see themselves as active and influential decision-makers. Nurses working on a busy medical admissions unit admitting 50 patients per day face a different set of decision challenges from those facing health visitors (HVs) or public health nurses, who may see 10 people per day. Consider the extent to which judgement and choices feature in this HV's consultation:

> She was breast-feeding but had a very sore cracked and bleeding nipple on her left breast and she did not know what to do about it. [What did the HV think?, the mother asked.] The HV thought and replied that she had not come across this problem before, but asked if it was painful. Mum said that it was and she had tried to feed her from this breast but it was so painful that she had not done so. She had only fed from the right breast and for the past three evenings the baby had fed continuously for six hours and then slept all night. Someone had suggested using Camillosan cream for her cracked nipple but it had not helped at all. However, she knew that chamomile was a relaxant and maybe that was why the baby had slept for so long the last three nights. The HV mentioned a nipple shield but said that she had no experience of using them. The mum said that she wondered if she should just stop feeding from that breast altogether until it had healed, to which the HV agreed.

Table 30.1 Decision types and clinical questions/choices expressed by acute and primary care nurses

Decision type	Example of clinical questions/choices
Intervention/effectiveness: decisions that involve choosing between interventions	Choosing a mattress for a frail elderly man who has been admitted with an acute bowel obstruction
1. Targeting: a subcategory of intervention/effectiveness decisions outlined above, of the form 'choosing which patient will benefit most from the intervention'	Deciding which patients should get antiembolic stockings
2. Prevention: deciding which intervention is most likely to prevent occurrence of a particular health state or outcome	Choosing which management strategy is most likely to prevent recurrence of a healed leg ulcer
3. Timing: choosing the best time to deploy the intervention	Choosing a time to begin asthma education for newly diagnosed patients with asthma.
4. Referral: choosing to whom a patient's diagnosis or management should be referred	Choosing that a patient's leg ulcer is arterial rather than venous and merits medical rather than nursing management in the community
Communication: choosing ways of delivering information to and receiving information from patients, families or colleagues. Sometimes these decisions are specifically related to the communication of risks and benefits of different interventions or prognostic categories	Choosing how to approach cardiac rehabilitation with an elderly patient who has had an acute myocardial infarction and lives alone, with her family nearby
Service organization, delivery, and management: these types of decisions concern the configuration or processes of service delivery	Choosing how to organize shift handover so that communication is most effective
Assessment: deciding that an assessment is required and/or what mode of assessment to use	Deciding to use the Edinburgh Postnatal Depression screening tool
Diagnosis: classifying signs and symptoms as a basis for a management or treatment strategy	Deciding whether thrush or another cause is the reason for a woman's sore and cracked nipples
Information seeking: the choice to seek (or not to seek) further information before making a further clinical decision	Deciding that a guideline for monitoring patients who have had their ACE inhibitor dosage adjusted may be of use, but choosing not to use it before asking a colleague
Experiential, understanding, or hermeneutic: relates to the interpretation of cues in the process of care	Choosing how to reassure a patient who is worried about cardiac arrest after witnessing another patient arresting

The HV then said that if she was having pain in her breast, that could indicate that she had a thrush infection on her breast. She then asked if she had seen any white patches on the baby's tongue or in her mouth and mum replied that she had not. No more was said about that. They agreed that mum would not feed from her left breast and only use her right until it healed up. The HV said that as the baby was feeding well from her right breast then that was OK. (Field notes, health visitor)

This quote illustrates at least five judgement or decision challenges for the HV, all of which generate potential information needs: (1) ascertain the likely causes of sore and cracked nipples; (2) choose a management strategy in the context of little or no experiential knowledge; (3) judge whether the baby is getting sufficient breast milk; (4) choose between the merits of Camillosan, chamomile, or a nipple shield; and (5) identify the cause of pain (possibly thrush).

Decisional complexity

Three elements of decisional complexity that permeated nurses' accounts of their decisions are described below.

Time-limited decision-making activity
Nurses described situations in which rapid decisions were expected (a phenomenon known as *implied response time*).[16] Consequently, opportunities for seeking information beyond what was readily available were perceived as severely restricted. Limited time was a primary reason for the 'separation' of day-to-day decision-making from information seeking and appraisal. Despite these constraints on information use, some nurses felt that, as their expertise developed, they managed to reduce contact time with patients by virtue of having to spend less time seeking information to reduce uncertainty in decision-making. Decision-related information seeking was associated with novice rather than expert performance.

Multiple and diverse decision goals
The stepwise nature of information gathering and decision-making in patient encounters, as well as the need to foster patient perceptions of trust and credibility in the nurse, meant that decisions often had multiple and conflicting decision goals. For example, one HV described the need to build confidence in a young mother, leading her to sanction weaning at 12 weeks rather than (for her) the more optimal 16 weeks (note, current best evidence suggests that the optimum time for weaning is 6 months).[17]

Conflicting decision elements
As well as making decisions more complex, conflict can also simplify decisions. The following example of conflict in nurse–doctor power relations demonstrates this point:

When S came back she cleaned the patient's left leg with gauze soaked in saline and then applied a dressing (Jelonet). She said that she felt Jelonet was not ideal but the patient's consultant preferred it despite the fact that 'when you take it off you are removing the good tissue as well. Even if I change the dressing, when the patient goes to the outpatients' department and sees the consultant they will come back with Jelonet and clear instructions that we are to use Jelonet.' (Field notes, district nurse)

The cognitive continuum: the decision as driver for information behaviour

Since the 1960s, cognitive psychologists and decision theorists have developed the idea of the cognitive continuum[16, 18, 19] This model suggests that the major determinants of whether a person engages in *intuitive decision-making* (i.e. less likely to engage in evidence-based decision-making) or *rational decision-making* (i.e. more likely to engage in evidence-based decision-making) relate to the point at which a decision task, such as selecting a nursing intervention, lies on a (cognitive) continuum (Figure 30.1). This cognitive continuum has three dimensions,[16] which are described below.

1. Complexity of the task: the number of information cues (the more cues required for a decision, the more likely it is that nurses will fall back on intuitive reasoning); the number of judgement steps required to make a choice (e.g. selecting interventions for patients with chronic and comorbid conditions and a lack of complete information readily available).
2. Ambiguity of the task: the task characteristics that induce rational information processing include the presence of easily available organizing principles for collecting and handling information and simplifying decisions (known as

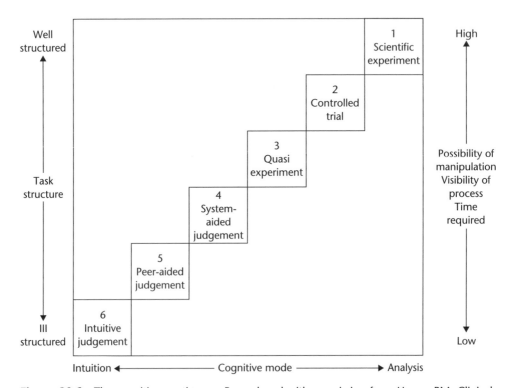

Figure 30.1 The cognitive continuum. Reproduced with permission from Hamm RM. Clinical intuition and clinical analysis: expertise and the cognitive continuum. In Dowie J, Elstein A, editors. *Professional Judgement: A Reader in Clinical Decision Making.* Cambridge: Cambridge University Press, 1988:87.

feedforward);[20] a familiar decision task with familiar content; the presence of an observable outcome for the task; and a degree of feedback on the likely success of the task. An example of a task that is more likely to induce rational processing (and draw on knowledge derived from research) is the assessment and treatment of people with chronic venous leg ulcers. Nurses assessing and treating people with leg ulcers identified the helpful role of the UK Royal College of Nursing Guidelines[21] in collecting the information required for a good assessment and decision, and the design of training, audit and feedback around the guidelines and decision-making in leg ulcer care.

3. Form of task presentation: very short time frames for exercising judgement are more likely to induce intuitive information handling. Alternatively, breaking the task down into components (*decomposition*) induces rationality in handling clinical information, as do information cues that are dichotomous or discrete (e.g. 'This Doppler reading indicates either venous or arterial aetiology'); similarly, the greater the need to make a decision visible to others, the greater the use of analytic reasoning.

The relative balance in the mixture of intuition-inducing and rationality-inducing task elements predicts the end of the continuum to which cognition is drawn. Correctly 'matching' information and the ways that it is processed (i.e. using more systematic, rational methods rather than intuition) to the nature of decision tasks results in better decision performance.[18]

Knowledge of a decision task alone, however, is not a sufficient basis for predicting whether a person will use analytic or intuitive reasoning, or indeed, whether they will even gather the information necessary to engage in analytic reasoning. Consider, for example, a primary care nurse who ignores the physical presence of a guideline during a consultation in favour of the more easily accessed (cognitively) knowledge of one's own memory and the advice of a colleague.

The reality of information behaviour

Two broad patterns of engagement among nurses, research-based information, and clinical decision and judgement tasks, were present in the studies.

Preference for humans as information sources

Both primary and acute care nurses were characterized by reliance on human sources of information as the primary means of informing situations in which they were uncertain.[5] We identified seven distinct perspectives on accessibility, all of which stress the relative accessibility of experiential sources of information, such as clinical nurse specialists, experienced colleagues, and other primary and secondary care team colleagues. Notable exceptions were local protocols and guidelines in acute care (particularly in areas such as coronary care) and sources of drug-related information, such as the British National Formulary (the national drug formulary from which doctors, nurses and dentists can prescribe), drug information sheets, and pharmacists in primary care. Even when textual information was seen as accessible, human sources of information were highly rated in terms of their accessibility. We also found that simple demographic or biographical variables, such as clinical experience, educational attainment, or role in the primary care team, were weak predictors of perspectives of accessible information sources.

The scale of the relative lack of engagement with information sources can be gleaned from our observational data. During 90 hours of observing community nurses in practice, we found that use of an information source while actually making a decision in the presence of a patient occurred only once, in the form of a telephone call to another clinician. Similarly, in acute care, 180 hours of observation (c.1080 decisions) revealed only two forms of text-based information used 'in action': local protocols or guidelines (used four times) and the British National Formulary (used 50 times).

It would be wrong to infer, however, that research-based knowledge has no part in nurses' decision-making. Rather, nurses chose not to use the systematic search–appraise–implement cycle of evidence-based decision making in real time for real clinical decisions with rapid implied response times. Nurses accessed 'evidence-based' information sources – if they accessed them at all – in contexts other than immediate decision-making environments. Nurses described contact with research-based information sources in the context of continuing professional development and formal education or training. Other influences included being involved in the production of local protocols and guidelines and having to make sense of research such as clinical trials, or using research evidence to help resolve conflict between colleagues. Perceptions about the relative accessibility of human sources of information were mirrored when we asked nurses about the usefulness of different sources of information for clinical decision-making.

Useful information sources are grounded in clinical reality

As with accessibility, we identified several important perspectives on the relative usefulness of different sources of information for clinical decision-making. Each of these perspectives stressed the usefulness of sources that were based on experience rather than research. Colleagues, other members of the primary care team, or senior members of the clinical team were viewed as the most useful (and accessible) information sources. In acute care, the most useful source of information across all perspectives was the clinical nurse specialist, who seemed to embody the characteristics of useful information sources: directly answered the question posed; was seen to be authoritative and trustworthy; provided (or could potentially provide) a balance of 'background'[13] (factual) knowledge as well as foreground (management) knowledge; provided supportive and unchallenging information; and had no or minimal associated need for critical appraisal.

Given these characteristics, it is easy to understand the appeal of clinical nurse specialists (or other experience-rich sources) as a source of information. A community nurse described a link nurse colleague (a nurse who is responsible for a particular area of knowledge and practice, such as diabetes or wound care, and is often linked to the work of a clinical nurse specialist):

> They [link nurses] are specialists in the area that they cover, what's the point of reinventing the wheel? Me going to the library getting all the information and thinking, 'Oh I've done a good job there.' I can go to them and they've already got it . . . But it also gives you back-up in areas where I'm not a specialist . . . It's not just a short cut, it's that they're knowledgeable. They have the information there.   (Community nurse)

As with perceptions of accessibility, we found that demographic and biographic variables, such as age, clinical experience, and levels of educational attainment, were poor predictors of how useful an information source would be to a nurse.

Decision-making and models for the implementation of research knowledge

Many theoretical models of research utilization implicitly recognize the importance of decision-making as a vital step in the process of converting knowledge into action. Despite this implicit recognition, most models fail to account for the relation between decision characteristics, information use and information processing. For example, Lomas[22, 23] has proposed a coordinated model of research implementation, in which one endpoint of knowledge diffusion is negotiating the application of research findings with patients during the course of clinical practice. In other work, Lomas[23] also calls for researchers and decision-makers to have increased levels of understanding of each other's worlds if research and policy (or practice) are to be better linked. We would argue that, although clinicians are making efforts to understand research (through initiatives such as critical appraisal training or by reading journals such as *Evidence-Based Nursing*), researchers and disseminators often fail to fully understand the decisions to which their products are being applied. In relation to organizational policy decisions, Lomas[23] suggests that researchers should endeavour to understand the institutional structures for decision-making, the values (expressed as ideologies, beliefs, and interests), and the fact that multiple producers of evidence (i.e. information that actually gets used for decision-making) often exist within organizations.[23] Other theorists who have attempted to build 'context' into models of research utilization also neglect the 'micro' context of the actual decisions: their type, the time available, their perceived complexity, the amount of supporting (or challenging) information available, and the presence (or absence) of organizing principles for this information.[24]

Some researchers have used clinical questions generated by clinical decisions as expressions of (potential) information need[6, 15, 25]. We would argue that researchers need to delve deeper and begin to develop research exploring the relation between the information needs such questions represent and information behaviour by nurses. Moreover, we need to recognize that simply mapping the core choice at the heart of a decision (such as whether it arises from uncertainty about a diagnosis, treatment, or prognosis) is a necessary but insufficient condition for determining whether information is deemed relevant or rejected as irrelevant.

Thus far, we have focused on the links between information behaviour and clinical decision-making from a researcher's perspective. It is important to recognize that the strategies available to clinical decision-makers can also alter their relation to information. Using the principles of the cognitive continuum, it is possible to simplify decisions by removing some of their complexity in an effort to induce individuals to apply 'search and appraisal' behaviour. For example, several nurses recounted the usefulness of a structured approach to gathering information as a means of simply gathering the 'important' facts when faced with the complex judgement task of assessing a patient's chronic leg ulcer for venous or arterial aetiology. This structured bundle of facts (e.g. Doppler reading, ulcer area, and clinical history) formed the basis of management decisions that were sometimes informed by appropriate national evidence-based guidelines (albeit often internalized). Similarly, the single aspect of decision-making in which observable text-based information use was (relatively) common was uncertainty about medication use. Nurses' accounts clearly showed that the sources of information used fit the questions that arose from their decisions – decisions that were often focused and well structured (e.g. should I give this patient drug X or drug Y to achieve outcome Z?).

This simplification induces shifts towards the rational end of the continuum. From this perspective, it is easy to imagine how thinking about nurses' clinical decisions might have an impact on their information behaviour. Indeed, some basic elements of the evidence-based nursing process could serve to simplify decisions. Specifically, the development of focused clinical questions can be conceptualized as a mechanism for removing some of the 'noise' that surrounds choices and helping to focus attention on the relevant populations, outcomes and interventions, and on the core type of uncertainty (diagnostic, intervention, or prognostic). Croskerry[26] proposes other, slightly more sophisticated, techniques under the banner of *cognitive forcing*. These techniques involve retraining clinicians to think differently about problems by accounting for the effects of limited memory, erroneous perspectives (e.g. ignoring base rates of disease when making diagnoses), limited capacity for self-critique, and poor selection of strategies. The end result is a heightened sense of meta-cognition or 'thinking about thinking'. Research examining the potential of these types of approaches to reflection on action is missing in nursing.

Summary

Nurses are increasingly regarded as key decision-makers within the health care team. They are also expected to use the best available evidence in their judgements and decisions. The prescriptive model of evidence-based decision-making – and the search–appraise–implement process that accompanies it – is an active process. Clinicians who want to implement research in clinical settings sometimes forget that active information seeking is only one of several possible responses to the irreducible uncertainties of clinical practice. In fact, observation of nurses in practice suggests that when 'search and appraise' information behaviour occurs at all, nurses are far more likely to view colleagues (human sources of information) as useful and accessible sources of information than research in any form. Colleagues are perceived as delivering context-specific, clinically relevant information that takes into account the needs of the judgement or decision situation and requires minimal critical appraisal; and they are time efficient. We would argue that this implies a degree of 'fit' between the decision task and the information provided, although not necessarily the provision of high-quality (i.e. reliable or valid) information. Moreover, long-standing theoretical frameworks explain this lack of fit between traditional evidence-based sources of research information and the decisions that nurses encounter.

The cognitive continuum model offers a theoretical basis for a research agenda that is just emerging in nursing. Outlining the types of clinical decisions is only a starting point for this agenda. Future work should attempt to explore and explain the patterns of information use in decisions for which far more detailed maps exist. Moreover, there is a need for high-quality development and evaluation of interventions that target evidence-based information provision at those individuals most likely to influence professional choices (e.g. clinical nurse specialists). We feel that such knowledge will add a valuable, and hitherto missing, dimension to existing models of research utilization and knowledge transfer.

LEARNING EXERCISES

Exercise 1: some discussion/reflection questions

Think about the types of decisions you make in clinical practice. Write them down in order of frequency and then complexity.

1. What makes some decisions simple and others complex? You might like to look at Wilson T, Holt T, Greenhalgh T. Complexity science: complexity and clinical care. *BMJ* 2001;**323**:685–8 (available at www.bmj.com).
2. Does having research evidence available help simplify decisions or make them more complex? If so, what can you do about this?
3. Does the frequency with which you encounter decision challenges make a difference to the evidence you draw on to help when you are uncertain?

Exercise 2: clinical uncertainty and questions

1. Buy a notebook!
2. For the next month write down a key decision for which you were uncertain of the 'correct' choice for each patient you hand over to another nurse or professional.
3. Express each decision as a structured clinical question (see Chapter 3 on PICO).
4. At the end of the month, examine the questions. Do similar questions arise on more than one occasion?
5. Could you use this technique for training, helping target EBN activity, and reflecting on your own decisions and information behaviour, and if so how?

References

1 Chief Nursing Officer. *Developing Key Roles for Nurses and Midwives – A Guide for Managers.* London: Department of Health, 2002.
2 Department of Health. *Making a Difference: Strengthening the Nursing, Midwifery and Health Visiting Contribution to Health and Healthcare.* London: HMSO, 1999.
3 McCaughan D. What decisions do nurses make? In Thompson C, Dowding D, editors. *Clinical Decision Making and Judgement in Nursing.* Edinburgh: Churchill Livingstone, 2001:95–108.
4 McCaughan D, Thompson C, Cullum N, Sheldon TA, Thompson DR. Acute care nurses' perceptions of barriers to using research information in clinical decision-making. *J Adv Nurs* 2002;**39**:46–60.
5 Thompson C, McCaughan D, Cullum N, Sheldon TA, Mulhall A, Thompson DR. The accessibility of research-based knowledge for nurses in United Kingdom acute care settings. *J Adv Nurs* 2001;**36**:11–22.
6 Thompson C, McCaughan D, Cullum N, Sheldon TA, Mulhall A, Thompson DR. Research information in nurses' clinical decision-making: what is useful? *J Adv Nurs* 2001;**36**:376–88.
7 Thompson C. Qualitative research into nurse decision making: factors for consideration in theoretical sampling. *Qual Health Res* 1999;**9**:815–28.
8 Thompson C. Clinical experience as evidence in evidence-based practice. *J Adv Nurs* 2003;**43**:230–7.
9 Thompson C, McCaughan D, Cullum N, Sheldon TA, Raynor P. Increasing the visibility of coding decisions in team-based qualitative research in nursing. *Int J Nurs Stud* 2004;**41**:15–20.

10 Brown SR. A primer on Q methodology. *Operant Subjectivity* 1993;**16**:91–138.

11 DiCenso A, Cullum N, Ciliska D. Implementing evidence-based nursing: some misconceptions. *Evidence-Based Nursing* 1998;**1**:38–40.

12 Wilson T, Walsh C. *Information Behaviour: An Inter-disciplinary Perspective.* British Library Research and Innovation Report 10. London: British Library Research and Innovation Centre, 1996. http://informationr.net/tdw/publ/infbehav/cont.html (accessed 29 June 2006).

13 Sackett DL, Straus SE, Richardson WS, Rosenberg W, Haynes RB. *Evidence Based Medicine: How to Practice and Teach EBM.* Second edition. London: Churchill Livingstone, 2000.

14 Case DO. *Looking for Information: A Survey of Research on Information Seeking, Needs, and Behaviour.* London: Academic Press, 2002.

15 Cogdill KW. Information needs and information seeking in primary care: a study of nurse practitioners. *J Med Libr Assoc* 2003;**91**:203–15.

16 Hamm RM. Clinical intuition and clinical analysis: expertise and the cognitive continuum. In Dowie J, Elstein A, editors. *Professional Judgement: A Reader in Clinical Decision Making.* Cambridge: Cambridge University Press, 1988:78–105.

17 Pan American Health Organization and World Health Organization. *Guiding Principles for Complementary Feeding of the Breastfed Child.* Washington: PAHO/WHO, 2001. http://www.who.int/child-adolescent-health/New_Publications/NUTRITION/guiding_principles.pdf (accessed 20 June 2006).

18 Hammond KR, Hamm RM, Grassia J, Pearson T. Direct comparison of analytical and intuitive cognition in expert judgment. *IEEE Transactions on Systems, Man, and Cybernetics* 1987;**17**:753–70.

19 Thompson C. A conceptual treadmill: the need for 'middle ground' in clinical decision making theory in nursing. *J Adv Nurs* 1999;**30**:1222–9.

20 Cooksey RW. *Judgment Analysis: Theory, Methods, and Applications.* New York: Academic Press, 1996.

21 Royal College of Nursing. *Clinical practice guideline: the management of patients with venous leg ulcers.* RCN Institute, Centre for Evidence-Based Nursing, University of York and the School of Nursing, Midwifery and Health Visiting, University of Manchester. 1998, updated 2006. http://www.rcn.org.uk/publications/pdf/guidelines/venous_leg_ulcers.pdf

22 Lomas J, Haynes RB. A taxonomy and critical review of tested strategies for the application of clinical practice recommendations: from "official" to "individual" clinical policy. *Am J Prev Med* 1988;**4**(4 Suppl):77–94.

23 Lomas J. Connecting research and policy. *ISUMA* 2000;**1**:140–4. http://www.isuma.net/v01n01/lomas/lomas_e.shtml (accessed 29 June 2006).

24 Rycroft-Malone J, Kitson A, Harvey G, McCormack B, Seers K, Tichen A, Estabrooks C. Ingredients for change: revisiting a conceptual framework. *Qual Saf Health Care* 2002;**11**:174–80.

25 Ely JW, Osheroff JA, Ebell MH, Chambliss ML, Vinson DC, Stevermer JJ, Pifer EA. Obstacles to answering doctors' questions about patient care with evidence: qualitative study. *BMJ* 2002;**324**:710.

26 Croskerry P. Cognitive forcing strategies in clinical decision making. *Ann Emerg Med* 2003;**41**:110–20.

Chapter 31

COMPUTERIZED DECISION SUPPORT SYSTEMS IN NURSING

Dawn Dowding

Decision support systems integrate evidence (ideally from high-quality research) with the characteristics of individual patients, in order to provide nurses with advice during decision-making. When viewed this way, decision support systems, in general, may help nurses to make more evidence-based decisions. Decision support systems can provide information and advice in a variety of formats, including paper-based guidance and computerized systems. *Computerized decision support systems* (CDSSs) are examples of evidence-based clinical information systems, the apex of the 4S pyramid classification of evidence from research as discussed in Chapter 4. CDSSs match information about individual patients to a computerized knowledge base, using separate software algorithms to generate patient-specific recommendations.[1] CDSSs differ from other computerized clinical information systems, such as electronic patient records, in several ways. In particular, CDSSs use information about an individual patient to provide specific advice to a clinician about what to do *for that specific patient* (having integrated this information with a large, and hopefully evidence-based, knowledge database). By contrast, systems such as *electronic patient records* enable clinicians to consult the clinical information for an individual patient but provide little or no guidance on how to use that information to make a decision. Benefits of CDSSs, compared with paper-based approaches, include the large amounts of information that can be stored and processed efficiently and the capacity to readily update the evidence base. Some research has also suggested that computerized forms of decision support are more likely to improve clinical practice.[2]

Types of decisions suitable for the use of CDSSs

In Chapter 30, we described how nurses make different types of decisions in practice. Table 31.1 presents a typology of nursing decisions, with examples of relevant CDSSs identified in systematic reviews by Garg *et al.*[1] and Randell *et al.*[3] This table highlights that not all types of decisions made by nurses (or other clinicians) are currently supported by CDSSs. This could be because the types of decisions are not suitable for decision support or because systems have not yet been developed to help nurses make decisions in these areas.

Table 31.1 Types of nursing decisions matched to computerized decision support systems

Type of decision	Type of decision support system
Intervention/effectiveness	Computer-assisted anticoagulant dosing[1, 3]
	Computer-assisted drug dosing and prescribing[1]
• Targeting • Prevention • Timing • Referral	Reminder systems[1]
Communication	
Service organization, delivery, management	Computer-assisted disease management[1]
Assessment	Telephone triage systems[3]
Diagnosis	Computer-assisted diagnosis[1]
Information seeking	
Experiential, understanding or hermeneutic	

Decisions that require clinicians to undertake multifaceted tasks that integrate complex information, often of different types, and require several steps to process the information are most likely to be amenable to using decision support. Furthermore, the context in which the decision must be made should allow time for a system to be used. The framework of the cognitive continuum (Chapter 30) provides a valuable guide to situations where decision support may be useful. Decisions such as diagnosis, assessment and disease management require clinicians to consider many different types of information (e.g. a patient's symptoms, clinical test results, and the prevalences of particular diseases within a population). Clinicians must then integrate this information in order to reach a judgement about a patient's condition and appropriate treatment. These types of decision lend themselves to decision support. CDSSs, such as prescribing and reminder systems, have also been developed for situations where clinicians are known to have difficulties with decisions (sometimes measured by the number of mistakes or adverse events that occur)[4, 5] or may forget to deliver care.

Examples of CDSSs used in nursing

Two different types of decision support used by nurses are generic systems and nurse-specific systems. Generic systems used in the UK include PRODIGY, now known as Clinical Knowledge Summaries (www.cks.library.nhs.uk/clinical_knowledge), which provides support and guidance to practitioners on the management of conditions commonly seen in primary care. As nurses take on extended roles and responsibilities, such as the management of patients with chronic conditions and the prescription of medications, it is likely that the use of such systems will expand. Several CDSSs exist to help doctors with decision-making in the areas of chronic disease management and diagnosis,[6, 7] and these types of systems are also used by nurses and others as they assume these roles.

Good examples of nurse-specific CDSSs are the national first-contact telephone triage services used in the United Kingdom (NHS Direct in England and Wales and NHS 24 in Scotland) and elsewhere (e.g. Telehealth Ontario in Canada). These systems enable nurses to provide telephone health advice to callers. Individuals who call the service are triaged by nurse advisors using computerized decision support software and directed to the most appropriate service for their needs (e.g. self-help advice, a recommendation to contact their general practitioner, or advice to attend a hospital accident and emergency department).[8] Nurses access a relevant algorithm or guideline from the CDSS database based on the caller's symptoms. The system then prompts the nurse to ask the caller a series of questions and, based on the caller's responses, provides the nurse with a recommendation.[9]

Another area of practice where nurses use CDSSs to support practice is anticoagulation management.[10, 11] Warfarin dosing for patients requiring anticoagulation is carefully adjusted according to blood clotting time, a process that requires regular blood tests. Traditionally, this type of patient management has been carried out in specialist hospital outpatient clinics, with prescription decisions made by specialist physicians.[10] In some areas, nurses have taken on this role, using 'near patient testing' to establish a patient's blood clotting time; the clotting result is entered into a CDSS, which provides a warfarin dosage recommendation for the patient.[10, 11] This has allowed anticoagulation management to be relocated to primary care settings in some areas in the UK, reducing demand on more specialist hospital services without increasing the risk to patients.

Evaluations of CDSSs

We do not know whether using a CDSS to support decision-making in nursing has positive effects on how care is delivered or the quality of care patients receive. A recent systematic review on the use of CDSSs in nursing suggests that the evidence base is very limited.[3] The review identified eight trials, which focused on three areas of nursing practice: oral anticoagulation management, telephone triage, and glucose regulation in intensive care. The results suggest that nurses' use of CDSSs for oral anticoagulation management may improve the care received by patients.[10–12] Studies of telephone triage provide a more mixed picture, with some evidence that use of CDSSs may affect the way services are delivered (e.g. a decrease in the number of general practice appointments needed by patients who receive telephone advice).[13] However, the studies failed to provide evidence for the effects of CDSS use on patient outcomes. One study suggested that patients triaged by nurses using a CDSS were less likely to experience an adverse event.[13] Another study found that use of a CDSS had detrimental effects on all patient outcomes measured.[14] A study of the use of a CDSS to assist glucose regulation in intensive care showed that its use improved the number of samples taken on time.[15]

A broader review by Garg et al.[1] examined the effects of using CDSSs across health care disciplines and summarized the findings according to the type of decision a system was designed to support. The review showed that reminder systems for preventive health care generally had positive effects, with 16 of 21 studies (77%) indicating a beneficial outcome with the use of CDSSs. Similarly, systems designed to help clinicians with disease management appear to improve practitioner behaviour (62% of studies showed a positive effect on clinician behaviour), and drug dosing/prescribing systems appear to improve clinician prescribing practices (62% of trials of single drug dosing systems and 80% of trials of multi-drug prescribing systems showed improved outcomes). However, evidence for the effectiveness of CDSSs in assisting clinicians with diagnosis is less strong: 40% of studies showed improved clinician performance with CDSS use. The effect of using CDSSs on patient outcomes is also unclear. Most studies in the review by Garg *et al.*[1] either did not measure patient outcomes or were too small to be able to detect differences between groups. Of the 52 trials that examined patient outcomes, only seven (14%) found that patient outcomes improved with the use of CDSSs.

Overall, evidence for the benefits of using CDSSs to support nurse decision-making in practice is currently limited despite the fact that CDSSs have been integrated into the everyday practice of some nursing areas, such as telephone triage. Some evidence from trials that have examined the use of CDSSs in general suggests that they may improve what clinicians *do* when caring for patients in certain areas. In particular, use of CDSSs appears to assist clinicians in the organization of preventive health care, drug dosing/prescribing, and complex disease management. It is less clear whether improvements in how clinicians act have consequent effects on patient outcomes.

Summary

There is often a gap between what is known to be effective in nursing and what is practised. Evidence-based decision-making aims to ensure that decisions made about patient care use research evidence in an effective way. CDSSs have the potential to assist with this aim, as they can provide nurses with an organized database of current research evidence and help them to process information in a way that is individualized to specific patients. Evidence on the effects of CDSSs in health care in general suggests that their use may improve the way that care is delivered. In particular, use of CDSSs for reminders in preventive health (e.g. screening and vaccination programmes), chronic disease management and prescribing appears to improve the way that care is delivered. Nurses are increasingly taking on extended roles in areas such as chronic disease management and prescription of medications, and the use of CDSSs has the potential to help them with their practice in these areas. However, evidence is currently limited on how the use of CDSSs affects nursing practice and decision-making. It is also uncertain whether changes in the delivery of care resulting from the use of CDSSs actually translate into better patient outcomes. Despite these uncertainties, the use of CDSSs has the potential to encourage more evidence-based decision-making within nursing practice.

LEARNING EXERCISE

Identify an area of your practice where you perceive a difficulty in making decisions about patient management. Think about the types of decisions involved and why you might be having problems. A decision support system may already be available that could help with your decision problem (e.g. your hospital or trust may have a system in place that you don't know about, or one may be available on the Internet). If possible, try using the system to examine a patient case for which you have already made a decision. Do you think that using the system would have helped you in the decision-making for your patient case?

References

1 Garg AX, Adhikari NK, McDonald H, Rosas-Arellano MP, Devereaux PJ, Beyene J, Sam J, Haynes RB. Effects of computerized clinical decision support systems on practitioner performance and patient outcomes: a systematic review. *JAMA* 2005;**293**:1223–38.

2 Kawamoto K, Houlihan CA, Balas EA, Lobach DF. Improving clinical practice using clinical decision support systems: a systematic review of trials to identify features critical to success. *BMJ* 2005;**330**:765–72.

3 Randell R, Mitchell N, Dowding D, Cullum N, Thompson C. Effects of clinical decision support systems on nurse performance and patient outcomes: a systematic review. *J Health Serv Res Policy*, in press.

4 Kaushal R, Shojania KG, Bates DW. Effects of computerized physician order entry and clinical decision support systems on medication safety: a systematic review. *Arch Intern Med* 2003;**163**:1409–16.

5 Tamblyn R, Huang R, Perreault R, Jacques A, Roy D, Hanley J, McLeod P, Laprise R. The medical office of the 21st century (MOXXI): effectiveness of computerized decision-making support in reducing inappropriate prescribing in primary care. *CMAJ* 2003;**169**:549–56.

6 Eccles M, McColl E, Steen N, Rousseau N, Grimshaw J, Parkin D, Purves I. Effect of computerised evidence based guidelines on management of asthma and angina in adults in primary care: cluster randomised controlled trial. *BMJ* 2002;**325**:941.

7 Montgomery AA, Fahey T, Peters TJ, MacIntosh C, Sharp DJ. Evaluation of computer based decision support system and risk chart for management of hypertension in primary care: randomised controlled trial. *BMJ* 2000;**320**:686–90.

8 O'Cathain A, Nicholl J, Sampson F, Walters S, McDonnell A, Munro J. Do different types of nurses give different triage decisions in NHS Direct? A mixed methods study. *J Health Serv Res Policy* 2004;**9**:226–33.

9 O'Cathain A, Sampson FC, Munro JF, Thomas KJ, Nicholl JP. Nurses' views of using computerized decision support software in NHS Direct. *J Adv Nurs* 2004;**45**:280–6.

10 Fitzmaurice DA, Hobbs FD, Murray ET, Holder RL, Allan TF, Rose PE. Oral anticoagulation management in primary care with the use of computerized decision support and near-patient testing. *Arch Intern Med* 2000;**160**:2343–8.

11 Vadher BD, Patterson DL, Leaning M. Comparison of oral anticoagulant control by a nurse-practitioner using a computer decision-support system with that by clinicians. *Clin Lab Haematol* 1997;**19**:203–7.

12 White RH, Mungall D. Outpatient management of warfarin therapy: comparison of computer-predicted dosage adjustment to skilled professional care. *Ther Drug Monit* 1991;**13**:46–50.

13 Lattimer V, George S, Thompson F, Thomas E, Mullee M, Turnbull J, Smith H, Moore M, Bond H, Glasper A. Safety and effectiveness of nurse telephone consultation in out of hours primary care: randomised controlled trial. The South Wiltshire Out of Hours Project (SWOOP) Group. *BMJ* 1998;**317**:1054–9.

14 Richards DA, Meakins J, Tawfik J, Godfrey L, Dutton E, Richardson G, Russell D. Nurse telephone triage for same day appointments in general practice: multiple interrupted time series trial of effect on workload and costs. *BMJ* 2002;**325**:1214–17.

15 Rood E, Bosman RJ, van der Spoel JI, Taylor P, Zandstra DF. Use of a computerized guideline for glucose regulation in the intensive care unit improved both guideline adherence and glucose regulation. *J Am Med Inform Assoc* 2005;**12**:172–80.

Additional resources

Reading

Crouch R. Computerised decision support. In: Thompson C, Dowding D, editors. *Clinical Decision Making and Judgement in Nursing*. Edinburgh: Churchill Livingstone, 2002:165–81.

Websites

American Nursing Informatics Association (http://www.ania.org/). The mission of the ANIA is to provide networking, education and information resources that enrich and strengthen the roles of nurses in the field of informatics. The website provides news updates in the field and many useful weblinks.

British Computer Society Specialist Nursing Group (www.nursing.bcs.org/).The website of a UK organization for nurses and therapists interested in the management and use of information to improve care.

Clinical Knowledge Summaries (formerly PRODIGY Knowledge Service) (www.cks.library. nhs.uk/clinical_knowledge). Provides guidance on patient management for clinicians working in primary care.

Isabel (http://www.isabelhealthcare.com/). A computerized decision support system designed to aid in diagnosis.

NHS Direct (http://www.nhsdirect.nhs.uk/). Online guidance for patients.

Nursing Informatics Europe (http://www.nicecomputing.ch/nieurope/). This is the website of the nursing informatics section of the European Federation for Medical Informatics. The latest news and useful weblinks can be found here.

OpenClinical. (http://www.openclinical.org/dss.html). An overview of decision support systems.

4S DAWN Clinical Software (http://www.4s-dawn.com/dawnac/).Anticoagulation software site.

Chapter 32

BUILDING A FOUNDATION FOR EVIDENCE-BASED PRACTICE: EXPERIENCES IN A TERTIARY HOSPITAL

E. Ann Mohide, Esther Coker,
Jennifer Wiernikowski and Bernice King

This final chapter describes how nurses working in a tertiary hospital in Canada set about making evidence-based nursing a reality.

Hamilton Health Sciences (HHS) is a tertiary teaching hospital in a large city in southern Ontario comprising four hospitals (with over 1000 inpatient beds providing inpatient and outpatient acute and rehabilitation care across several health programmes) and a regional cancer centre. Approximately 3500 nurses (3044 Registered Nurses, 330 Registered Practical Nurses, and others in specialty positions, such as education) are employed by HHS and work across health programmes ranging from infertility services and obstetrics to ageing adults. HHS provides regional services to 2.2 million people in Hamilton and Central South Ontario.

In 2000, the Nursing Practice Committee (NPC)* was responsible for nursing strategy at HHS and was accountable to the Chief Nursing Officer. The NPC identified three priorities for development; one was to promote evidence-based nursing practice among nurses at the bedside. As a first step, an Evidence-Based Nursing (EBN) Committee was created and given the mandate of developing the use of evidence-based practice (EBP) at the patient care level and recommending processes that would promote EBP among direct care nurses. In 2000, the fledgling EBN Committee established a mission and set of responsibilities. In 2002, the original responsibilities were expanded and later slightly modified (Box 32.1).

Under the co-leadership of a clinical nurse specialist (BK) and a school of nursing faculty member with a track record in health services research (EAM), the EBN Committee membership was established, taking the following factors into account: hospital sites, health care programmes, major representation of direct care Registered Nurses and Registered Practical Nurses, academic and research representation from McMaster University School of Nursing, and links to community care. Two-hour EBN Committee meetings were scheduled monthly after Nursing Advisory Council (NAC) meetings for the convenience of members serving on both committees. Until 2002, funds were provided for direct nursing staff replacement costs so that EBN Committee members could complete preparatory work and attend meetings.

---

* The NPC has recently been re-named the Nursing Advisory Council (NAC), with responsibility for nursing decision-making. In line with the updated organizational structure and function of NAC, the Council is accountable to the Vice President Professional Affairs and Chief Nursing Executive.

Box 32.1 Terms of reference for Hamilton Health Sciences (HHS) Evidence-Based Nursing (EBN) Committee

Mission

- To foster evidence-based practice among HHS nurses

Responsibilities

- To advance knowledge about evidence-based practice
- To make recommendations about processes that promote evidence-based practice to appropriate decision-making bodies
- To develop communication mechanisms that inform nurses about evidence-based practices
- To collaborate with others to evaluate evidence-based trends in practice
- To facilitate the appropriate application of best practice guidelines and other evidence-based findings to practice
- To provide undergraduate and graduate nursing students with an opportunity to learn about the EBN Committee and the implementation of evidence-based practice in nursing

In the beginning, several barriers to the implementation of EBP by nurses were recognized and taken into account as the EBN Committee planned change.[1, 2] First, direct care nurses on inpatient units have little control over their clinical workloads, which can hamper involvement in non-direct care activities, such as learning about EBP or participating in evidence-based clinical projects.[2, 3] Compounding this, a continuing nursing shortage increased the amount of overtime nurses were working.

An earlier merger of different health care facilities brought differing cultures and organizational challenges to the fledgling, albeit large, hospital. Early on, the merger itself created the need to forge a unified organization, and numerous merger goals became priorities for action. New organizational priorities, such as the development of post-merger organizational structures, had primacy over nursing goals. This meant that the promotion of EBP by nurses had been on hold. Another early barrier to the implementation of EBP was the limited access to research journals and other research resources within or close to the clinical areas of the hospitals. Even if research resources are readily available, most nurses lack the training and skills in effective literature searching and critical appraisal.[1] Furthermore, experiential knowledge is often favoured by nurses over empirical evidence.[4] A critical issue is lack of support by ward managers for the concept or application of EBP.[5] At the outset, some HHS nursing staff reported a lack of support, although infrequently. In these cases, nursing staff reported that information seeking and critical appraisal were not valued as a part of the nursing culture on the unit, and limited access to computer resources exacerbated the problem. Communication with nursing staff across sites was problematic because of the lack of a common electronic communication system and incomplete electronic address listings for nursing staff; however, this situation has been rectified. Finally, the complexities of modern health care organizations can create a formidable barrier to creating change in clinical practice. The sound administration of today's health care organization depends on the interrelatedness of administrative bodies within the agency. This interrelatedness creates professional interdependencies that require considerable communication, negotiation, and collaboration and can result in protracted change processes that consume both energy and time.

Despite the barriers identified at the outset, several opportunities for change were identified:

- The nursing organization had identified EBP as a priority for planning and action
- The EBN Committee volunteers were motivated to learn about EBP and effect change
- The partnership between the clinical and academic organizations within the EBN Committee encouraged clinical scholarship, a concept utilizing inquiry and reflection to scrutinize practice[6]
- At an early stage, the EBN Committee viewed the journal *Evidence-Based Nursing* as an important resource for research dissemination[7, 8]

In 2002, site-specific chiefs of nursing practice were appointed, and the NAC was restructured to include important council committees, one of which focused on nursing research. The question was then how to relate the Research and EBN Committees. Although the EBN Committee mandate and responsibilities fell within the larger research portfolio, it was also seen to focus on the performance of discrete post-research production activities. With this in mind, the EBN Committee was positioned as a subcommittee of the Research Committee, reporting to NAC through the Research Committee. To promote communication and collaboration, one Chair of each Committee sits as a member of the other's Committee.

Selecting a model for EBN practice and an EBP model for implementing change in nursing practice

As a first step in developing a foundation for EBP by nurses at HHS, the EBN Committee members agreed on a conceptualization of a model for EBN practice.[9] Initially, the model of the three intersecting circles representing best research evidence, clinical expertise, and patient/family values was examined.[10] Then, an adapted version of the model, which added a circle representing the influence of resources, was considered.[11] However, as Committee members discussed the merits of the two models and applied them to different clinical situations, it became clear that an additional element representing 'overarching contextual issues' was needed. In addition to resource allocation, other issues and factors were raised, including program mandate, characteristics of the practice setting, socio-political atmosphere, and cultural diversity. As a result of these discussions, the Committee ratified the Hamilton Health Sciences Model for Evidence-Based Nursing Practice (Figure 32.1), which subsumed the three-element model within an overarching concept called 'context'.[9]

Once the model for EBN practice had been described, members synthesized current literature about models of evidence-based practice in order to recommend a specific EBP model for use by HHS nurses. Literature searches of several databases, including CINAHL and MEDLINE, were done using terms such as 'diffusion of innovation' and 'evidence-based medicine'. Other search techniques included reviewing reference lists and Internet sources and consulting with the Canadian Centre for Evidence-Based Nursing.[12] From these sources, 78 titles relevant to EBP models were retrieved, and 23 distinct models were identified.

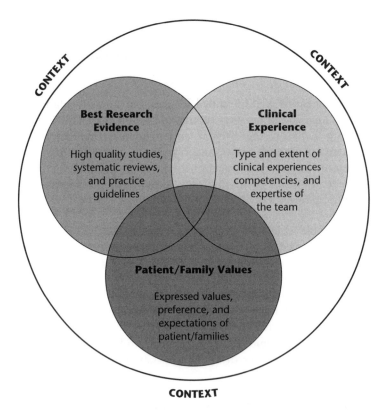

Figure 32.1 Hamilton Health Sciences Model for Evidence-Based Nursing Practice. Reprinted with permission from Mohide EA, Coker E. Toward clinical scholarship: promoting evidence-based practice in the clinical setting. *J Prof Nurs* 2005;**21**:372–9.

Five criteria for relevance to clinical nursing in tertiary care hospitals were established based on HHS needs and those cited in the literature. First, the model had to be clear and concise so that diagrammatic representation would allow quick assimilation of the concepts and organization of steps. Secondly, it required comprehensiveness from the beginning stages to implementation and evaluation. Thirdly, ease of use when applying the concepts to direct health care issues was needed. Fourthly, the model had to be applicable across the varied HHS health care programmes. Finally, published evidence evaluating the use of the model in practice was considered to be a strength.

Each model was rated independently by four people (EAM, BK, an emergency room nurse, and an occupational health nurse). Each criterion was scored on a 6-point scale (0 = lowest rating, 5 = highest rating). Data were entered and analysed using SPSS. Total rating scores, mean ratings, and standard deviations were generated for each model. The preferred implementation model was selected based on the highest mean scores for the total rating of each model. The data were re-analysed excluding the fourth and fifth criteria, as few empirical studies assessing the effectiveness of the models were identified in the published literature, and the ratings showed little variation in the scoring of the generalizability criterion. Table 32.1 shows the results for

Table 32.1 Ratings for the top eight evidence-based practice implementation models

Total rating for 5 criteria*		Total rating for 3 core criteria*†	
Model	Mean (standard deviation)	Model	Mean (standard deviation)
Rosswurm and Larrabee[13]	20.00 (3.74)	Rosswurm and Larrabee[13]	13.25 (1.26)
Iowa[16]	16.75 (6.02)	Iowa[16]	10.25 (3.77)
Children's Hospital of Philadelphia[17]	16.25 (6.80)	Children's Hospital of Philadelphia[17]	9.25 (4.50)
Stetler[15]	16.25 (2.22)	Aurora[14]	8.80 (2.05)
Aurora[14]	15.20 (2.78)	Stetler[15]	8.75 (1.26)
Diffusion of Innovation[18]	14.00 (8.79)	Diffusion of Innovation[18]	8.75 (4.99)
Research Nurse Intern Program[19]	14.00 (7.35)	Research Nurse Intern Program[19]	8.75 (4.27)
Process of Research Utilization[20]	12.75 (2.63)	Process of Research Utilization[20]	8.75 (1.70)

* Highest possible total mean score is 25 for five criteria and 15 for three criteria.

† Core criteria: clear and concise; comprehensive; ease of use by clinicians.

the top eight rated models,[8–15] with mean total scores for the five criteria and three core criteria (clear and concise, comprehensive, and ease of use by direct care nurses).

Using either set of criteria, the mean total rating for the Rosswurm and Larrabee model[13] was well above those of the other models. Only one minor difference in the two sets of rankings was found: the comparison showed a reversal in the rank order of the Aurora and Stetler models.[14, 15] The analyses enabled a clear decision to adopt the Rosswurm and Larrabee model.[13]

The EBN Committee made several adaptations to the framework to better reflect the needs of HHS nurses and the context in which the model would be used. First, the linear framework was re-oriented to a feedback loop so that the model is viewed as a cycle (Figure 32.2). This emphasizes the need for continuing examination of clinical questions over time and permits application of the EBP process or examination of projects at discrete steps in the cycle. When data are insufficient to support a decision about whether to maintain a specific practice or adopt a new one, the added step, 'stimulate inquiry', encourages nurses to seek out colleagues (e.g. nurses with advanced research training) to assist in developing an answerable research question and possibly lead a research project. In its current form, this model is dynamic, iterative, and clinician-friendly in that it mirrors the nursing process. It is clear, concise, and easily depicted as a diagram, and is applicable to clinical care. The Hamilton Health Sciences Model for Implementing Change in Nursing Practice is being used by the EBN Committee to focus its work and to orient staff nurses to the EBP concept and the sequence of steps used to implement it. For dissemination purposes, the model is incorporated into posters and a brochure to reinforce EBP concepts.

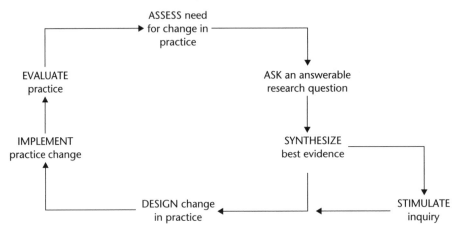

Figure 32.2 Hamilton Health Sciences Model for Implementing Change in Nursing Practice. Adapted from Rosswurm MA, Larrabee JH. A model for change to evidence-based practice. *Image J Nurs Sch* 1999;**31**:317–22.

Prioritizing and disseminating research findings to health care programmes

A lack of critical appraisal knowledge and skills and the clinical demands of providing direct care are barriers to HHS nurses participating in EBP projects to search for, appraise, disseminate, and apply relevant high-quality research. With these barriers in mind, the EBN Committee decided to develop a system to identify, rate and disseminate important research findings to health care programmes in the organization. In addition, the project set out to shorten the time lag between research dissemination and clinical uptake of the findings.[9]

Recognizing the journal *Evidence-Based Nursing* as a powerful tool in harnessing EBP, especially during the early development of the concept at HHS, the EBN Committee developed a project to determine the usefulness and feasibility of recommending research findings to relevant HHS health care programmes. This abstraction journal was selected as the source of scientific evidence because it produces user-friendly synopses of high-quality, current clinical studies and reviews with balanced commentaries.[21]

As a first step, an abstract rating form was developed to rate abstracts of primary studies and systematic reviews from the latest issue of *Evidence-Based Nursing*. The rating form identified the *Evidence-Based Nursing* citation, the citation for the original research article, and the major finding, as stated in the declarative title of the abstract. A series of checklists followed. First, raters (i.e. EBN Committee members) indicated whether the research was primarily applicable to clinical care or some aspect of health care administration and specified the HHS programmes to which the findings would likely be relevant. Raters then checked off a series of factors that might increase or decrease the perceived importance of the research findings, including the magnitude of the health problem, the burden of illness, and the extent of variation in clinical practice. Finally, raters assigned a score indicating the importance of disseminating the findings of each abstracted study. Raters assigned scores on a scale of 1–7, where 7 was the highest priority, and 1 was the lowest priority. Using the 7-point scale, raters were also asked to indicate their confidence in assigning the rating, and the extent to which the accompanying commentary helped in their prioritization. A glossary of terms and examples was developed.

The Committee refined the rating form over several iterations, and then seven *Evidence-Based Nursing* abstracts of quantitative studies were randomly selected for rating. Six EBN Committee members independently reviewed each abstract and commentary before completing the rating form. Raters completed each review in 20 minutes or less. Three of the seven abstracts received high mean global ratings for implementation (6–7 points), and four received moderate mean global ratings (4–5 points). Global ratings had moderate inter-rater reliability (intra-class correlation coefficient = 0.60). The Committee decided to disseminate the findings and accompanying information for abstracts that received an average global rating of 5 or above by three or more raters.

In a pre-test of the dissemination of research findings, programme managers,[22] Advanced Practice Nurses, and educators [23] (all of whom can assist in creating change by virtue of their positions in the organization) were receptive to receiving the abstracts, and most provided specific details about how the information could be used in clinical practice. The process has been refined and continues quarterly. Clinical areas report on whether the findings have been implemented. Where practice is not consistent with the disseminated research findings, the contact in the clinical area either provides an explanation for why a practice change is not appropriate or is helped to devise an implementation strategy. Implementation interventions were developed from the typology described by Stone *et al.*[24] (e.g. education, reminders, audit and feedback). When this prioritization/dissemination cycle had been conducted over five consecutive issues of *Evidence-Based Nursing*, we assessed that most abstracts of quantitative research are relevant to HHS programmes, and half received average global ratings of 5 or more by our priority raters. In almost two-thirds of cases, we found that clinical practice was already in line with the research findings before the EBN Committee dissemination. This finding gives positive reinforcement to the programmes in question and provides the EBN Committee with data to monitor trends in research uptake. In cases where research findings were not taken up, some success has been achieved in helping programmes to use specific strategies to implement the findings. Several recommendations for continuation of the process have been reported elsewhere.[25]

Evaluating an important EBP application in direct patient care

During the process of reviewing *Evidence-Based Nursing* abstracts, the EBN Committee identified a study that concluded that chlorhexidine was a more effective skin antiseptic than two other cleansing agents in preventing peripheral intravenous catheter-related infection.[26] This finding resonated with EBN Committee members because confusion existed among them as to which of the two cleansing agents, chlorhexidine or alcohol, was required at HHS for this purpose. Confusion on this issue became more evident when the clinical policy was reviewed. Although the approved policy for skin cleansing before intravenous initiation was changed to chlorhexidine in 2000 by a regional infection control committee, the written policy statement was non-specific, stating only that the 'recommended' cleansing agent should be used, without explicitly naming the agent.

This topic presented an excellent example for the evaluation of adherence to EBP as it relates to the 'evaluate practice' and 're-assess the need for a change in practice' steps in the model (see Figure 32.2). Importantly, the effectiveness of chlorhexidine was clearly established, showing consistency across a number of studies. In fact, Mermel[27] published a systematic review in 2000, which indicated the need to change practice to the use of chlorhexidine based on Level IIa evidence from randomized trials. Secondly, the issue is relevant, as most intravenous therapy is initiated by nurses. Thirdly, morbidity and mortality associated with intravenous catheter infections made this a critical patient safety issue. Furthermore, because chlorhexidine swabs are more costly than alcohol swabs, the appropriate use of chlorhexidine swabs is a cost containment issue. Finally, examination of this clinical EBP issue presented an opportunity for interactive learning involving HHS nursing staff.[7]

With these issues in mind, the EBN Committee conducted a one-day census survey of all Registered Nurses and Registered Practical Nurses (excluding those without the skills in question). A short, pretested, closed-ended questionnaire was administered by Committee members or their delegates. A total of 324 HHS nurses responded: a response rate of more than 90%. The findings indicated that less than 75% of nurses reported using chlorhexidine (the proper agent for asepsis before intravenous initiation), whereas 42% reported using chlorhexidine for asepsis before venipuncture (where alcohol was the recommended aseptic agent).

This exercise led to several interventions designed to change practice. An explicit policy statement about the cleansing agent to be used for peripheral intravenous cannulation was disseminated. A one-page description of the study and its results was disseminated to all clinical unit nursing staff. The EBN Committee members acted as champions within their clinical areas, doing one-to-one teaching with staff. Advanced Practice Nurses and nurse educators were asked to teach appropriate chlorhexidine use. In areas where large numbers of intravenous cannulations were initiated, unit-specific survey results were provided (audit and feedback). Furthermore, a poster presentation of the study was included at the annual HHS nursing conference.

In keeping with managerial responsibilities for effecting change and ensuring implementation of high-quality, current research in practice, clinical managers were asked to identify and reduce or eliminate barriers to appropriate chlorhexidine use on their units.[22] In areas identified as having low adherence to the policy of chlorhexidine use, a diagrammatic prompt illustrating 'best practice' was placed above alcohol and chlorhexidine swab containers. A follow-up survey was completed 14 months after implementation of the last strategy to effect change. The absolute difference in self-reported adherence to the chlorhexidine policy was examined in the first and second surveys. The results showed a 10% improvement in correct usage of chlorhexidine as a cleansing agent before intravenous cannulation.

Other progress

To date, the EBN Committee has been assessing the stage of adoption of nursing-related clinical practice guidelines, such as the Registered Nurses Association of Ontario (RNAO) Best Practice Guidelines.[28–30] Seasoned clinical nursing experts with credibility among their peers have been invited to present their clinical programme's/unit's progress in implementing guidelines to the EBN Committee.[9] In addition, the EBN Committee acknowledges what is sometimes a lengthy and complicated journey and encourages further progress on the 'evidence pipeline'.[31] Furthermore, the presentation process helps to increase the visibility of the work and allows the Committee to identify groups of nurses in the organization who are conducting exemplary EBP activities. Each successful group can be viewed as role models for staff in areas where there is less progress along the guideline adaptation process.[9]

Most recently, HHS has been chosen by RNAO to implement two RNAO Best Practice Guidelines:[30] 'Prevention of falls and fall injuries in the older adult' and 'Risk assessment and prevention of pressure ulcers'. In order to support the project, the manager of the implementation initiative has been invited to become a member of the EBN Committee. The EBN Committee will work with the manager to increase awareness about the project throughout the organization and provide educational material on the EBN Committee intranet site.

A number of ongoing activities have been initiated to market the shift to an EBP culture.[9] The Committee developed its own logo, with an accompanying slogan, 'We are proud to practise EBN'. The logo and slogan appear on all posters, information flyers, correspondence, and general communication. The importance of linking the EBP rationale to specific decision-making about policies and procedures is recognized. As Valente[32] described, wherever possible, the link between scientific evidence and practice recommendations should be clear; therefore, the Committee uses the EBN branding to reinforce the link.

The Committee produced a brochure called 'What is evidence-based practice?' to increase awareness of the concepts and to promote the shift to an EBP culture.[9] The brochure describes how to use the HHS model for EBN practice using a stepwise progression of illustrations and includes the model for implementing a change in nursing practice. Some strategies to promote the implementation of changes are noted, and information about the EBN Committee is included on the back cover. Based on the brochure material and layout, an EBN Committee site has been constructed within the HHS intranet.

Over the past two years during the HHS Nursing Week celebrations, the Committee has hosted an HHS intranet-based contest to increase awareness about the HHS electronic library access to *Evidence-Based Nursing*.[9] Using a process similar to that described by Mohide *et al.*[33] four hypothetical patient-care scenarios are developed using abstracts from the most recent issue of *Evidence-Based Nursing*. Respondents are required to correctly answer the question embedded in the scenario using the research data found in the abstract and the supporting material. The nurses draw a conclusion and make a patient care recommendation based on the information provided in the hypothetical scenario and the research evidence. One correctly answered response for each scenario is drawn, and prizes are awarded.

The EBN Committee strives to use principles derived from experience to guide its activities. Some of these have been described here and elsewhere.[9] Box 32.2 outlines the principles that have helped to shape the HHS EBN Committee experience.

Summary

The rapidity of change and the reorganization of nursing services within the health care sector present challenges for the advancement of EBP. Managers and administrators should facilitate the uptake of practice based on current, high-quality research by formalizing the expectation that nursing care *be* evidence-based.[21] Health care

Box 32.2 Guiding principles used in the development and continuing evolution of the HHS EBN Committee[9]

- Organizational endorsement is an essential prerequisite in the cultural movement towards EBP.
- A nursing partnership between the health agency and an academic institution strengthens clinical scholarship.
- Committee membership reflecting the organization's diverse nursing roles increases the credibility of the Committee's activities and encourages involvement of the groups represented by the members.
- Communication with other nursing and interdisciplinary bodies, accountability to administration, and opportunities to influence decision-making can be achieved by positioning the EBN Committee within the organization's nursing committee structure.
- Working together on the development of the Committee mission and responsibilities creates a shared vision and sense of ownership.
- Articulating the preferred EBP conceptualization promotes a common understanding of beliefs, key terms, and concepts.
- The selection of an evidence-based model for implementing change in nursing practice should be readily understandable, practical, and easy to apply.
- The Committee's use of an evidence-based approach to decision-making serves to model the desired behaviours.
- Achieving and sustaining a desired change in practice may be optimized by using multiple implementation strategies targeted to individual, group and organizational levels.
- The use of readily available, high-quality research sources, in conjunction with a systematic mechanism for determining the priorities for dissemination, conserves resources and maximizes efforts.
- Ultimately, clinical programmes are responsible for assessing the relevance, importance, and applicability of high-quality research and/or practice guidelines and for closing the implementation cycle.
- By recognizing, properly acknowledging and supporting EBP efforts throughout the organization, the cultural movement towards EBP can be enhanced.
- Multiple approaches to marketing EBP are likely to increase frontline nurses' awareness of the intellectual aspects of nursing practice.

and professional organizations must pursue systems that facilitate easy access to research evidence and educational EBP materials. Researchers need to assume more responsibility for EBP by helping clinicians to implement current research findings.[34] This also holds true for health professionals with research expertise, whether based in practice or academic settings, or both.

This chapter illustrates one tertiary hospital's evolving experience in shifting the nursing culture towards EBP and implementing EBP in nursing. The EBN Committee strives to respond to the needs and capabilities of nurses and the organization, to apply a series of important principles for closing the research gap, and to use systematic and varied approaches to create change in practice.

LEARNING EXERCISES

1. Using the Hamilton Health Sciences Model for Evidence-Based Nursing Practice (Figure 32.1), apply the elements of the model to a patient issue or situation. Identify how the application of the elements assisted you to make an evidence-based clinical decision.

2. Select a topic related to your current clinical practice. Identify a clinical question addressed by a recently published systematic review that suggests a change in practice is warranted. Check to see if the finding has been integrated into clinical practice. If not, use the Hamilton Health Sciences Model for Implementing Change in Nursing Practice (see Figure 32.2) to develop a plan for changing the practice.
3. Think about a health care organization in which you have worked or work currently and the extent to which nursing, in that context, has embraced a culture of EBP. Consider the factors that may have influenced the culture of EBP in the organization.

References

1 Funk SG, Tornquist EM, Champagne M. Barriers and facilitators of research utilization. An integrative review. *Nurs Clin North Am* 1995;30:395–407.
2 Fink R, Thompson CJ, Bonnes D. Overcoming barriers and promoting the use of research in practice. *J Nurs Admin* 2005;35:121–9.
3 Royle J, Blythe J. Promoting research utilisation in nursing: the role of the individual, organisation, and environment. *Evidence-Based Nursing* 1998;1:71–2.
4 Estabrooks CA. Will evidence-based nursing practice make practice perfect? *Can J Nurs Res* 1998;30:15–36.
5 Newman M, Papadopoulos I, Melifonwu R. Developing organisational systems and culture to support evidence-based practice: the experience of the Evidence-Based Ward Project. *Evidence-Based Nursing* 2000;3:103–5.
6 Sigma Theta Tau International. Clinical scholarship white paper: Knowledge work, in service of care, based on evidence. Indianapolis: Sigma Theta Tau International, 1999.
7 Moulding NT, Silagy CA, Weller DP. A framework for effective management of change in clinical practice: dissemination and implementation of clinical practice guidelines. *Qual Health Care* 1999;8:177–83.
8 DiCenso A, Cullum N, Ciliska D. *Evidence-Based Nursing*: 4 years down the road. *Evidence-Based Nursing* 2002;5:4–5.
9 Mohide EA, Coker E. Toward clinical scholarship: promoting evidence-based practice in the clinical setting. *J Prof Nurs* 2005;21:372–9.
10 Haynes RB, Sackett DL, Gray JM, Cook DJ, Guyatt GH. Transferring evidence from research into practice: 1. The role of clinical care research evidence in clinical decisions. *ACP J Club* 1996;125:A14–16.
11 DiCenso A, Cullen N, Ciliska D. Implementing evidence-based nursing: some misconceptions. *Evidence-Based Nursing* 1998;1:38–40.
12 Ciliska D, DiCenso A, Cullum N. Centres of evidence-based nursing: directions and challenges. *Evidence-Based Nursing* 1999;2:102–4.
13 Rosswurm MA, Larrabee JH. A model for change to evidence-based practice. *Image J Nurs Sch* 1999;31:317–22.
14 Van Mullem C, Burke LJ, Dohmeyer K, Farrell M, Harvey S, John L, Kraly C, Rowley F, Sebern M, Twite K, Zapp R. Strategic planning for research use in nursing practice. *J Nurs Adm* 1999;29:38–45.
15 Stetler CB. Refinement of the Stetler/Marram model for application of research findings to practice. *Nurs Outlook* 1994;42:15–25.
16 Titler MG, Kleiber C, Steelman V, Goode C, Rakel B, Barry-Walker J, Small S, Buckwalter K. Infusing research into practice to promote quality care. *Nurs Res* 1994;43:307–13.
17 Barnsteiner JH, Ford N, Howe C. Research utilization in a metropolitan children's hospital. *Nurs Clin North Am* 1995;30:447–55.
18 Pearcey P, Draper P. Using the diffusion of innovation model to influence practice: a case study. *J Adv Nurs* 1996;23:714–21.
19 Warren JJ, Heermann JA. The Research Nurse Intern program. A model for research dissemination and utilization. *J Nurs Adm* 1998;28:39–45.

20 Hunt JM. Barriers to research utilization. *J Adv Nurs* 1996;**23**:423–5.
21 Haynes RB. Of studies, summaries, synopses, and systems: the "4S" evolution of services for finding current best evidence. *Evidence-Based Nursing* 2005;**8**:4–6.
22 Browman GP, Snider A, Ellis P. Negotiating for change. The healthcare manager as catalyst for evidence-based practice: changing the healthcare environment and sharing experience. *Healthc Pap* 2003;**3**:10–22.
23 Krugman M. Evidence-based practice. The role of staff development. *J Nurses Staff Dev* 2003;**19**:279–85.
24 Stone EG, Morton SC, Hulscher ME, Maglione MA, Roth EA, Grimshaw JM, Mittman BS, Rubenstein LV, Rubenstein LZ, Shekelle PG. Interventions that increase use of adult immunization and cancer screening services: a meta-analysis. *Ann Intern Med* 2002;**136**:641–51.
25 Coker ME, Mohide EA, Fairfield BL, Lee RN, Phillips LA, Wiernikowski J. Prioritizing and disseminating research findings to clinical programs. Montreal: Sigma Theta Tau International Honor Society of Nursing, 2006.
26 LeBlanc A, Cobbett S. Traditional practice versus evidence-based practice for IV skin preparation. *Can J Infect Control* 2000;Spring:9–14.
27 Mermel LA. Prevention of intravascular catheter-related infections. *Ann Intern Med* 2000;**132**:391–402.
28 Kearsey K. Launch of nursing Best Practice Guidelines: envisioned as next step to more effective patient care. *Registered Nurse* 2001;November/December:8–11.
29 DiCenso A, Virani T, Bajnok I, Borycki E, Davies B, Graham I, Harrison M, Logan J, McLeary L, Power M, Scott J. A toolkit to facilitate the implementation of clinical practice guidelines in healthcare settings. *Hosp Q* 2002;**5**:55–60.
30 Registered Nurses Association of Ontario (RNAO). http://www.rnao.org
31 Glasziou P, Haynes RB. The paths from research to improved health outcomes. *Evidence-Based Nursing* 2005;**8**:36–8.
32 Valente SM. Research dissemination and utilization: improving care at the bedside. *J Nurs Care Qual* 2003;**23**:114–21.
33 Mohide EA, Matthew-Maich N, Cross H. Syllabus selection: innovative learning activity. Using electronic gaming to promote evidence-based practice in nursing education. *J Nurs Educ* 2006;**45**:384.
34 Waddell C. So much research evidence, so little dissemination and uptake: mixing the useful with the pleasing. *Evidence-Based Nursing* 2002;**5**:38–40.

GLOSSARY

Absolute risk difference (ARD): the arithmetic difference in event rates between experimental and control groups (i.e. obtained by subtracting the one event rate from the other); usually reported as a percentage (%). Also referred to as the 'absolute benefit increase' if the rate of a 'good' outcome (e.g. remission) is larger in the experimental group than the control group and the 'absolute benefit reduction' if the rate is smaller in the experimental group. Also referred to as the 'absolute risk reduction' if the rate of a 'bad' outcome (e.g. mortality) is lower in the experimental group than in the control group and as the 'absolute risk increase' if the rate is higher in the experimental group.

Adjusted analysis[1]: statistical modification of outcome data to account for group differences in baseline characteristics (e.g. age).

Analysis of covariance[2]: a statistical procedure to test the mean difference between groups on a dependent variable while controlling for one or more extraneous variables (covariates), such as age, sex or baseline differences.

Ascertainment bias[3]: occurs when the results of a trial are systematically distorted by knowledge of which intervention participants receive; when participants are not 'blind' to the intervention.

Axial coding[4]: second level of coding in a grounded theory study, which involves categorizing, recategorizing and condensing first-level codes by connecting categories and subcategories.

Before–after design: data are collected from the same participants both before and after the introduction of an intervention.

Bias[5]: a systematic error or deviation from the truth in results or inferences. See Ascertainment bias, Expectation bias, Performance bias, Surveillance bias, Selection bias.

Binary data: see Dichotomous data. Blinding (masking): refers to whether patients, clinicians providing an intervention, people assessing outcomes, and/or statisticians were aware or unaware of the group to which patients belonged.

Case–control study[1]: an observational study that begins by identifying patients who have the health problem (cases) and control participants who do not have the health problem and then looking back in time to identify the existence of possible causal factors, for example, identifying patients with and without lung cancer and looking back in time to determine past smoking behaviour (exposure to tobacco).

Case study research[6]: an empirical enquiry that investigates a contemporary phenomenon within its real-life context. Case studies may involve collection and analysis of both qualitative and quantitative data and may focus on single or multiple cases.

Causal relationship: a 'cause and effect' relationship in which an exposure (to a particular intervention or some other agent) increases the probability of experiencing a particular outcome. A causal relationship is more likely to exist if several criteria are met, including the existence of a temporal relationship (i.e. the exposure precedes the outcome) and the existence of a dose–response relationship (i.e. the outcome is more likely when the amount of exposure is greater).

Cluster randomization[3]: randomization of groups of people rather than individuals; this approach is often used to avoid 'contamination' when the way in which people in one group are treated or assessed is likely to modify the treatment or assessment of people in other groups.

Cohort analytic study: two or more groups of people who do not have the outcome of interest are assembled; one group is exposed to a particular factor or set of factors (i.e. a potential causative agent for a particular disease or an intervention), and then all groups are followed up for a specified time period to compare the incidence of the outcome of interest.

Cohort study: a group of people with a common characteristic or set of characteristics are followed up for a specified period of time to determine the incidence of an outcome; there is no comparison group.

Concealment of randomization: in a randomized controlled trial, the extent to which those involved in participant recruitment could have foreknowledge of the group to which prospective participants would be allocated. *Concealed allocation* occurs when researchers are deemed to have taken adequate measures to conceal allocation to study group assignments from those responsible for assessing patients for entry in the trial (e.g. central randomization; sequentially numbered, opaque, sealed envelopes; coded bottles or containers; drugs prepared by the pharmacy).

Confidence interval (CI): quantifies the uncertainty in measurement; usually reported as 95% confidence interval, which is the range of values within which we can be 95% sure that the true value for the entire population lies.

Confounder[7]: a variable that affects the observed relationship between two other variables. For example, alcohol consumption is related to lung cancer but does not cause the disease; instead, both alcohol consumption and lung cancer are related to smoking (the confounder), which causes lung cancer.

Confounding bias: see Performance bias.

Consensus dialogue[8]: in qualitative research, multiple concepts are analysed simultaneously, drawing on the scientific and clinical expertise of more than one person through extensive discourse.

Constant comparison: an analytic approach in qualitative research, characterized by comparing and contrasting incidents to discern conceptual similarities and differences, formulate categories, establish their boundaries and properties, and thereby discover patterns amenable to theorizing.

Contamination: study participants in the control group accidentally receive the experimental intervention, thereby minimizing potential differences in outcomes between groups.

Continuous data[5]: data with a potentially infinite number of possible values along a continuum (e.g. weight, blood pressure).

Control event rate (CER): rate (%) of the outcome of interest observed in the control group.

Convenience sampling: participants are selected on the basis of ease of access and, secondarily, for their knowledge of the subject matter.

Conversation analysis[9]: examines the organization and structure of conversation, including all that is said.

Cost–benefit analysis: a type of economic evaluation that measures both costs and effects in monetary terms to estimate the net social benefit of a strategy

Cost–consequences analysis: an economic evaluation in which incremental costs and consequences are merely listed without any attempt to aggregate them.

Cost-effectiveness analysis: a type of economic evaluation in which incremental costs and effects are aggregated into a ratio, and effects are measured in a common natural unit such as 'cost per pressure ulcer free day'.

Cost-minimization analysis: a type of economic evaluation in which the outcomes associated with competing strategies (e.g. interventions) are regarded as equal, and only the costs are compared; the aim is to choose the least costly alternative.

Cost–utility analysis: a specific type of cost effectiveness analysis in which effects are measured in terms of subjective measures of well-being (utilities), commonly quality-adjusted life-years (QALYs); the results of such an analysis would be presented in terms of cost per QALY.

Covariate[1]: a potentially confounding variable that is controlled for in an analysis of covariance.

Criterion standard: see Diagnostic standard.

Critical ethnography[10]: a qualitative research approach concerned with relationships and power inequities between individuals and the sociopolitical framework, transformation of these relationships, and attention to the research process as a form of action.

Crossover trial: a method of comparing two interventions in which patients are switched to the alternative intervention after a specified period of time.

Cross-sectional study[1]: an observational study that examines a characteristic (or set of characteristics) and a health outcome in a sample of people at one point in time.

Data saturation: see Saturation.

Deductive reasoning: a process of logic often used in quantitative research, whereby general or universal premises are used to derive inferences about particular instances of a phenomenon. Contrasts with inductive reasoning, in which inferences about specific instances of a phenomenon are used to derive generalized conclusions about the phenomenon.

Dependent variable: a variable, the value of which is related to the value of another variable (the independent variable). For example, in aetiological study, the outcome is the dependent variable and the exposure is the independent variable.

Detection bias: see Surveillance bias.

Diagnostic standard: the current best available measure of an outcome; used for assessing properties of a new diagnostic or screening test. The results from a new test are compared with the results from the diagnostic standard to assess the usefulness of the new test (i.e. its sensitivity, specificity, and likelihood ratios). Also known as Gold standard or Criterion standard.

Dichotomized data[5]: data that can take one of two values (e.g. dead or alive, present or absent). Sometimes, continuous or ordinal data can be converted to dichotomous data. For example, blood pressure values ≥140/90 mmHg might be classified as high blood pressure and those <140/90 mmHg might be classified as normal blood pressure. Also known as Binary data.

Discounted[11]: in an economic analysis, an adjustment based on the assumption that people place greater value on something they have today than on something they will have in the future.

Discourse analysis[12]: a qualitative method of investigation focused on the representation and creation of meaning through language and visual imagery. A discourse is defined as a patterned way of representing phenomena in social and material worlds.

Dose–response[13]: indicates that a relation exists, such that increasing doses or duration of treatment results in increased frequency or intensity of outcomes (i.e. as the dosage of a medication increases, so does the magnitude of pain reduction). This is one of the criteria to support the existence of a causal relationship between a potential exposure and an outcome.

Effect size[5]: a measure of effect that is typically used for continuous data when different scales are used to measure an outcome (e.g. pain measured using different scales). It is usually defined as the difference in means between the intervention and control groups divided by the standard deviation of the control group or both groups. It can be used to combine results across studies in a meta-analysis.

Effectiveness: the extent to which an intervention does more good than harm for participants who receive the intervention *under usual conditions*. It answers the question *Does it work?*

Efficacy: the extent to which an intervention does more good than harm for participants who receive the intervention *under optimal conditions* (e.g. complete compliance with treatment). It answers the question *Can it work?*

Epistemology: the branch of philosophy that considers the nature of knowledge and ways of knowing.

Ethnography (ethnographic study)[2]: an approach to inquiry that focuses on the culture or subculture of a group of people, with an effort to understand the world view of those under study.

Ethnomethodology: an approach to inquiry that focuses on the way people make sense of their everyday lives.

Expectation bias[14]: knowledge about a patient influences a data collector's 'expectation' of finding an exposure or outcome. In clinical practice, a clinician's assessment may be influenced by previous knowledge of the presence or absence of a disorder.

Experimental event rate (EER): rate (%) of the outcome of interest observed in the experimental group.

Exposure: contact with something that influences a person's outcome. This might be exposure to a causal agent that increases the risk of developing a disease or, in people who already have a disease, reaching a particular endpoint. It may also refer to exposure to something that improves outcomes, such as a beneficial intervention.

Factorial design[4]: a design where two independent variables are simultaneously manipulated; permits analysis of the main effects of the independent variables separately as well as the interaction of these variables. For example, in a 2×2 factorial study, patients were allocated to aspirin or no aspirin and to vitamin E or no vitamin E for prevention of cardiovascular events.

False negative result[14]: a test result that incorrectly identifies people as not having the target disease when they actually have the disease.

False positive result[14]: a test result that incorrectly identifies people as having the target disease when they actually do not have the disease.

Fisher exact test (2-tailed)[1]: a test for 2×2 contingency tables, used to test the null hypothesis that proportions are equal or that characteristics are independent or not associated with each other. It is used if the sample size is too small to use the chi-squared (χ^2) test.

Fixed effect model[5]: gives a summary estimate of the magnitude of effect in meta-analysis. It takes into account within-study variation but not between-study variation and hence is usually not used if there is significant heterogeneity.

Generalizability[14]: the degree to which the results of a study can be applied to patients or settings other than those included in the study.

Giorgi's method[15]: an approach to the analysis of phenomenological data that involves four steps: (1) reading the text to get a sense of the whole; (2) dividing the text into meaning units; (3) transforming the language of participants into disciplinary language (e.g. nursing); and (4) synthesizing the structure to describe its essence.

Gold standard: see Diagnostic standard.

Grounded theory[2]: an approach to collecting and analysing qualitative data with the aim of developing theories 'grounded' in real world observations.

Hazard ratio[16]: the weighted relative risk over the entire study period; often reported in the context of survival analysis.

Hermeneutics[2]: a qualitative research tradition that draws on interpretive phenomenology and uses the lived experiences of people as a tool for understanding the social, cultural, political and historical context in which those experiences occur.

Heterogeneity[5]: the degree to which the effect estimates of individual studies in a meta-analysis differ significantly.

Heterogeneity sampling: see Maximum variation sampling.

Homogeneous sampling: an approach to purposive sampling in qualitative research aimed at selecting a small sample of people who share some characteristic of interest, for the purpose of describing some subgroup in depth.

Immersion/crystallization analysis method[2]: in qualitative research, an interpretive style of analysis that involves the analyst's total 'immersion' in and reflection of the textual material and results in an intuitive 'crystallization' of the data.

Inception cohort: a defined, representative sample of patients assembled for a study at a common (ideally early) point in their disease or condition and followed up over time.

Incidence[1]: the proportion of people who develop a specific disease or condition within a specified time frame (new cases).

Independent variable: a variable that is believed to influence the value of another variable (the dependent variable). For example, in an aetiological study, the exposure is the independent variable and the outcome is the dependent variable.

Inductive analysis: often used in qualitative research, this type of analysis begins with specific observations from which generalizations are developed; opposite to deductive analysis, often used in quantitative research, which begins with the abstract (e.g. general laws or hypotheses), from which logical deductions about specific phenomena are made.

Inductive reasoning: a process of logic whereby inferences about specific instances of a phenomenon are used to derive generalized conclusions about the phenomenon. Contrasts with deductive reasoning, whereby general or universal premises are used to derive inferences about particular instances of a phenomenon.

Information bias: see Surveillance bias.

Intention to treat analysis (ITT): in a randomized controlled trial, all patients are analysed in the groups to which they were randomized, even if they failed to complete the intervention or received the wrong intervention.

Interpretative interactionalism[17]: a qualitative method that aims to bring out subjective and personal experience through the development of thick description, which illuminates context, meanings and interpretation instead of just reporting facts; it was developed to examine the relation of personal troubles to the resources available to address those troubles.

Inter-rater agreement[14]: the degree to which two or more independent observers assign the same ratings/values to an attribute being measured or assessed.

Interrupted time series[18]: involves multiple observations over time on the same units (e.g. particular individuals) or on different, but similar, individuals (e.g. same community or worksite); requires knowing when an intervention took place in order to compare outcomes before and after the intervention.

Interval variable: data that arises in ordered categories; the categories have equivalently sized intervals between them, but a zero value does not imply the absence of the phenomenon (e.g. temperature measured in Celsius or Fahrenheit; date of birth).

Kappa: a statistic that indicates the extent of agreement between two or more observers beyond that expected by chance. A kappa of 1.0 indicates perfect agreement.

Life history research: an approach to qualitative research that uses life stories as a route to understanding and illustrating particular phenomena.

Life-years saved: difference (in years) in life expectancy with an intervention (e.g. in smokers who receive a smoking cessation programme and stop smoking) and without an intervention (e.g. in smokers who do not receive the programme and continue smoking); often considered in economic analysis.

Likelihood ratio (for positive and negative results)[19]: a way of summarizing the findings of a study of a diagnostic test for use in clinical situations where there may be differences in the prevalence of the disease. The likelihood ratio for a positive test is the probability that a positive test result comes from a person who really does have the disorder rather than one who does not have the disorder [sensitivity/(1-specificity)]. The likelihood ratio for a negative test is the probability that a negative test result comes from a person with the disorder rather than one without the disorder [(1-sensitivity)/specificity].

Linear analysis (regression): a statistical technique for determining the relation (prediction equation) between continuous variables.

Log rank test[1]: a statistical method for comparing two survival curves when censored observations exist.

Logistic regression[1]: a statistical technique that determines the probability of a dependent dichotomous variable (outcome) occurring when the independent (explanatory) variables are present or absent. It determines whether a model that includes the variable(s) explains more about the outcome variable than a model that does not include the variable(s).

Markov Monte Carlo simulation model[20]: a decision analysis that tries to more accurately represent the complex processes involved in transitions into and out of various states of health.

Maximum variation (heterogeneity) sampling: a type of purposive sampling aimed at capturing differences in cases. Also known as Heterogeneity sampling.

Median: the values of the middle observation in a sample. That is, if the data from 99 people were ordered from high to low, the median would be the value of the 50th observation.

Meta-analysis[1]: a method for combining the results of several independent studies that measure the same outcomes so that an overall summary statistic can be calculated.

Meta-study (meta-synthesis): a process that involves the analysis and synthesis of qualitative findings, methods and theories or frameworks from different studies to develop overarching or more conclusive ways of thinking about phenomena.

Mixed methods studies: studies that involve the collection of both qualitative and quantitative data.

Multiple case study approach: a non-experimental study design involving a series of cases (e.g. individuals, groups or organizations); data are collected and analysed from these multiple sources (cases).

Multiple regression: a statistical technique to determine the probability of a dependent variable (outcome) occurring when the independent (explanatory) variables are present or absent. It determines whether a model that includes the variables explains more about the outcome variable than does a model that does not include the variables.

Multivariate analysis[1]: analysis involving several independent or dependent variables.

Narrative analysis: an analytical technique that uses people's stories to gain insight into their lived experiences.

Naturalistic inquiry[4]: the goal of this research is to understand how individuals construct reality within their own natural setting and context.

Negative predictive value: a measure of the performance of a diagnostic test; it is the proportion of participants with negative test results who do not have the disease or condition being evaluated.

Nested case-control study: a case-control study done within a prospective cohort study.

Network sampling: see Snowball sampling.

Nominal group technique[21]: a highly structured group process that provides an orderly procedure for obtaining qualitative information from specific groups who are closely associated with the area of interest.

Nominal variable: data that exist as unordered, qualitative categories (e.g. sex, ethnicity or religion).

Non-probability sampling: a method of sampling that does not use random selection (e.g. purposive sampling, snowball sampling).

Number needed to harm (NNH)[22]: number of patients who, if they received the experimental treatment, would lead to one additional person being harmed compared with patients who receive the control treatment; this is calculated as 1/absolute risk increase (rounded to the next whole number), accompanied by the 95% confidence interval.

Number needed to treat (NNT): number of patients who need to be treated to prevent one additional negative event (or to promote one additional positive event); this is calculated as 1/absolute risk reduction (rounded to the next whole number), accompanied by the 95% confidence interval.

Objective outcome: an outcome that is measurable and requires no judgement (e.g. dead or alive).

Odds: the ratio of the probability of an event occurring to the probability of it not occurring.

Odds ratio (OR): describes the odds of a patient in the experimental group having an event divided by the odds of a patient in the control group having the event *or* the odds that a patient was exposed to a given risk factor divided by the odds that a control patient was exposed to the risk factor.

Ontology: philosophical considerations of the nature of existence, reality and ways of being.

Open coding[4]: first level of coding in a grounded theory study, consisting of basic descriptive coding of narrative content.

Opportunity costs: the value of the benefits foregone from using resources for an alternative purpose, for example, reducing number of nursing staff in the hospital in order to provide care in the home following discharge.

Ordinal variable: data that exist in ordered categories (e.g. social class or pressure ulcer grading tools).

Participant observation: a method of data collection, rooted in anthropology, which involves the researcher as an observer of a group or case under study. The extent to which the researcher acts as an observer or participant can vary.

Participatory action research: action-oriented research in which the researchers and participants are partners in developing the question, intervention and evaluation.

Performance bias[5]: occurs when the results of a trial are distorted by systematic differences in the care provided to participants, other than the intervention being evaluated. Also known as Confounding bias.

Phenomenological reduction: an analytic technique introduced by Edmund Husserl that involves suspension ('bracketing') of our natural attitudes and commonly held beliefs about the world so that our understanding of objects within the world becomes a window into describing the events of consciousness.

Phenomenology[4]: an approach to inquiry that emphasizes the complexity of human experience and the need to understand that experience holistically, as it is actually lived.

Positive predictive value: a measure of the performance of a diagnostic test; it is the proportion of participants with positive test results who actually have the disease or condition being evaluated.

Post-test probability[14]: the probability that a target condition is present after the results of a diagnostic test are available.

Power[1]: the ability of a study to detect an actual effect or difference between groups; it has to do with the adequacy of sample size. Before a study begins, researchers often calculate the number of participants required to detect a specified difference between two groups. If a study has insufficient power (i.e. the sample size is too small), actual differences between groups may not be detected.

Pretest probability[14]: the probability that a target condition is present before the results of a diagnostic test are available.

Prevalence[1]: the proportion of people who have a given disease or condition at a specified point in time.

Probability[14]: a quantitative estimate of the likelihood that a condition exists (as in diagnosis) or the likelihood of subsequent events(such as in an intervention study).

Probability sampling: a method of sampling that uses some type of random selection to ensure that different units in the population being sampled are equally likely to be selected. Also known as random sampling.

Prognosis: the possible outcomes of a disease or condition and the probabilities that they will occur.

Prognostic factors: variables that help to predict future health outcomes (e.g. cancer staging systems).

Purposeful (purposive) sampling: the process of selecting information-rich cases, participants, or settings for study. Information-rich cases are those from which we can learn a great deal about the phenomena of interest.

p-value: a statistical value, which relates the probability that the obtained results are due to chance alone (type I error); a p-value <0.05 means that there is less than a 1 in 20 probability of that result occurring by chance alone under the null hypothesis that there is no difference in the populations.

Qualitative research: research that aims to generate an understanding of complex, unquantifiable phenomena, such as people's experiences or perceptions. (Also, see specific types of qualitative research: Ethnography, Grounded theory, Phenomenology).

Quality-adjusted life-years gained: difference (in years) in life expectancy with an intervention versus without an intervention, taking into account not only the additional years but also the quality of life during the period of extended life. This measure is often used in the context of economic analysis.

Quasi-randomized study: participants are not randomly allocated to groups, but some other form of allocation is used (e.g. day of the week, month of birth).

Random effects model[5]: gives a summary estimate of the magnitude of effect in meta-analysis. It takes into account both within-study and between-study variance and gives a wider confidence interval to the estimate than a fixed effects model if there is significant between-study variation.

Random sampling: see Probability sampling.

Randomized controlled trial (randomized clinical trial, randomized trial) (RCT): a study in which individuals are randomly allocated to receive alternative preventive, therapeutic, or diagnostic interventions and then followed up to determine the effect of the interventions (one of the alternatives might be no intervention).

Ratio variable: has all of the features of an interval variable (i.e. ordered categories with equivalent-sized intervals between each) but also has an absolute zero (e.g. absolute temperature, weight, height).

Receiver operating characteristic (ROC) curve[23]: an analysis used to assess the clinical usefulness of a diagnostic or screening test. It yields a score that has the highest rates of both sensitivity and specificity with respect to a diagnosis – that is, a score that will give the maximum rate of accurate classifications.

Redundancy: see Saturation.

Relative benefit increase (RBI): the proportional increase in the rates of good events between experimental and control participants; it is reported as a percentage (%).

Relative benefit reduction (RBR): the proportional decrease in rates of good events between experimental and control participants; it is reported as a percentage (%).

Relative risk (RR): proportion of patients experiencing an outcome in the treated (or exposed) group divided by the proportion experiencing the outcome in the control (or unexposed) group.

Relative risk increase (RRI): the proportional increase in bad outcomes between experimental and control participants; it is reported as a percentage (%).

Relative risk reduction (RRR): the proportional reduction in outcome rates of bad events between experimental and control participants; it is reported as a percentage (%).

Reliability[24]: the extent to which a measurement is replicable. Lack of reliability can be due to differences in technique between observers, instability of the measurement instrument, or because the phenomenon being measured is itself changing.

Representative sample: the sample taken reflects the characteristics of the population from which it was taken.

Saturation: a point reached in qualitative research at which no new information is yielded by further data collection. Also known as Data saturation or Redundancy.

Screening[14]: services designed to detect people at high risk of a disease or condition that is associated with a modifiable adverse outcome. Offered to people who do not have symptoms or risk factors (other than age or sex) for the disease or condition.

Selection bias[3]: occurs when the results of a trial are distorted by systematic differences in the way in which participants are assigned to one group or another.

Sensitivity[22]: a measure of a diagnostic test's ability to correctly detect a disorder when it is present in a sample of people.

Sensitivity analysis: tests the robustness of the observed results relative to sensible modifications in important variables. For example, in a meta-analysis, one can test to see if results differ based on the quality of individual studies.

Snowball sampling[4]: sometimes used in qualitative research; participants are identified by earlier participants in a study. Also known as Network sampling.

Specificity[22]: a measure of a diagnostic test's ability to correctly identify the absence of a disorder in a sample of people who do not have the disorder.

Standard error: standard deviation of the mean values computed from repeated samples drawn from the same population; i.e. it is the error associated with the calculated mean.

Standardized mean difference[5]: in a systematic review, a way of combining the results of studies that may have measured the outcome (e.g. pain) in different ways, using different scales; effects are expressed as a standard value, with no units (difference between 2 means / estimate of within-group standard deviation).

Stepwise multiple regression: a statistical technique that determines the probability of a dependent variable (outcome) occurring with the independent (explanatory) variables present or absent. In stepwise regression, the independent variables are selected sequentially for the prediction equation. It determines whether the model that includes the variable(s) explains more about the outcome variable than does the model which does not include the variable(s).

Stratified randomization[5]: used in trials to ensure that equal numbers of participants with a particular characteristic (e.g. age) are allocated to each comparison group.

Subjective outcome: an outcome that requires judgement rather than the direct measurement of an observable phenomenon (e.g. degree of support provided to the patient by a spouse).

Surveillance bias[14]: the tendency to search more (or less) diligently for an outcome in a comparison group because of knowledge of exposure or intervention/control status. Also known as information bias or detection bias.

Symbolic interaction[2]: a qualitative research method that focuses on the way in which people make sense of social interactions and the meanings they attach to social symbols such as language.

Theoretical sampling[2]: in qualitative studies, selection of study participants based on emerging findings to ensure adequate representation and full variation of important themes.

Time series[2]: a study design that involves collection of data at multiple time points before and after the introduction of an intervention. It is often used to compare outcomes before and after the introduction of new treatment policies or legislation.

Trend: an estimate that approaches a predefined level of statistical significance.

Triangulation[2]: use of multiple methods or perspectives to collect and interpret data about some phenomenon, to converge on an accurate representation of reality.

U-shaped curve: describes the shape of the data when they are plotted on a graph; denotes a relation that is not linear, but increases at both ends of the graph (e.g. mortality is high when body mass index is very low or very high).

Validity[24]: indicates whether a measurement measures what it is supposed to measure.

Verification bias[14]: the results of a diagnostic test influence whether patients are assigned to an intervention group. Also known as Work-up bias.

Wald test[25]: used to evaluate the significance of individual predictors in a logistic regression equation.

Washout period[3]: in a crossover design, a period of time between patients receiving the first and second intervention; it is used to ensure that patients are free of the influence of the first intervention before they begin receiving the second intervention. For example, in a crossover study comparing aspirin and acetaminophen, before crossing over to the alternative treatment, patients go through a 'washout period' where they receive no medications.

Weighted: statistical analysis accounts for differences in certain important variables.

Weighted mean difference[5]: in a meta-analysis, used to combine outcomes measured on continuous scales (e.g. height), assuming that all trials measured the outcome on the same scale; the mean, standard deviation and sample size of each group are known; and weight given to each trial is determined by the precision of its estimate of effect.

Work-up bias: see Verification bias.

References

1 Dawson-Saunders B, Trapp RG. *Basic and Clinical Biostatistics.* Second edition. Norwalk: Appleton and Lange, 1994.
2 Polit DF, Beck CT, Hungler BP. *Essentials of Nursing Research: Methods, Appraisal, and Utilization.* Fifth edition. Philadelphia: Lippincott, 2001.
3 Jadad AR. *Randomised Controlled Trials.* London: BMJ Books, 1998.
4 Polit DF, Hungler BP. *Essentials of Nursing Research: Methods, Appraisal, and Utilization.* Fourth edition. Philadelphia: Lippincott, 1997.
5 Green S, Higgins J, editors. Glossary. Cochrane Handbook for Systematic Reviews of Interventions 4.2.5 (updated May 2005). http://www.cochrane.dk/cochrane/handbook/handbook.htm (accessed 5 October 2006).
6 Yin RK. *Case Study Research: Design and Methods.* Second edition. Thousand Oaks: Sage, 1994.
7 Crombie IK. *The Pocket Guide to Critical Appraisal: A Handbook for Healthcare Professionals.* London: BMJ Publishing Group, 1996.
8 Leidy NK, Haase JE. Functional status from the patient's perspective: the challenge of preserving personal integrity. *Res Nurs Health* 1999;**22**:67–77.
9 Kettunen T, Poskiparta, Liimatainen L, Sjogren A, Karhila P. Taciturn patients in health counseling at a hospital: passive recipients or active participators? *Qual Health Res* 2001;**11**:399–422.

10 Varcoe C. Abuse obscured: an ethnographic account of emergency nursing in relation to violence against women. *Can J Nurs Res* 2001;**32**:95–115.

11 Stone P. A brief smoking cessation intervention for adults in hospital was cost effective. *Evidence-Based Nursing* 1999;**2**:58. Comment on: Meenan RT, Stevens VJ, Hornbrook MC, La Chance PA, Glasgow RE, Hollis JF, Lichtenstein E, Vogt TM. Cost-effectiveness of a hospital-based smoking cessation intervention. *Med Care* 1998;**36**:670–8.

12 Barclay L, Lipton D. The experiences of new fatherhood: a socio-cultural analysis. *J Adv Nurs* 1999;**29**:1013–20.

13 Adler AS, Clark R. *How it's Done: An Invitation to Social Research*. Scarborough: Wadsworth, 1999.

14 DiCenso A, Guyatt G, Ciliska D, editors. *Evidence-Based Nursing: A Guide to Clinical Practice*. St Louis: Elsevier Mosby, 2005.

15 Webb C. Information point: Colaizzi's framework for analysing qualitative data. *J Clin Nursing* 1999;**8**:576.

16 Guyatt G, Rennie D, editors. *Users' Guides to the Medical Literature. A Manual for Evidence-Based Clinical Practice*. Chicago: American Medical Association, 2002.

17 Hall BA. Patterns of spirituality in persons with advanced HIV disease. *Res Nurs Health* 1998;**21**:143–53.

18 Cook TD, Campbell DT. *Quasi-Experimentation: Design and Analysis Issues for Field Settings*. Chicago: Rand McNally, 1979.

19 Streiner D, Geddes J. Some useful concepts and terms used in articles about diagnosis. *Evidence-Based Mental Health* 1998;**1**:6–7.

20 Beck JR, Pauker SG. The Markov process in medical prognosis. *Med Decis Making* 1983;**3**:419–58.

21 Van de Ven AH, Delbecq AL. The nominal group as a research instrument for exploratory health studies. *Am J Public Health* 1972;**62**:337–42.

22 Sackett DL, Haynes RB, Guyatt GH, *et al*. *Clinical Epidemiology: Basic Science for Clinical Medicine*. Second edition. Boston: Little, Brown and Company, 1991.

23 Steer RA, Cavalieri TA, Leonard DM, Beck AT. Use of the Beck Depression Inventory for Primary Care to screen for major depression disorders. *Gen Hosp Psychiatry* 1999;**21**:106–11.

24 Last JM, editor. *A Dictionary of Epidemiology*. Fourth edition. Oxford: Oxford University Press, 2001.

25 Polit D. *Analysis and Statistics for Nursing Research*. Toronto: Prentice-Hall, 1996.

INDEX

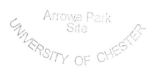

Page numbers in *italics* refer to figures; those in **bold** to tables or boxes.